You. Supercharged!
The Exact Formula for Fitness, Weight Loss, and Longevity

Fitz Koehler, MSESS
Fitzness Books

A division of Fitzness International LLC
Fitzness is a registered trademark of Fitz Koehler
and Fitzness International LLC
Gainesville, FL
You. Supercharged! The Exact Formula for Fitness, Weight Loss, and Longevity
Copyright @2025 by Fitzness International LLC
First Edition
All rights reserved, including the right to reproduce this
book or portions thereof in any form whatsoever.
For information or large orders, visit Fitzness.com
@Fitzness on Instagram, Facebook, and YouTube

Manufactured in the United States of America
Library of Congress Cataloging-in-Publication Data Available

Koehler, Fitz
You. Supercharged! The Exact Formula for Fitness, Weight Loss, and Longevity

★Fitzness International LLC non-fiction original paperback★
1. HEA019000 **HEALTH & FITNESS** / Diet & Nutrition / Weight Loss
2. HEA010000 **HEALTH & FITNESS** / Healthy Living
3. HEA007000 **HEALTH & FITNESS** / Exercise / General

Cover Designer: Alexander von Ness
Cover and Author Photographer: Eden Hetzroni Makeup: Rozie Weeks
Layout Designer: Alen Čar - Slim Rijeka
Editing Team: Doug Thurston, Rudy Novotny, Jennifer Jeffres Senn, Cade Leone, Anna McKinney, Meredith Moldawsky, Brady Freidkes, Isabelle Torres, Camila Corvalan, Emily Gill, Grant Meece, Sean Thompson, Tara Steinberg, Melany Flores, Nicole Becerra, Emilie Jaen, and Danica Lustberg.
Everything Exercise Photographer: Phil Stokes

ISBN: 978-1-7355998-9-2

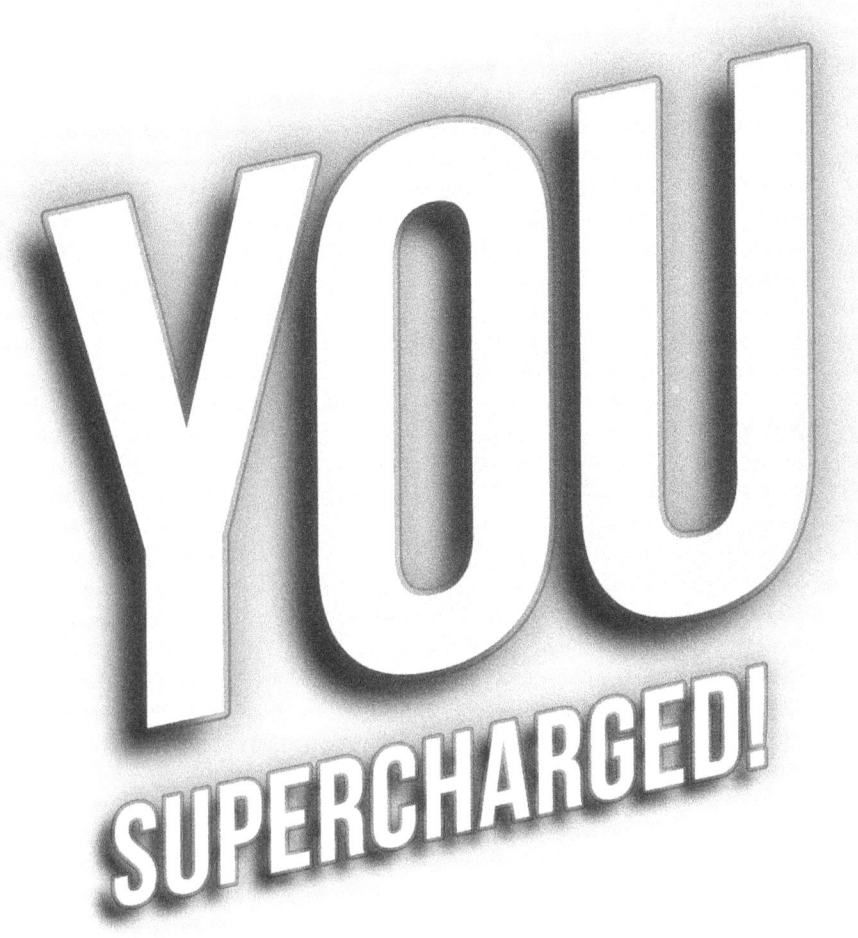

The Exact Formula for Fitness,
Weight Loss, and Longevity

Fitz Koehler, MSESS

I dedicate this book to every person I've ever had, and will have, the privilege of guiding, supporting, and harassing into a fitter body and mind. Helping you live better and longer is my driving force, and each milestone you accomplish makes my life more meaningful. Thanks for showing up, putting in the work, and proving what you're capable of. I love you...

NOW GET TO WORK!

Contents

Introduction 1

CHAPTER 1
High-Performance Health 7

CHAPTER 2
Who Do You Want to Be? 13

CHAPTER 3
The Exact Formula for Weight Loss 19

CHAPTER 4
Supercharged Nutrition: Rocket Fuel for Your Body 29

CHAPTER 5
Liquid Gold vs. Liquid Garbage 53

CHAPTER 6
Chop It Like It's Hot 65

CHAPTER 7
The Case Against Diets 73

CHAPTER 8
Four Pillars of Fitness & The F.I.T.T. Principle 83

CHAPTER 9
Everything Exercise 91

CHAPTER 10
Sleep Like an Angel 179

CHAPTER 11
Motivation vs Discipline 185

CHAPTER 12
Ripped Abs & Gorgeous Glutes 195

CHAPTER 13
Breaking Up with Body Shame 199

CHAPTER 14
Get Comfortable Being Uncomfortable 205

CHAPTER 15
Flawless-ish 211

CHAPTER 16
Obesity is Scary Stuff 225

CHAPTER 17
Health During Hardship & Mental Health 231

CHAPTER 18
Persevering Through Pain 247

CHAPTER 19
Brain Gains 257

CHAPTER 20
Full-Throttle Femininity 263

CHAPTER 21
Man Mode 273

CHAPTER 22
Supercharge Your Family 281

CHAPTER 23
Built to Last: Aging Like a Badass 291

CHAPTER 24
So Busy Yet So Successful 297

CHAPTER 25
High Tech Health 303

CHAPTER 26
Workday Workouts 311

CHAPTER 27
Traveling Fit 319

CHAPTER 28
Holiday Hacks 325

CHAPTER 29
Running, Walking, and Racing 333

CHAPTER 30
Why Your Excuses Are Lame 343

CHAPTER 31
Questions and Answers 355

CHAPTER 32
Do's and Don'ts of Supercharging 367

CHAPTER 33
Get it Together! The Tough Love Chapter 375

CHAPTER 34
You Did It! Now What? 381

You Can Do Hard Things! 387

Acknowledgements 391

INTRODUCTION

You. Supercharged!

Stronger, more energetic, flexible, creative, confident, intelligent, and high-freaking-powered: that's Y-O-U—Supercharged!

It's time to transform your body, mind, soul, and life into the most capable, joyful, and resilient version possible. You still get to be you, just infinitely better in every imaginable way.

Let's make your body the powerhouse it was born to be, enhancing your strength, stamina, flexibility, mobility, and balance. You can be leaner, harder, more athletic, resilient—and yes, curvy too! If you're one of the bazillions of people who want to lose anywhere between one and 1,000 pounds while looking, feeling, and performing better, you picked up the right book. Your goals are valid, and they're absolutely attainable. Aside from changing your height, the possibilities for physical upgrades are virtually endless. And, as a powerful bonus, when your physical health improves, your mental health does too.

Introduction

That's the beauty of this supercharging process: the same effort you put into building a better body also rebuilds and recharges your mind. With a better body, stress subsides, toxic feelings fade, and confidence takes center stage. That stronger mental state makes it easier to stay committed to the healthy habits that got you there: consistent movement, smart nutrition, and high-quality sleep. If you start loving your body right now, you can exchange shame for excitement, moving forward with only positivity. Combine a healthy body with an energized mind, and you become a force to be reckoned with. Friends, I am also going to turn you into a full-blown joy addict!

I'm stoked to help you unlock that greatness. You won't find any snake oil here. No fad diets. No gimmicks. I teach simple, sustainable habits that work. I often joke that I have a master's degree in the simplest science on Earth, and, as you read these pages, you might shake your head and think, "It can't be that easy." But it is. And once you start, you may wonder why you didn't do this sooner. But don't waste a minute on regret. Just absorb what you learn and move forward with fierce commitment. Control what you can, when you can, starting now.

The stars of this supercharged show are:

The Exact Formula for Weight Loss—so customizable, it works just as brilliantly for weight maintenance and even weight gain. Get excited to discover just how much control you can wield over your weight.

The Four Pillars of Fitness—four essential focus points of exercise to prepare your body for anything.

The Everything Exercise Chapter—packed with pictures and designed to demystify all forms of exercise so you know exactly how to get to work.

The F.I.T.T. Principle—teaching you the frequency, intensity, time, and type of exercise you should be doing for optimal results.

Quality Nutrition—eat more foods that help and fewer that hurt.

Health During Hardship and Mental Health—because your body and mind need each other to be at their best.

Motivation vs Discipline—empowering you to do what needs to be done on any day and every day.

Why Your Excuses Are Lame—cutting you off before you begin with any nonsense that makes you worse, not better.

Sleep Like an Angel—an eye-opener (and, hopefully, eye closer), inspiring you to prioritize and attain the rejuvenating sleep your body and brain need.

Full-Throttle Femininity—harness the power of being a woman while navigating menopause, menstruation, bone density, incredible curves, and satisfying sex!

Man Mode—bro time to talk testosterone, muscles, Dad Bods, sports, MANopause, heart health, and supercharged shlongs.

Raising Fit Families—change your family's culture by adopting healthy habits that ensure you and your children have long and happy lives together.

Workday Workouts—learn to use healthy habits as a boost to your professional power and productivity.

I'll also tackle goal-setting, aging like a badass, obesity, body image, navigating vacations and holidays without gaining weight, building a better brain, managing stress, sex, executing discipline,

Introduction

high-tech health tools, running, and so much more. The *Question and Answer* chapter is packed with golden nuggets galore.

This is your life we're talking about! Exercise, nutrition, and sleep aren't optional if you want to enjoy a long, active, and vibrant future. Getting older can be a beautiful thing, unless you spend your golden years trapped in a body riddled with pain or disease, reliant on others. That's not the retirement dream.

You are not stuck! You are not doomed to be overweight, weak, or unfit. With very few exceptions, humans were built for movement. Our bodies–this wild system of muscles, bones, and joints–were made to lift, run, jump, stretch, and endure. Think about what athletes across 10 different sports can do. Your body was made to move like theirs, too. Modern life may have left you sedentary, but it's time to awaken the strength and agility you were born with.

And here's the best part: I'm going to dump all of the fitness expert content from my big brain into yours, making fitness feel understandable, attainable, and fun. Because it is, and you're going to learn how to do it without suffering, starving, or draining your bank account. You'll realize that becoming supercharged isn't as complicated as you thought, and that better version of yourself you've been wishing for? Totally within reach. I'm coming with you every step of the way. In fact, you will soon live each day with a bossy Lil' Fitzy on your shoulder. She'll serve as a potent tool to keep you on track.

Your body and mind were built for greatness. Let's get to work!

Disclaimer: *My editors have warned that I often sound harsh. Yep, I can. I'm passionate and intense because I love you and know that if you hear the truth from a wise, bossy woman who genuinely cares, you'll receive it warmly and get serious about your health. I am frequently thanked for my brutal honesty, but I genuinely know no other way. I* *refuse to sugarcoat things because your time, body, and energy are too valuable to beat around the bush. So when you read something that resonates but makes you think, "ouch!", know it was written with love because your health is in my heart.*

Chapter 1

HIGH-PERFORMANCE HEALTH

You. Supercharged!

Supercharge your body and mind with both tiny and major efforts today to radically transform your entire world tomorrow. You know that refreshing feeling you get walking out of a barber shop or salon after a haircut? That's what's about to happen daily as you update, upgrade, and revitalize your insides and outsides. But before sculpting your dream body, let's zoom out and get a clear vision for your overall health. Hitting your goal weight is just one piece of the puzzle. When you can truly wrap your head around living better and longer, you're far more likely to get and stay on track for the long haul.

Think of your body like a car. Your heart is the engine. Your joints? The suspension system. Your brain? The onboard computer. Cars are composed of various parts and systems that need to work in harmony to keep cruising. Some parts are essential, while others you could technically live without. However, driving becomes awkward, uncomfortable, or downright impossible when even small things start failing.

If you shift your focus beyond the number on the scale and commit to keeping all of your systems and parts in tip-top shape, your body won't just run like a hot rod today, it'll age like a classic car worthy of the car show.

Chapter 1 | High-Performance Health

Cars need regular driving, quality fuel, oil changes, tire rotations, brake checks, and the occasional spa day with a good wash and wax. Smart car owners don't ignore these needs because breakdowns and repairs are inconvenient and expensive. But if the car completely falls apart? Well, you can always trade it in. Not so with your body. You get one model—no returns, no trade-ins. Sure, you can swap out a knee or buy a fresh set of boobs, but your original model is mostly permanent. The "VIN" stamped on your butt is for life.

The Perks of Peak Health

When you hit your ideal weight *and* build a fit body, the list of benefits is absurdly long. Let's rattle off a few (and yes, you're going to want all of these):

Cardiovascular health: A strong heart means a lower risk of disease, stroke, and blood pressure issues.

Metabolic function: Better blood sugar control and reduced risk of type 2 diabetes.

Immune power: Your body becomes a fortress against infections.

Mental health: Lower depression and anxiety, with a brighter, more stable mood.

Energy: Goodbye, fatigue. Hello, stamina!

Quality Sleep: More Zzz's, fewer disruptions.

Longevity: You don't just add years to your life, you add life to your years.

Mobility, strength, balance, and flexibility: You move better, fall less, and hurt less.

Bone and muscle health: You stay strong and avoid frailty.

Brain power: Sharper memory, better focus, clearer thoughts.

Skin, digestion, and reproductive health: Yep, those get a glow-up, too.

Athletic performance: If you've got game, it'll show.

Lower medical bills: Because prevention is a whole lot cheaper than treatment.

Confidence: Fit feels good, and looks even better. Better jobs and extra friends included!

I trust that as you read that list, you found yourself nodding in approval. Who *wouldn't* want better skin, longer life, and a more exciting social calendar? Only weirdos, that's who! And here's the clincher: *There is nothing else on earth that can offer all of those benefits besides your own healthy actions.* You could try pills, potions, or biohacks, but none of them come close to the power of simple healthy habits.

The Price of Inaction

Now, let's flip the script. The burdens that come with being overweight and unfit aren't just about tight pants or unflattering photos. They're serious, dangerous, and all-too-common.

Heart disease, stroke, and high blood pressure

Type 2 diabetes and insulin resistance

Sleep apnea and breathing issues

Joint damage, arthritis, and mobility loss

Depression, anxiety, and lowered self-worth

Certain cancers (breast, colon, kidney, etc.)

Liver, kidney, and gallbladder problems

Hormonal chaos, infertility, and sexual dysfunction

Digestive issues and acid reflux

Chronic inflammation and cognitive decline

Reduced length and quality of life

The worst part? These issues are often self-inflicted. And every single one of them *sucks*. They cost you energy, comfort, happiness, and precious time. I'm thrilled that you're reading this book, because it means you're choosing better. We're going to upgrade your life, one awesome habit at a time.

Mental Health Matters Too

Pair a strong body with a strong mind, and you become unstoppable. Yet, efforts to promote mental fitness are often neglected or stigmatized, reserved for those labeled "crazy." What a load of nonsense! Your brain is your command center. And just like your body, it requires training, nourishment, rest, and care. The great news? You have influence. You can *absolutely* become more focused, optimistic, joyful, resilient, and emotionally agile.

A cranky, foggy, pessimistic mind can become bright, sharp, and hopeful just like an overweight, sedentary body can become lean and athletic. It's all about effort and intention.

Even better? The connection between your physical and mental health is a two-way street. Improve one, and the other rises with it. Take care of your brain, and you'll make better choices with your body. Take care of your body, and your brain will reward you with feel-good chemicals and mental clarity.

As one particularly boisterous American president once said, *"We're going to win so much, you're going to get sick of winning!"* Brace yourself. That kind of extraordinary success is just ahead.

Chapter 2

WHO DO YOU WANT TO BE?

You. Supercharged!

Knowing what you want from any situation is crucial to getting it. If you don't know what you want, you'll likely be stuck accepting whatever you get, like when a Southern mama tells you, "You get what you get, and you don't get upset!" Not fun to hear, and, let's be honest, the results rarely rock. Accepting fate blindly is a no-can-do scenario for me. I want as much control as possible over my life, and I take control 93% of the time. When it comes to *your* life, there should be zero other captains, navigators, or head honchos. Advisors? Sure: input from doctors, coaches, and experts can be helpful. But don't get it twisted: *you* are the supercharged CEO of Y-O-U, and it's time to make some executive decisions.

Take a moment to think about what you want to accomplish with your weight, shape, strength, muscle mass, endurance, mobility, and balance. How do you want your body to *feel*, *perform*, and *look*? Decide exactly who you want to be, because if you don't know where you're going, how on earth will you figure out how to get there? Can you imagine poking "somewhere" into your GPS? Heck no! Instead, you enter a specific address and get clear instructions, even when you make wrong turns and hit traffic along the way. Your health works the same way when you have a precise destination. I like the S.M.A.R.T. framework which states that goals should be: Specific, Measurable, Achievable, Relevant, and Time-bound.

Chapter 2 | Who Do You Want to Be?

Your Target Weight

You might be wondering what to choose as your ideal weight. Fair enough, but I have a hunch that most of you already know what it is. Or, you're darn close. Sure, you can look at generic charts and graphs, but since they ignore your shape and muscle-to-fat ratio, I find them borderline useless. Some are laughably off. Instead, trust your intuition and what you already know about yourself. You know your fighting weight, the weight or range where you've felt your best. Who knows your body better than you? No one.

Think back. Was there a time when you felt amazing, or is there someone of a similar height whose physique inspires you? Use that as a reference point. Then, get real with your current stats: weight, measurements, and body fat percentage. These numbers will help you set meaningful goals. If your situation is more complex, consult a doctor; just keep a few things in mind.

Aim for greatness. If you've got a lot of weight to lose, don't aim halfway because you're scared of failing. Be more afraid of *not* going all the way. Shoot for your best-case scenario. You can always reassess once you get close.

Set a deadline. "Someday" is not a plan. If you aim to lose one to two pounds weekly, it's easy to calculate a timeline that keeps you on track.

Your Shape

While genetics plays a role in your starting point, it shouldn't dictate your outcomes. You may have to adjust based on your natural body type, but make no mistake, progress is always possible. You've got control here, and it's crucial that you know it. Body types are broken down into three categories:

Endomorph: Rounder, softer, may struggle with weight loss but builds muscle easily;

Mesomorph: Naturally athletic, builds muscle quickly;

Ectomorph: Lean and slender, has trouble gaining weight.

I'm sharing these body type classifications, not as limitations, but to cancel your excuses. I know some of you are yelling at the page, "But I'm an endomorph, I *can't* lose weight!" or "I'm an ectomorph, I'll *never* gain muscle!" Nonsense. You *can*. Everyone can build strength and lose fat. Some folks just have to hustle harder to move the needle, but physical progress is achievable for all.

And guess what? Choosing your shape can be fun! Want a slimmer waist and broader shoulders? Fabulous. Dreaming of a rounder tush? I love that for you. Hoping your calves or triceps pop? Great goal. Fitness goes way beyond appearance, but let's be honest: caring about how you look is *totally* okay. Most of us care about how our homes, cars, and outfits look, so why wouldn't we care about our bodies?

Now, here comes the fun/scary/courageous part. I want you to stand in front of a mirror nude. Yep, naked, and take a close look. Did I just tell you to strip down? Indeed, I did. Your body is YOURS. It's *you*. Don't think I'm creepy, but I love your body. It houses your mind and soul and can do amazing things. I'm grateful for it. I hope you are, too.

So as you fling your top and drawers on the floor, do it joyfully. No nitpicking, just observing. Be kind. Start by writing down five things you love: maybe your strong legs, your sparkly eyes, curvy shoulders, firm booty, and yes, your adorable weenus (look it up). Then, make a list of things you'd like to enhance. Be detailed, and again, be kind. This list becomes your action plan. If you don't know where you're going, how can you possibly know how to get there?

While designing your future look, build in performance goals. After all, what good is a sculpted body if it's not capable?

Strength

You'll be better off when all your muscles are powerful, period. I'm not giving you the option to choose weak, squishy, or injury-prone muscles. And no cherry-picking a strong upper body with a sad lower half (or vice versa). Sorry, not in this book. All your muscles should support you through daily life, unexpected tumbles, and oodles of fun. You can aim for firm and functional, or push for visible strength, the kind that makes people say, "Whoa, you work out!" And, just to be clear, *all* muscles matter. Don't just focus on your triceps and tush. From head to toe, every muscle should be supported.

Endurance

Do you prefer to grow winded on a casual hike, or breeze through your day with gas in the tank? Endurance is your ability to power through life without burning out. Want to climb stairs, chase kids, or play pickleball without wheezing? Then put in the work with cardio. Set your sights high!

Flexibility

When I say "flexibility," think "mobility." You should be able to bend, twist, reach, and move comfortably in all directions, without pain or restriction. Start small: maybe just getting your socks on without tweaking your back. Then, dream big. Scratch your own back, swim the breaststroke with ease, or land a karate kick square to someone's head (in class, of course).

Balance

Balance gets ignored way too often, but it's *vital*. At the very least, you need it to stay upright on flat earth, but you can do better. Aim for the type of balance that keeps you safe on cobblestone streets, heels, or even rollerblades. Better balance means fewer falls and enhanced athletic performance. Want to move gracefully in sports and life? This is your secret weapon.

Mental Health

A strong, clear mind is a mighty tool. If positivity and discipline don't come naturally to you, guess what? You can *build* them. Mindsets can be made like muscles, and they are trainable with effort and repetition. Don't skip this part when mapping out who you want to be. Do you want to be more creative, punctual, focused, patient, or supportive? Write it all down. Make a list using pen and paper, your phone, a vision board, or whatever floats your motivational boat. This is your most important project: the reinvention of YOU. Give it a cool name like these (but not mine, make it yours) and get started!

- Fitz 2.0
- Fitz But BETTER!
- The Fitzness Project
- New Gen Fitz

Chapter 3

THE EXACT FORMULA FOR WEIGHT LOSS

Weight loss isn't rocket science. In fact, it's quite simple. I promise that if you follow The Exact Formula for Weight Loss, you will never have to diet, suffer, or waste your money buying nonsense like pills, supplements, shakes, or wraps again. And when supercharging your body and life, the impact of getting to and remaining at your ideal weight can not be overstated. It will make a ginormous, mind-boggling difference every day.

Your body needs calories to function. Humans burn about 10 calories per pound of body weight per day. So, if you weigh 200 pounds, your body will likely burn about 2,000 calories to maintain its size and normal body function. That's not counting exercise. It's just the amount of calories your body will burn doing essential tasks like digesting food, pumping blood, processing oxygen, walking around the house, brushing hair: the standard stuff. Every move we make requires energy, and thus, calories are burned. If you burn about 2,000 calories a day and you're not losing weight, we know you're also consuming at least 2,000 calories daily.

3,500 extra calories consumed = one pound gained

3,500 extra calories burned = one pound lost

Chapter 3 | The Exact Formula for Weight Loss

If you presently weigh 200 pounds but have a healthy or preferred weight of 150 pounds, it's safe to say that you'll need to lose 50. If you'd like to weigh 150 pounds, you should eat the proper amount of calories to sustain a person no larger than 150 pounds! 150 X 10 calories per day = 1,500. At 200 pounds, you're consuming at least 2,000 calories per day, likely way more if you exercise regularly. That's why you aren't losing weight. But the good news? Adjusting your intake can reverse it.

Customizing The Formula to your personal needs is easy. Decide what your healthy weight is, and then tack a ZERO onto the end of it. That provides you with 10 calories per pound of ideal body weight. By sticking to this caloric formula, your body will shrink down to your ideal weight. You will be feeding it enough to function well at your ideal weight, but won't be feeding it enough to remain at its larger size.

Examples:

Want to weigh 214 pounds? Keep your intake under 2,140 calories per day.

Want to weigh 132 pounds? Keep your intake under 1,320 calories per day.

This Formula works EVERY TIME! It's NOT a diet; it's just a method of managing your consumption habits (both food and beverage) to ensure you're providing your body with the ideal amount of energy (calories) and not too much.

Now: you can do this the smart way or the dumb-dumb way. The dumb-dumb way would have you eat four doughnuts each day and nothing else. Yes, you can consume 1,500 calories with just a few doughnuts and still lose weight. However, with this methodology, you'd have no energy, feel hungry, have headaches, grow cranky, and quit. This dumb-dumb plan is not built for success.

The smart way? Fill your plate with foods that give you energy, satisfy you, and taste good. Think colorful fruits and veggies, lean proteins, and whole grains. These foods are packed with tons of nutrients and are usually lower in calories. Avoid high-calorie beverages, too. You don't have to be perfect, but yes, I am suggesting that you have really high standards most of the time.

This is not a diet! You're simply going to start becoming particular about what you put in your mouth. Fill up on the great stuff and scrutinize the high-calorie, high-fat non-essentials. Could you grill that chicken breast without all of the oil? Sure, you can! Can you dip your salad in a side cup of dressing instead of letting the restaurant dump ladles full on top of it? Of course! Can you choose another way to relax each night besides having that glass of wine or beer? Unless you've got a problem, skip the alcohol and go for a walk or take a bath instead.

And if you're trying to gain weight, the Exact Formula works in reverse. You just tell it how much you want to weigh, by eating a minimum, and eventually the pounds will come. Want to gain weight to become 220 pounds? Consume at least 2,200 calories daily! Note: This is not the time to shovel unhealthy garbage into your mouth. Instead, choose nutritious foods, pair them with exercise, and the weight you gain will make you better, not worse.

The Formula works for weight maintenance, too. Once you make it to your goal weight, if you would like to stay there, continue with your daily caloric budget. Veer from it, and so will your weight. The Exact Formula works for life. If you were dieting, you would eventually go "off" your diet, go back to eating whatever you ate pre-diet, and gain a bunch of weight. Since The Formula is not a diet and not restrictive, you can and should

Chapter 3 | The Exact Formula for Weight Loss

maintain it for life. Want to weigh 160 pounds forever? Your daily caloric budget will always be around 1,600 calories. It's a simple strategy for maintenance that works.

Folks, weight management isn't about suffering. It's about fueling your body the right way, making smart swaps, consuming reasonable portions, and staying consistent. Master that, and the results will come. Positive changes often come with an adjustment period. Even though The Formula is both genius and simplistic, escaping your previous eating habits will still require thought and discipline. Stay the course. The Formula works every time. You've just got to stick with it.

*If you're trying to lose weight, your caloric budget is the maximum. If you're trying to gain weight, your caloric budget is a **minimum**.*

Frequently Asked Questions

When I lose weight, can I go back to eating more calories?

No. To be a smaller person for the long haul, you'll have to continue eating like a smaller person. You may be able to eat a bit more on occasion if you exercise vigorously for extended periods of time, but if you veer too far from your formula, you'll eventually gain weight.

How do I keep track of calories?

I recommend using an app. You can plug in every bite and sip you take each day to ensure you don't go over your daily caloric budget. You can also jot down notes with a pen and paper to keep track. I advise you not to take the advice of apps, though, as they're historically known to give terrible guidance. Stick with your formula and exclusively use the app for calorie tracking. You'll find plenty that are free and easy to use.

What if I hate counting?

Counting calories isn't fun. But neither is being frustrated with your weight. Think of it like budgeting money: tracking just enough to stay in control.

What if I hate scales?

That's like saying you hate thermometers or rulers. Scales are simply tools of measurement. They don't love you, hate you, or care if it's the holidays. They just tell you the truth and let you make decisions based on that information. Your weight is not the only important factor in health, but you're likely reading these words because you care about your weight. Don't put your head in the sand. Check in with a scale regularly; I recommend weekly. You know you've been doing well if the scale moves in the right direction. If the number is sticking or going the wrong way, you'll know to tighten up and put in more effort. Plus, if you were religious about checking in with the scale, do you think you'd have gained a bunch of weight in the first place?

What if I love my scale too much?

Obsessing over your weight can be a real problem. This is why I heartily recommend that you only weigh yourself once weekly. Doing so daily can drive you batty. Our weight fluctuates over time depending on how much food is being digested, whether salty items are making us retain water, and more. Weighing in multiple times per day may actually drive you insane. Of course, you will weigh more after eating breakfast and lunch and drinking a bunch of water. And you will certainly weigh less after using the potty, toilet, loo, etc. Duh! Why do you need this information? You don't. So instead, weigh yourself weekly. If you are sticking with The Formula, your weight should be going in the right direction. If you don't get a huge result immediately, stay the course, and good news will come. If you're working to lose weight, you're looking for a downward trend over time. Don't obsess.

What about the 1,200-calorie-a-day message I've always heard?

It's preposterous to think that a random amount of calories would suit everyone. Every professional football player would starve if that's all they were fed daily. That utterly random number does not take into account various heights, weights, body types, or goals. With the Exact Formula for Weight Loss, you choose your goal weight, and your caloric budget is specific to you.

What if I can't lose weight?

It may feel impossible, but it's not. If you were stranded at sea for a week, would you lose weight? Of course you would! It's not that you can't lose weight; the reality is you haven't yet done what it takes to be successful. I'm obviously not suggesting you strand yourself somewhere in the middle of the ocean. What I am telling you is that you definitely can lose weight if you stick with The Formula, over time, your unwanted weight will come off.

What if my weight gets stuck?

If you've been losing weight and your scale gets stuck for a while, that could be attributed to a few different causes. It's possible you're consuming more calories than you think and need to tighten up on your calorie management. Perhaps some of your favorite foods contain more calories than you think. Measuring or weighing them might help you achieve the accurate serving size. It's also possible that your body is just taking its sweet time letting go of the weight. I wish I had a brilliant explanation for this phenomenon, but I don't. Sometimes we can be doing all the right things, and our body just won't let go, but then, it does. Your body actually has no choice but to respond to The Formula, because if you are not feeding it enough to maintain its size, it will shrink.

Most importantly, if you're trying to lose weight, you should be looking for a downward trend over time. You don't need to lose exactly two pounds weekly. You may lose four in the first week, three in the second, and then nothing in the third. Just stay the course. If you stick with The Formula, your body will eventually shrink down to the size you're telling it to be.

Do I have to avoid all unhealthy foods? Absolutely not. Aim for 80-90% of your food and beverage choices to come from the healthy category and have a little fun with the rest if you choose. The key to eating less-healthy foods is keeping portions reasonable without going overboard. Have a little, take a deep breath, share a big smile, and move on.

Should I add exercise?

Of course! You can be trim without exercise, but you CANNOT be fit without it. Exercise is a powerful force in weight management, but more importantly, it is the only way to become strong, flexible, resilient, with good balance and endurance! Skinny is no prize! Your goal should be to become lean and strong!

If I exercise, do I eat those calories to compensate for the calories burned?

NO! Purposely re-consuming the calories you just burned to lose weight would be completely counterproductive! That would be like quickly spending the $1,000 you just earned on a fancy purse, when you were trying to save up to buy a $15,000 car! If you're training intensely for over an hour, think marathon training or high-intensity sports, you may need extra fuel. Otherwise, let your workout boost your calorie deficit. Many apps and diets mistakenly tell you to eat the burned calories. But unless you're doing extreme workouts, you don't need to. If you burn an extra 500 calories daily through exercise, you will lose an extra pound a week. You will lose zero extra pounds weekly if you burn 500 calories and quickly re-consume them. Don't do it.

Can I splurge?

It's your caloric budget! You don't have to be perfect. Perfect is boring! Make great choices and stick to your budget 80-90% of the time. I eat a small piece of milk chocolate every single day. It makes me happy.

It's not fair that my husband gets to eat more than I do!

Larger spouses often get way more calories than their smaller spouses. If you want to eat as much as he does, prepare to weigh as much as he does. Food is fuel. He needs more. You do you and mind your plate.

What if I have an enormous amount of weight to lose?

Use The Formula in stages. If you need to lose 100+ pounds, it's best to break it into phases. Start with a caloric budget for a 50 pound loss. Once you lose the first 50, adjust your caloric budget to lose even more weight.

Do I have to count calories forever?

Only if you would like to remain at your goal weight forever, because I certainly do. I used to weigh 45 pounds more than I do now. When I was overweight, I was teaching two intense group fitness classes a day, and my weight never budged. What changed? My eating habits! Once I learned the math and science behind managing my calories, I began keeping track meticulously, and my excess weight started disappearing. When I reached the weight that elated me, I continued to track calories using pen and paper for years. I no longer write it all down, but I always do the math in my head. I'm not willing to gain weight again, so this simple method is mandatory. The Exact Formula has allowed me and many others to reach our ideal weight and maintain it for life.

How long will it take?

That depends on how much weight you have to lose. If you have a large amount to lose, it'll likely take a significant amount of time. If you're only trying to shed five-to-ten pounds and you're disciplined with The Formula, it shouldn't take long. Losing two to three pounds per week is a desirable pace, but if you're obese and trading unhealthy habits for The Formula, don't be surprised if you drop pounds more rapidly.

Weight loss isn't about luck. It's about using a system that works. Stick to The Formula, stay consistent, and you'll see results that last a lifetime.

Chapter 4

SUPERCHARGED NUTRITION: ROCKET FUEL FOR YOUR BODY

Contrary to popular belief, eating wisely can be simple, fun, tasty, and affordable. In fact, you probably learned almost everything you need to know in kindergarten. Exciting, right? I just have to deprogram you. Deprogram? What? Yup. So, any confusion concerning proper nutrition is likely the result of some nasty shenanigans by evildoers and lying liars who have been preying on you and everyone else. These vultures target people trying to lose weight, pushing expensive diets, bogus supplements, and quick fixes that don't work. They've screwed up this simple science for many big time! But you're here now, and I'm pumped to set things straight. The real solution is to eat the right amounts of the right foods for the size you'd like to be. It's simple: eat a colorful mix of fruits, veggies, whole grains, lean proteins, and healthy fats. Drink your water. Avoid overly processed, sugary, or fat-laden products as well. Boom! You're on your way to feeling better, looking better, and living longer.

Everything you put into your mouth has the ability to help or do harm, so I'm hoping to convince you to choose more healers than harmers. And I declare right now that you do not have to be perfect! In fact, my motto, "Perfect is boring," works in every area of life, and I'm happy to share it with you. The mental taxation, stress, and suffering brought on by extreme approaches to nutrition will only set you up for failure. So take a deep breath. We

Chapter 4 | Supercharged Nutrition: Rocket Fuel for Your Body

will break it all down into simple concepts, and your responsibility will be to do the best you can. Like with exercise, start where you are and aim to get one percent better every day. To make this as simple as possible, I recommend combining the Exact Formula for Weight Loss with a commitment to quality, aiming for 80-90% of your calories to come from whole, nutrient-dense sources. Do this, and enjoy some wiggle room and flexibility when you'd like to indulge.

Fueling your body with healthy foods will enhance all of your efforts with exercise, serving as a rocket booster for your workouts. Want them to count more? Healthy food has the power to make your exercise more impactful. Downing unhealthy foods and beverages will have the opposite effect. Easy choice, right? It'll also help you sleep better, think better, and improve energy, digestion, skin, hair, and all sorts of things we discussed in the introduction. The Exact Formula is your recipe for weight management. Quality nutrition is the necessary ingredient for function, performance, and health. Two very important but separate things.

Let's break it down and discuss how truly *doable* it is to eat well and why each type of food is worth inviting to your plate. I recommend using a highlighter and marking up the sections that make you think, "Yeah, I could use more of that!" Instead of looking for nutrition in pill or powder form because everyone you know is pushing supplements, consider which real foods could do your body good and make an effort to consume them more often.

Supercharge Your Insides

Fruits & Veggies

Fruits and vegetables are basically superheroes in disguise. They're packed with essential vitamins, minerals, fiber, and antioxidants. Low in calories, high in benefits, what's not to love? They're packed with magic nutrients like:

- **Vitamin C** helps repair tissues and keeps your immune system in beast mode.

- **Potassium** keeps your blood pressure and heart in check.

- **Folate** helps with cell growth and repair.

Plus, fiber is your digestive bestie. Fiber keeps things moving, helps you feel full longer, and keeps blood sugar steady. Fiber should be your closest ally if you want to avoid getting "hangry" or stuck on the potty.

Let's not forget antioxidants like flavonoids and carotenoids. These powerhouses fight inflammation, slow aging, and help prevent chronic diseases.

Color matters, too! Different colors offer different nutrients. So go wild with greens, reds, oranges, purples, and everything in between. Doing so will benefit different areas of your body, like your vision and memory. From spinach to strawberries, from bell peppers to blueberries, variety equals vitality.

It's okay to have favorites, but don't be afraid to try new things, because trying new foods can be a game-changer. Case in point: when I was 21, a guy I was dating made me broccoli, cauliflower, and onions for dinner at his place. I'd never eaten them before, was grossed out by the prospect, and cringed when I saw them hit my plate. But because I liked him (and had manners), I gave them a shot, and loved them! That dinner changed my future in a significant way. I went from a gal who considered iceberg lettuce, tomatoes, and cucumbers big deal veggies to one who eats almost all of the veggies all of the time.

Chapter 4 | Supercharged Nutrition: Rocket Fuel for Your Body

Of course, there will naturally be healthy food items you genuinely dislike, and that's okay. I hope you will try most things at least a few times, prepared in different ways. When it comes to produce, you will be hard-pressed to find anything else so rich in nutrients while typically low in fat and calories. They will be one of your most excellent tools in losing weight while avoiding hunger pains.

Don't rely on juicing.

I do not recommend leaning on juicing for nutrition. Even though some juices are made of fruits and veggies, the process removes much of the fiber, which reduces their ability to make you feel full. Juices can also be very high in sugar and calories. Apples vs apple juice is a fantastic example. You could likely drink an 800-calorie gallon of fiber-destroyed apple juice and still feel hungry. But you could also consume one medium 70-calorie fiber-filled apple and feel stuffed. Fiber is an essential component of weight management. When it comes to nutrition, whole foods will always be the undeniable champions. So, unless it's a rarity, skip the juice; or, make sure your choice is low in both calories and sugar.

Veg Out!

It's strange how many people claim to dislike veggies, when they come in so many colors, textures, and tastes. Really? Do you dislike them all? How can that be? It probably can't. Vegetables are more than just broccoli and salad. These low-calorie, nutrient-dense, low-sugar phenoms include sweet potatoes, carrots, and garlic! Nom nom nom. You're not six anymore. Be brave and give veggies a try. If you can't do it on your own, ask a hottie to prepare them for you. That'll do the trick!

Leafy Greens

Packed with vitamins A, C, K, folate, iron, and fiber, leafy greens fight inflammation, boost energy, and can make your skin glow! They can also help keep your brain young and smart! Check out spinach, kale, romaine lettuce, Swiss chard, collard greens, and arugula.

Root Vegetables

Root veggies are loaded with complex carbs for long-lasting energy, plus tons of antioxidants and minerals. Roasting them brings out their natural sweetness. They're your tasty ticket to better digestion and stronger immunity. Examples include carrots, beets, sweet potatoes, turnips, parsnips, and radishes.

Cruciferous Vegetables

These veggies help your body detox like a boss and may reduce the risk of certain cancers. They're rich in fiber, vitamin C, and sulforaphane (a fancy word for "natural body armor"). Enjoy broccoli, cauliflower, Brussels sprouts, cabbage, and bok choy.

Fruiting Vegetables

Technically fruits, they are juicy, colorful, rich in antioxidants like lycopene and vitamin C, and great for heart health and glowing skin. The brighter the color, the better the benefits! Think tomatoes, cucumbers, bell peppers, eggplant, zucchini, and okra.

Allium Vegetables

These zesty, aromatic veggies are good for your heart and immune system. They fight inflammation, help lower cholesterol, and are so tasty that many add them exclusively for flavor. They may

Chapter 4 | Supercharged Nutrition: Rocket Fuel for Your Body

not keep vampires away, but they can fend off diseases. Examples include garlic, onions, leeks, shallots, and scallions.

Starchy Vegetables

These are your fuel foods, also known as nature's energy bars! High in healthy carbs and fiber, they give you energy to crush workouts, deadlines, and dance floors. Get down with corn, green peas, potatoes, butternut squash, and yams.

Fungi

Mushrooms may not be veggies, but they're earthy, meaty, and full of immune-boosting goodness. They've got vitamin D and antioxidants to help you thrive. Try white button, portobello, shiitake, cremini, and oyster mushrooms if you dare.

Stem Vegetables

Stem veggies like celery and asparagus are crunchy, hydrating, and low-calorie. Packed with water, they're great for digestion, hydration, and snacking without guilt. Go wild on celery, asparagus, rhubarb, kohlrabi, and bamboo shoots.

Fun fact: asparagus may make your urine smell funky, and not the fun kind of funky. It doesn't happen to everyone, but many of us will enjoy a bizarre, sulfur-laden stench in the loo for about half a day post-consumption. Asparagus is still worth it, but I wanted to warn you because the first time I experienced this I thought I might be dying.

Tutti Frutti: Nature's Candy

Fruit is like dessert without the guilt, the absolute queen of pleasing our taste buds and bodies. I bet you can already make a list of fruits you adore, and that's awesome. Now double that list to target all the goals on your "who do I want to be?" game plan. Nom nom nom your way to better skin, a stronger immune system, a sharper brain, and more. Also, if a complete ignoramus tells you to avoid fruit because it has sugar, poke them in the nose and run away. These natural sugars are not your enemy. If you're cutting back on sweets, start with pies, pastries, and cookies, not grapefruit. Yeesh!

Citrus Fruits: The Immune Boosters

Citrus fruits are bursting with vitamin C, antioxidants, and flavonoids that support your immune system, skin health, and heart. They're hydrating, tangy, and can be sweet or sour. You'll love the zesty punch from oranges, grapefruits, lemons, limes, and tangerines, all stars in the immunity Olympics!

Berries

Tiny but mighty, berries are packed with antioxidants, fiber, and brain-boosting power. They help fight inflammation, support your skin, and even improve memory.

Enjoy the goodness of strawberries, blueberries, raspberries, blackberries, and cranberries in your smoothies, oatmeal, parfaits, or toss them into your mouth straight from the carton.

Pome Fruits

These fruits grow around a core and are typically high in fiber and vitamin C. They're filling and crunchy and help regulate blood sugar and digestion. An apple a day? Yes, please. Try pears and quince for their sweet, juicy crunch, too!

Stone Fruits

Stone fruits get their name from the single hard pit in the center. They're loaded with vitamins A and C, potassium, and hydration, improving skin and energy levels. Peaches, nectarines, plums, apricots, and cherries are so sweet, they're often the base for dessert!

Tropical Fruits

Rich in natural sugars, enzymes, and hydration, tropical fruits support digestion, immune function, and overall vitality. They also taste like vacation. Think bananas, pineapples, mangoes, papayas, and guavas.

Melons

These fruits are made up of over 90% water, making them perfect for hydration, especially during hot days or workouts. They're also low in calories and full of vitamins A and C. Watermelon, cantaloupe, and honeydew are like nature's sports drinks.

Grapes & Vine Fruits

Vine fruits are known for their polyphenols, which promote heart health and fight oxidative stress. They're convenient, bite-sized, and oh-so-satisfying. Grapes, kiwifruit, and even passionfruit are perfect for snack trays or pretending you're fancy.

Fatty Fruits

These fruits are unique because they're rich in healthy fats like omega-3s and loads of fiber, potassium, and folate. Shrewd choices for brain function and heart health. Avocados and olives are the main characters, big scores for those who love guacamole and Italian foods.

Challenge time!

- Try a bite of as many produce items as you can.
- Make a list of those you've tried and rate each from 1-5 on taste.
- Try each in various forms, raw, cooked, or mixed into a dish; you never know what you'll fall in love with.

Whole Grains

Whole grains like oats, quinoa, brown rice, and whole wheat are nutritional MVPs. They are often villainized as "evil carbs", but nothing could be further from the truth. Complex carbohydrates give you steady energy (no sugar crash!), and they're packed with fiber to keep you full and your digestive system happy.

They also bring B vitamins, iron, magnesium, and selenium to the table, nutrients that support everything from brain function to strong bones and immune health. Whole grains even contain plant compounds that may help lower the risk of chronic diseases, including heart disease and some cancers. If you or a loved one is navigating cancer recovery, check out my book, Your Healthy Cancer Comeback: Sick to Strong, where I dive deeper into nutrition and strength-building strategies for patients and survivors.

So, what's the difference between **whole** and **refined** grains? Whole grains have all the good stuff: bran (fiber central), germ (nutrient-packed core), and endosperm (starch and protein). Refined grains toss out the bran and germ, leaving behind...well, not much. And don't be fooled by "brown" bread, rice, or pasta. Some companies just dye refined grains brown to trick you. How rude! Right? But now you're too smart for that. Look for the word "whole" in the ingredients list, *whole wheat, whole oats, whole grain anything*. That's how you know it's the real deal.

Cereal Grains

These grains are the foundation of many healthy cultures around the world. They're packed with fiber, B vitamins, and complex carbohydrates that give you long-lasting energy and help manage blood sugar. Cereal grains include familiar favorites like whole wheat, oats, corn, brown rice, barley, and rye. You'll find them in everything from bread and pasta to oatmeal and grain bowls, keeping you fueled and full.

Pseudo-grains

While technically not true grains, pseudo-grains act like them in cooking and nutrition. They're high in protein, fiber, and essential amino acids, making them a favorite among plant-based eaters and ancient grain fans alike. Quinoa, amaranth, and buckwheat top the list here, each one gluten-free and surprisingly versatile, whether you're whipping up salads or baked goods.

Sprouted Grains

Sprouted grains are regular whole grains that have just begun germinating, boosting their nutrient content and making them easier to digest. This process can enhance the availability of vitamins and minerals and give the grains a slightly sweet, nutty flavor. Sprouted wheat, barley, and brown rice are common choices, often found in specialty breads and cereals that taste great and are easier on the gut.

Gluten-Free Whole Grains

For those with gluten sensitivities or preferences, there's a whole world of nutritious grains that don't include gluten but still bring all the benefits. Brown rice, millet, sorghum, teff, and certified gluten-free oats are in this group. They're perfect for baking, cooking, or mixing into power bowls for a satisfying crunch and a boost of fiber and minerals.

Heirloom and Heritage Grains

These are traditional grains that haven't been altered through modern agricultural breeding, preserving their original nutrition and character. They're typically more nutrient-dense and rich in flavor than their modern cousins. Einkorn, farro, spelt, and freekeh are among these heritage stars, offering chewy textures and nutty flavors that make your meals feel both gourmet and traditional.

Incorporating these whole grains into your meals will keep you fueled, full, and feeling fantastic. So next time you're grocery shopping, skip the white bread trickery and go for the real deal. Get down with brown!

Proteins

Protein isn't just for bodybuilders. It's essential for everyone, as it is necessary to repair tissue, make hormones, support immunity, and keep muscles strong (especially as we age). Plus, it's a secret weapon for feeling full longer and keeping cravings at bay. Note: Fiber and protein are the best at providing that feeling of fullness. When you feel full, you're likely to put the fork down. So, use both to prevent yourself from overeating and ingesting too many calories.

Animal Proteins

Easy to incorporate into any meal, animal proteins contain complete amino acid profiles. Just go easy on the fatty cuts and processed meats, they come with lots of saturated fat and sodium you don't need. Ideal animal-based options include skinless chicken, turkey, fish (especially salmon, tuna, and sardines for those heart-healthy omega-3s), eggs, and low-fat dairy products like Greek yogurt, cottage cheese, and milk.

Plant-based Proteins

Beans, lentils, tofu, tempeh, quinoa, nuts, and seeds are packed with protein, fiber, and healthy fats. They also come with phytonutrients and antioxidants, fancy words for natural chemicals that reduce inflammation, boost immunity, and may protect against cancer and heart disease.

Vegetarians and vegans can absolutely get enough protein. If you're a skeptic, fear not. It requires effort, but wonderful things usually do. Most plant-based proteins are naturally low in saturated fat and cholesterol. They're great for your heart and help keep blood sugar steady. Nuts and seeds are higher in fat, but it's the good kind, heart-healthy and brain-boosting. Soy and quinoa are complete proteins, and mixing different plant proteins (like rice + beans or hummus + whole-grain pita) will get you everything you need.

Endless research proves that exchanging animal products for whole plant-based nutrition can increase your chances of aging in good health, free of major disease, with a sharp mind and a strong body. If you're inspired to move in this direction, I encourage you to avoid labeling yourself "vegan" or "vegetarian" right away. Instead, start exchanging animal products for plant-based meals and snacks. You can become more disciplined over time without the pressure of failing in front of friends. I'm a vegetarian, but my commitment to this lifestyle was instigated by my love for animals; the health benefits are truly an added benefit for me. Whether you choose to be a vegetarian, vegan, or just avoid animal products as often as possible, the benefits to your health can be significant.

Dairy Proteins

Dairy products offer protein, calcium, and vitamin D, making them excellent for bone health and recovery. Greek yogurt stands out for its high protein content and probiotic boost, while cottage cheese is a go-to muscle-maintenance snack. Depending on your needs, milk, whether skim, low-fat, full-fat, or dairy-free (soy, almond, or oat), delivers a smooth protein punch and blends easily into meals and shakes. Cheese can be part of the lineup too, especially options like mozzarella or reduced-fat cheddar, which offer protein without excess saturated fat.

Seafood Proteins

Seafood is one of the best protein sources for supporting brain and heart health. Fatty fish like salmon, mackerel, and trout are rich in omega-3 fatty acids, which reduce inflammation and support cardiovascular health. Shellfish like shrimp, scallops, and crab are low in fat and high in protein. White fish such as cod, haddock, and tilapia are mild in flavor and quick to cook, making them perfect for healthy meals in a hurry.

Red Meats

Of course, many of you are shouting at me through the pages of this book because you love red meats like beef, pork, and lamb. Okay, okay: I hear you! They are indeed powerful sources of protein and iron. However, as your friendly neighborhood fitness pro, it's my responsibility to steer you toward the best options. Research from organizations like the World Health Organization and the American Institute for Cancer Research links frequent red and processed meat consumption to an increased risk of colorectal cancer. While some people enjoy red meat in moderation, experts recommend prioritizing options like poultry, fish, and plant-based proteins for long-term health benefits.

When to Eat Protein

Whatever type of protein you choose, start your day with it, and keep it coming! A protein-packed breakfast (think eggs, Greek yogurt, nuts, or beans) sets the tone and keeps you full and focused. To feel stronger and more energized throughout the day, add protein to salads, soups, and sandwiches, make it the focus of your entrees, and snack on it often.

How Much?

People always ask me how much protein they should consume daily. The Recommended Dietary Allowance is 0.36g per pound of body weight (time to break out your calculator). Still, many experts recommend higher intakes, closer to 0.6 -- 0.9g/lb, if you are highly active, an athlete, pregnant, breastfeeding, over 65, recovering from an injury or surgery, or trying to pack on muscle. You may need less if you suffer from kidney or liver disease, are sedentary (you better not be!), or are under a doctor's orders to consume less. If an exact amount of protein is a serious priority, I recommend discussing it with your doctor or a registered dietitian. Know this, though: eating absurd amounts of protein won't make you more muscular. Your body can only utilize a certain amount; the rest gets expelled or stored as fat.

Do you need protein shakes and bars?

Not likely. Most carnivores do not. Nor do disciplined vegetarians. I recommend doing your best to get what you need nutritionally from real food. Start there. Supplementing that with quality bars or shakes if you fall short is fine, like during illness, extreme physical activity, or if you need something prepackaged with a longer shelf life for athletic adventure. I lost a ton of weight during chemotherapy and turned to protein shakes for added calories and nutrition. I've also used bars on very long runs. That's when supplementation has made sense to me; they are a backup. Read labels and choose options with high-quality ingredients you recognize and can pronounce. Avoiding chemicals and dyes is wise. My favorite protein bar is made of nuts and seeds, dried fruit, and bits of chocolate. Whole foods in bar form. Perfection!

No matter what your choices look like, getting enough protein is key for strength, satiety, and overall health. Prioritize real food, mix up your sources, and fuel your body for success.

Fats

Fat is not your enemy, at least not healthy fats. And consuming them will not make you fat. For decades, fats were demonized, leading to the rise of fat-free diets, which made billions for those promoting them. But we now know that not all fats are bad! Science has prevailed, and we no longer have to treat avocados like criminals. Healthy fats provide energy, support cell function, help the body absorb important vitamins, and give your skin that glowy "I woke up like this" look. Oh, and they can make food taste amazing. Did I mention that when avocados grow up, they can become guacamole? Yum.

There are four different types of fats in food; two are good for you, and two you can do without. The good kinds of fats are polyunsaturated and monounsaturated, and both decrease your risk for heart disease while lowering your bad cholesterol LDL (low-density lipoprotein). They also boost your good cholesterol HDL (high-density lipoprotein). To help myself memorize which type of cholesterol is good vs bad, I imagine the L in LDL to stand for "lousy" and the H in HDL to represent "healthy." Keep in mind that consuming fats does not make you "fat". Fats have a vital role in your body's ability to function, so do not avoid the good kind.

Monounsaturated Fats

These fats are good fats, helping lower bad cholesterol (LDL) and raise good cholesterol (HDL), thus reducing your risk of heart disease. They're also anti-inflammatory and can help regulate blood sugar, which is a big win. Monounsaturated fats are liquid at room temperature and harden when chilled. They can be found in plant foods such as nuts, avocados, and olive oil.

Polyunsaturated Fats

These include omega-3 and omega-6 fats, which the body needs for brain function and cell growth. They are found in plant and animal foods, including fatty fish (salmon, tuna, mackerel, sardines, and trout), walnuts, soy milk, tofu, sunflower, sesame, and pumpkin seeds.

Trans Fats

Artificial trans fats have been banned in the U.S., but trace amounts may still appear in some processed foods, especially imported items or older products still on shelves. Common culprits are commercial baked goods, frozen pizza, fried foods, and margarine.

Saturated Fats

Mostly found in animal products, with some exceptions, these menaces are typically solid at room temperature. The American Heart Association recommends that they be limited to no more than six percent of your daily caloric intake, as they can raise your LDL cholesterol. Saturated fats are commonly found in beef, lamb, pork, poultry skin, lard, butter, cheese, ice cream, coconut oil, palm oil, palm kernel oil, and anything baked or fried with these ingredients. While HDL cholesterol is delivered directly to your liver to be removed from your bloodstream, LDL cholesterol travels straight to your arteries, where it can build up.

It's a common misconception that eating foods high in dietary cholesterol (like eggs and shrimp) directly causes high blood cholesterol. For most people, it does not. I know, this is crazy confusing, but the bigger culprits for high blood cholesterol levels are eating saturated and trans fats. These troublemakers can affect how your liver processes fats, raising LDL (or bad) cholesterol. That excess has the potential to build up in your bloodstream and stick to the walls of your arteries, narrowing them and increasing your risk for a heart attack or stroke. Some cholesterol is essential for cell structure and hormone production, but your body actually produces enough, so it's not necessary to eat any dietary cholesterol.

It's important to know the difference between fats you call friends and fats you call foes! If you avoid trans and saturated fats with vigor, you should certainly see significant upgrades in your health. This is the kind of thing that gets doctors pumped; improved blood work leads to serious fist bumps in an exam room.

Processed Foods

Not all processed foods are evil, but some deserve a hard pass. Processing simply means changing food from its original form, sometimes for convenience (like pre-cut veggies), but other times at the cost of nutrition. The problem isn't processing itself; it's the ingredients being added. When preservatives, hydrogenated oils, and mountains of sugar or salt sneak in, a once-nutritious food becomes something else entirely. These additives can turn a nutritious raw food item into an unhealthy choice in a hurry. It's pretty sad when quality food is completely bastardized. Frozen peaches, for example, are a fantastic choice because they are quickly peeled and frozen soon after being picked, maintaining most of their nutrition. On the other hand, canned peaches in sugary syrup are far less wonderful. A plain potato is packed with vitamin C and potassium, but those benefits take a serious hit once fried in oils or turned into salty chips.

Ready-to-eat snacks and meals like crackers, deli meats, and frozen dinners are often loaded with preservatives and sodium. Some studies have found a link between high intake of ultra-processed foods and increased risk of certain cancers. While more research is needed, choosing whole, minimally processed foods is a safe bet for long-term health

Limit these processed foods:

- Sugary soft drinks
- Shelf-stable meals (boxed mac & cheese, canned pastas)
- Packaged baked goods & breads
- Instant noodles & soups
- Packaged snacks (sweet or savory)

- Processed meats (bacon, hot dogs, pepperoni, deli meats)
- Anything made mostly from sugar, oils, or artificial fats

Choose foods and ingredients in their most natural form or as close to it as possible. Read labels. If the ingredient list looks like a science experiment, your body probably doesn't need it. Stick to real, recognizable foods whenever possible.

To Dessert or Not to Dessert

Getting fit doesn't mean you must say goodbye to all things sweet. In fact, dessert can totally be part of your wellness journey; the key is balance, not deprivation. If it fits into your exact Formula and daily caloric budget, have it! Choose balance and know that it's okay to enjoy without guilt. Just don't be reckless. If you've been treating yourself to multiple desserts daily, taper back to reach your goals. Ideally, 80-90% of your calories will be nutritious, so going overboard on desserts could damage that effort. Unless, of course, fruit salad is your chosen sweet treat. And if it is, go to town on it!

Occasionally enjoying a cookie, candy bar, or slice of cake won't ruin your progress; it's all about moderation. But if you can find or bake healthier versions of your favorites using whole grains and healthy fats, you should. I'll ignore the threat of being redundant here: perfect is boring! Unless medically or morally necessary, you don't have to lock yourself into any sort of weird "no sugar ever" box. Just be reasonable. I'm an incredibly-healthy eater and have no issues sticking with my Formula (I used to be 45 pounds heavier, by the way), but I have a small bit of milk chocolate almost every day. And if a day goes by without it, I consider it a sad day. Show both grit and grace when it comes to dessert.

Sugar

Sugar is so addictive! Of course, this sweet little tyrant comes with little quality nutritional value because, darn it, it tastes great! Listen, I can't tell you that refined, granulated, white, or brown sugar is good for you. It's not. But I'm also not going to recommend that you never have it. Instead, I'm going to encourage you to limit it because excessive sugar consumption is connected to all sorts of nasty health issues, including obesity, type 2 diabetes, cardiovascular disease, and poor oral health. Remember your mom telling you not to rot your teeth out? Ding! Ding! Ding! She was right.

So limit sweets like donuts, candy, and soda, but liberally enjoy natural sugars in whole foods like fruits, veggies, and whole grains. The good stuff contains fiber, vitamins, and minerals that help slow digestion and stabilize blood sugar, unlike refined sugars, which cause quick spikes and crashes. Sugar is also easy to over-consume, leading to excess calorie intake that can contribute to weight gain over time.

Is brown sugar better than white sugar? Nah. Brown sugar is just refined white sugar with dyes and/or molasses added. But hey, sugar is a carbohydrate, and carbs fuel our bodies, so it can be used as a quick energy source. It's just wiser to pursue natural sugars found in fruits, veggies, and whole grains. Sugar substitutes can dramatically decrease caloric intake, but some are better than others. These sweeteners are considered safe by regulatory agencies like the FDA when consumed in moderation, though some people prefer natural alternatives for taste or personal preference. Plant-based substitutions like Stevia and monk fruit are ideal because they offer natural options without the added calories.

Blood sugar, or glucose, is your body's energy source. Ideally, blood sugar remains steady, helping you feel energetic, think clearly, and avoid crashes. The best way to keep blood sugar stable is by eating healthy, whole foods like fruits, veggies, and whole grains, which release sugar at a slow pace into your bloodstream, causing a gradual rise in blood sugar levels. Unhealthy foods like sodas, candies, and processed foods can cause drastic highs and lows in your blood sugar levels, because refined sugars are quickly absorbed into your bloodstream. Spiked blood sugar can feel good at first, but then may leave you feeling jittery, anxious, or dizzy. This often causes an overproduction of insulin, which sends your blood sugar levels crashing in the opposite direction. Fatigue, crankiness, and hunger usually accompany these crashes. Instead of focusing purely on taste when deciding what to eat or drink, consider how your choices will make you feel. Blood sugar should be a key factor in that decision-making process.

Fast Food

I have nothing against getting my food quickly, especially when I'm hungry. I imagine you feel the same way. So, instead of vilifying all fast foods, let's steer clear of highly processed, sugar-infested, or fried foods. Easy, right? Times have changed, and restaurants have evolved to meet our demands. There are a ton of drive-throughs dishing out fresh veggies, grilled meats, whole grains, and fruit; the onus is on you to choose those restaurants and order healthy options. You can also choose fast foods at the grocery store, like bagged salads, pre-chopped and mixed fruit bowls, and packages of fresh sushi. Please don't allow time constraints to be your lame excuse for eating poorly. Fast food comes in all varieties; you now know how to differentiate the good from the bad. Choose wisely!

Chapter 4 | Supercharged Nutrition: Rocket Fuel for Your Body

Doing better with nutrition is absolutely attainable. Fueling your body well isn't about perfection; it's about making better choices more often. You don't need to overhaul your life overnight. You just need to start. Add more fruits and veggies. Swap white bread for whole grain. Add beans to your salad. Choose water over soda. Be intentional!

Keep it simple. Keep it colorful. Keep it real. And remember: your body is always paying attention to how you treat it. Feed it with care, and it'll thank you with energy, strength, and vibrant health for years to come.

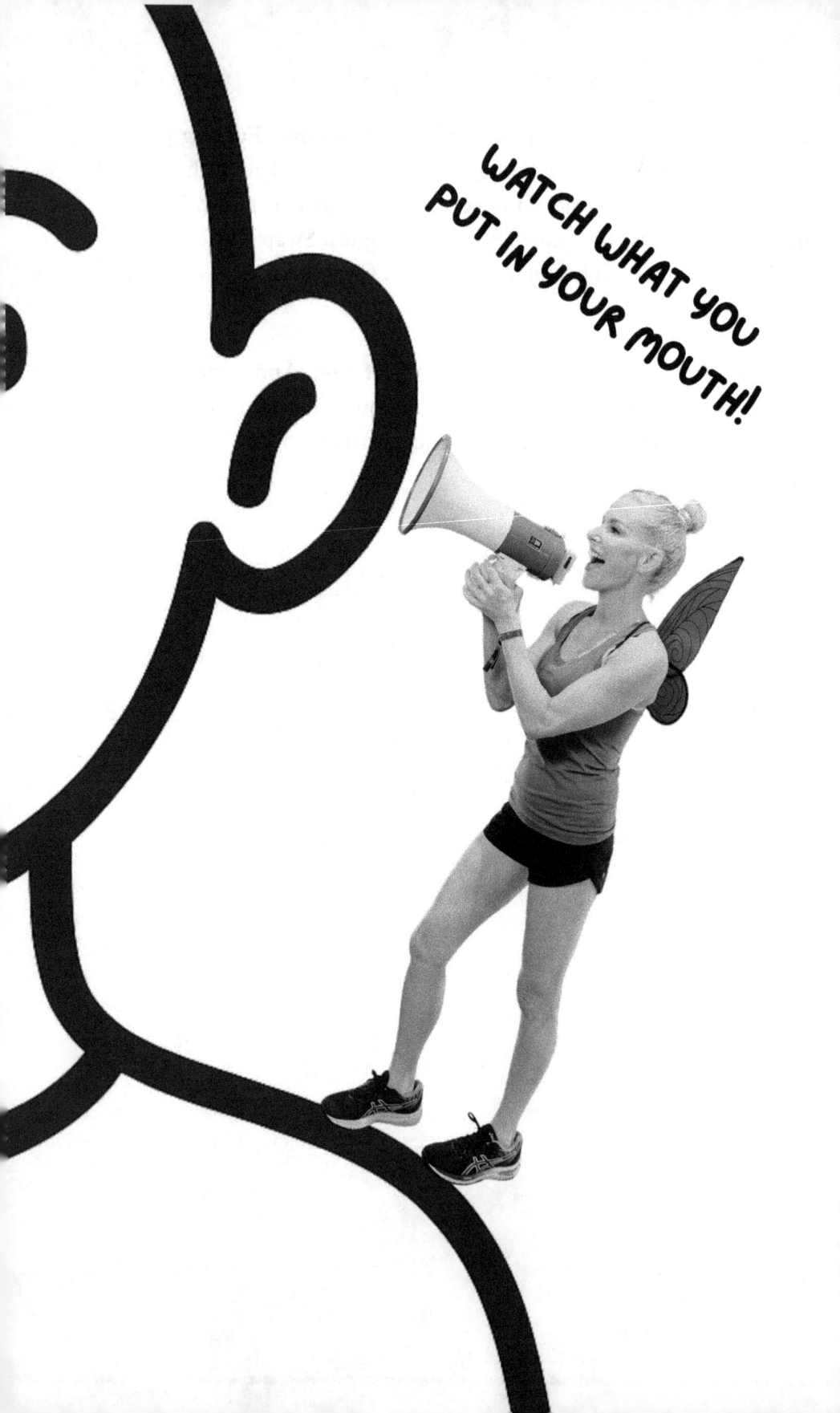

Chapter 5

LIQUID GOLD VS. LIQUID GARBAGE

Water

Water isn't just a thirst-quencher; it's the magic elixir that makes you tick. You're practically a walking can of soup, with water making up about 60% of your body. Fascinating and kinda weird, right? But this clear, calorie-free magic potion keeps every part of you working properly, from your organs to your brain, your muscles to your skin. Just as soup wouldn't be soup without water, neither would you. It's your main ingredient. The most effective, convenient, and affordable way to supercharge the way you look, perform, and feel is to drink water. Let's review.

Free AC

Water serves as your body's internal air conditioner. It regulates your temperature through sweat and breath, helping you keep cool during workouts, hot weather, or intense air guitar jams. Without enough water, your internal thermostat can get wonky, and overheating becomes a real risk.

Chapter 5 | Liquid Gold vs. Liquid Garbage

Regular = Excellent

Water aids digestion, moves nutrients, and keeps everything flowing smoothly, so you can proudly sport your #TeamRegular jersey. Staying hydrated softens stools and prevents the kind of constipation that makes you rethink your life choices.

Fuller Faster

Drinking water before and during meals can help you feel fuller, which means you might eat less without even trying. Studies back it up! Plus, swapping soda, sugary drinks, and boozy beverages for water can help slash hundreds of calories a day. Many folks lose weight just by switching to water. So easy!

Organ MVP

Every organ in your body, every *single* one, counts on water to do its job. Your kidneys? They need it to flush out toxins and keep kidney stones at bay. Your liver? It uses water to metabolize and detoxify. Your heart? Water helps keep your blood pressure steady and your ticker pumping smoothly.

The Ultimate Glow Up!

Water helps your skin stay elastic, hydrated, and healthy-looking. It's basically a beauty filter in a bottle (or a glass, or a reusable cup with a silly straw, whatever makes you sip more often). Combined with moisturizing creams applied to your outsides, water can boost your shine from your insides!

The Brainiac

Your brain loves water almost as much as your mouth loves coffee. Hydration supports hormone production, neurotransmitters, and cognitive function. Even slight dehydration can make you foggy, forgetful, and cranky. So, if you're feeling off or a headache is setting in, maybe don't blame the news. Grab some H2O instead.

Power-Up

Water enhances physical performance, keeps your mind sharp, focus steady, and helps you crush goals on every level. Hydration boosts endurance, strength, and stamina. Dehydration, however, can sabotage your session, increase your injury risk, and leave you feeling like a slug in the desert.

Don't Dehydrate

Dehydration might start with subtle signs like dry mouth and thirst. If ignored, it can spiral into fatigue, dizziness, and even life-threatening conditions like kidney failure. Don't let it sneak up on you. It's easy to avoid!

Drink Up, Buttercup

Water is cheap, accessible, and life-giving. While other low- or no-calorie drinks can help keep you hydrated, nothing beats good ol' H_2O. Aim to make at least every other beverage you sip plain water; it's the gold standard with zero downsides. Think of it as your secret weapon for better health, sharper focus, clearer skin, smoother digestion, and more productive workouts. So fill up that water bottle and give your body the love it deserves. Cheers!

Percentage of human body parts comprised of water:

Brain 73%

Heart 73%

Skin 64%

Pancreas 73%

Liver 71%

Muscles 79%

Kidney 79%

Lungs 83%

Bones 32%

According to H.H. Mitchell, Journal of Biological Chemistry, 1930; 158(3):625–637

Liquid Calories

Liquid calories are the ultimate source of weight loss sabotage. Drinking your calories sounds innocent, maybe even convenient. After all, sipping your way through your day can't be that bad! But here's the hard truth: 100 calories of soda is no different than 100 calories of candy. You might think it's a harmless habit, but your waistline disagrees! Imagine skipping a meal to consume a 300-calorie drink and wondering why you're still hungry an hour later. Spoiler alert: sugary drinks slip through the radar unnoticed. They never trigger your stomach's satisfaction sensors, so hunger pains start kicking in even though you've already downed hundreds of calories. Hunger will probably drive you to have a snack, and maybe another. The calories in that soda or juice? They might as well have vanished into thin air as far as your body's hunger signals are concerned. It's like magic, but the bad kind. Sugary drinks disappear into your system, but the calories don't trigger any of the satisfaction signals that solid food would, leaving you hungry again and reaching for more to eat.

Sugar Bombs

Let's talk about sugary drinks: soda, sweet teas, juices, flavored lattes, you name it. They're often the poster children for "empty calories," but that doesn't mean you should feel empty after drinking them. Oh no, you're actually full of sugar! These drinks pour refined sugars into your system at an alarming rate, throwing your body into a panic to process the sudden onslaught. Your waistline? Well, it's having a growth spurt. All those "refreshing" sugary sips come with a side of extra pounds, plus a heightened risk for heart disease and diabetes. And don't forget about fructose, the sneaky little sugar that loves to camp out in your liver and set up a fat storage facility.

Sports Drinks

Invented for athletes, electrolyte beverages are essential for anyone taxing their body through exercise, sports, or physical labor. What are electrolytes, and why do they need replacing, you ask? They're essential minerals (magnesium, potassium, and sodium) that regulate fluid balance, muscle contractions, and nerve function. When fluids leave the body through sweat, urine, diarrhea, or vomiting, electrolytes go with them. Replacing these minerals becomes necessary when we lose a bunch quickly.

I'm going to not-so-humbly brag that the original sports drink, Gatorade, was invented by a University of Florida physician, Dr. Robert Cade (a kidney specialist), in 1965. He created it to help the Florida Gator football team withstand training in Gainesville, Florida's hot, sticky, swamp-like summer climate. Made of sugar, salt, water, and eventually lemon juice, it effectively helped put pep back in the step of orange-and-blue-clad athletes, replacing the energy they'd burned through exercise and sweat. They soon discovered it was also superb for those dehydrated by illness. As a two-time Gator graduate, I must inform you that you're required to say "Go Gators!" each time you take a swig of this magical potion. Bonus points for doing the Chomp with your arms.

Chapter 5 | Liquid Gold vs. Liquid Garbage

Sports drinks are fantastic for hydration and balancing these essential minerals. But if you're not doing endurance activities, sweating profusely, or sick, they're mostly unnecessary, and may even be harmful. They're often loaded with sugar, salt, chemicals, caffeine, and artificial colors. Sure, many taste great, but you've got goals, and downing a bottle of calories and content you don't need may do more harm than good. Overdosing on excessive amounts of sports drinks can cause dizziness, blood pressure issues, nausea, and kidney, heart, and muscle problems. Sports drinks get a big thumbs up if you're working or playing on a hot day, exercising vigorously, or are ill. Stick to water if you're watching a movie on the couch or walking the mall.

Not So Smooth

Smoothies and fruit juices often masquerade as the "good guys" in the beverage world. After all, they've got fruit in them! Must be healthy, right? Newsflash: just because it's made with fruit doesn't mean it's free of consequences. A large smoothie could easily pack 500-800 calories, and your hunger may remain. The problem? Blending fruit disrupts the fiber structure, which makes the goal of satisfying your stomach a lot harder. But smoothies are not all bad. You just have to use legit discretion when choosing ingredients. Stick with whole fruits and veggies, add Greek yogurt or nut milks for satisfying protein, and avoid added sugar or syrups. Leave your produce chunky to preserve some fiber. A healthy smoothie with quality ingredients can be a fantastic alternative dessert.

Coffeeeeeee!

Coffee is actually pretty good stuff, and I'm not just saying that to get on your good side. Coffee alone is calorie and sugar-free, which is awesome, and certain types (depending on the beans it's made with) are filled with antioxidants and nutrients like riboflavin. Some studies show it may help fend off certain types of diseases, which is incredible. Caffeinated coffees can boost energy, which can be fab when you want it, but bad when you don't. If you want to avoid the jitters often associated with java, choose decaf throughout your day or as the perfect after-dinner drink to enjoy before bed. If you love coffee, I give it my full blessing; just don't load it up with sugar and cream.

Tea Time, Y'all

Whether you drink it hot or cold, black, green, oolong, or white, tea is a satisfying alternative to coffee. It packs plenty of antioxidants and is linked to improved heart and brain health and decreased chances of stroke. Tea is a quality option for those averse to caffeine as it packs 50% less than coffee. Avoid loading it with sugars and creams. Most importantly, if you drink it hot, hold your tea cup with a pinky finger pointed straight up toward the sky. Declare things around you to be "brilliant" and "lovely" while laughing with your lips together. If you prefer tea cold, use plenty of ice, and shout the word "y'all" with your outside voice as much as possible, even if you're inside.

Low and No-Calorie drinks. Water is the gold standard, and you should ideally make it at least 50% of your liquid intake, but if you want to enjoy some flavored or sparkling waters, so be it. I do! Aim for natural ingredients, which are better than the chemical ingredients you cannot pronounce.

Caffeinated DrAnks!

Caffeine is the world's most commonly used drug. It occurs both naturally and artificially in many drinks and some foods. Small amounts can generate some good feelings as they increase the circulation of adrenaline and cortisol, improving alertness, focus, and energy. Too much can cause headaches, insomnia, bladder

Chapter 5 | Liquid Gold vs. Liquid Garbage

irritation, chest pain, and anxiety. Figuring out how little or how much is right for you can be tricky.

Highly caffeinated energy drinks scare me. I've heard too many horror stories of people (often teenagers) suffering consequences that include cardiac and neurological issues, as well as behavioral changes. It's best to avoid these drinks entirely or consume them sparingly and with caution. With healthy habits, you shouldn't need to lean on caffeine as a crutch.

Here's a full disclosure message that goes along with my "perfect is boring" mantra. I drink decaffeinated Diet Coke, and you'll often see me on social media with it. Just know I drink a ton of water and decaffeinated hot tea, too. When adding a sweetener, my go-to is stevia. I consume mostly fresh produce, nuts, seeds, beans, and soy. I rarely consume things on the harmful list, so a decaf Diet Coke here and there isn't a big problem. Remember, if 80-90 % of your caloric intake is nutritious, you can have a little fun with the rest.

Alcohol

Unless it's pretty rare, alcohol consumption can kill your weight loss and fitness goals. First, alcohol is calorie-dense with very little nutritional value, and this alone can easily derail your efforts with the Exact Formula. It also slows down the body's ability to burn fat, as the liver prioritizes metabolizing alcohol over other nutrients. Additionally, alcohol can impair judgment and lead to overeating or poor food choices. Think about how many millions of pounds of nachos supreme and pizza have been devoured thanks to beer and cocktails. Once alcohol takes effect, discipline often goes out the window, and reckless consumption kicks in. The same goes for wine and champagne. Perhaps viewed as more civilized, the effects are the same.

The Domino Effect of One Drink

Alcohol can wreck your workouts, either by making you skip them altogether or by seriously reducing your effort when you do show up. It also ruins recovery by dehydrating your body and messing with your sleep. For some people, once it starts, the spiral can be hard to stop—kind of like that children's book *If You Give a Moose a Muffin*, but messier.

If you give Candace a cocktail, she'll probably decide to order a bunch of appetizers. And when she orders too many appetizers (likely onion rings or chicken poppers), she'll order another cocktail and completely blow her Exact Formula for the day. Oops! She might even give her phone number to Angus, the guy her friends have told her to steer clear of for weeks.

When Candace finally gets a rideshare home (smart move, Candace!), she's probably not going to brush or floss before bed (eww), and she definitely won't wash her face. Cue the breakouts! After passing out from the effects of all that alcohol, she'll toss and turn around 3:00 a.m., sweating and feeling queasy from her overindulgence. She'll make a few trips back and forth to the bathroom before things settle down.

Unfortunately, in the middle of all the bathroom runs, she'll bonk her head on the doorframe, leaving a bruise. How is she going to explain *that* to her boss, Tisha, at tomorrow's marketing strategy meeting?

When her alarm goes off at 6:15 a.m. for her morning bike ride with her training buddy Max, she tries to hit snooze but accidentally stops the alarm altogether. Poor Max shows up at the bridge, ready for their ride, but when Candy no-shows, he gets worried. Instead of his usual ride, he pedals over to her house to check on her. After knocking, then pounding on her door, he finally yells, "Candooo! Candooo!" (That's his nickname for her.)

Chapter 5 | Liquid Gold vs. Liquid Garbage

When Candooo finally stumbles to the door, Max is so upset he tears up and tells her they can't be workout partners anymore because she's just too unreliable. Ouch!

Disoriented, Candy checks her phone and realizes she's going to be late for her meeting with Tisha. In a hurry to get ready, she steps on the scale and notices she's four pounds heavier than last week. Dang! After trying on a few outfits, she realizes her favorite skirt is too tight. Hello, bloat! Finally, she rushes out the door and makes it to the office, only to be met by Tisha, hands on hips and a less-than-pleased expression.

With her mind too foggy to come up with any fresh ideas, Candy blurts out, "Let's do a campaign on MySpace.com!" Tisha stares at her in disbelief because, well, MySpace has been dead for decades. And just like that, Candy is fired.

Feeling defeated, Candy clears out her desk and heads straight to the bar to drown her sorrows in, you guessed it, another cocktail.

You see, even just one drink can set off a domino effect. It might lead to overeating, a bad night's sleep (or a sketchy night with Angus), and a foggy, cranky morning, skipped workouts, and poor decision-making. It's a slippery slope. For those serious about losing weight and getting fit, cutting back on or eliminating alcohol can make a world of difference.

Many of the people I guide have shared how they casually slid into having multiple drinks daily without even realizing it. This led to weight gain, problems at work and home, and depression. However, once they cut back or quit, they'd drop significant weight, feel sharper and more energetic, and return to rebuilding their relationships.

This isn't to say that enjoying an adult beverage once in a while has to be off-limits, but if you're serious about losing weight and improving your fitness, cutting back on alcohol can make a world of difference. Perhaps you could reserve it for weddings, holidays, or occasional nights with old friends? This is truly a case where less is more. Don't let one drink spiral into a series of poor choices; take control of your habits and reclaim your health. If you need support, Alcoholics Anonymous is a great place to start.

Without a doubt, your drinks do count. Instead of chalking them up as inconsequential freebies, consider them a valuable part in your health outcomes. Drink enough to stay hydrated, avoid refined sugars and excess calories, while enjoying the benefits that come from coffees, teas, and the occasional smoothie. If you start with water, end with water, and drink some water in between, both your insides and outsides will thank you. Cheers!

Chapter 6

CHOP IT LIKE IT'S HOT

Think cooking healthy is hard? Think again! Whipping up nutritious meals can be just as simple, and way more rewarding, than eating junk food, for real! Healthy cooking doesn't have to be complicated; it can be easy, quick, and downright delicious. With a little bit of planning and preparation and ginormous combination of whole ingredients, cooking styles, seasonings, and sauces to choose from, I'm eager to share all of the yummy options with you.

What's for Dinner?

Stuck on what to eat? Don't worry, your next meal is a choose-your-own-adventure story! Remember all the things we discussed in Chapter 4: Supercharged Nutrition? Welp, you can use any combination of those items to make breakfast, lunch, dinner, snacks, appetizers, desserts, and any other category of food I'm forgetting! Eat produce, whole grains, lean proteins, and low-fat dairy products in any combination you choose. Take a peek in your fridge right now. What healthy combos can you create? Maybe a veggie-packed omelet for breakfast or a whole-grain wrap with lean protein for lunch. Get creative and mix it up!

What's for Breakfast? Absolutely anything you want! Did you know eating chicken, asparagus, and quinoa in the morning is legal? I'm not talking crazy, friends. You are not stuck eating pancakes and bacon. Of course, typical breakfast foods like eggs, fruit, and steel-cut oatmeal can be healthy choices, but you shouldn't feel confined. Expand your options if you want to kick things up a notch in the A.M., and supercharge the rest of your day. Want a shrimp cocktail before work? Go for it.

Cooking Styles

Cooking doesn't have to be complicated. A world of easy and delicious options exists that don't require drowning your food in oil, butter, or sauces. You can bake, broil, boil, roast, toast, grill, air fry, steam, or microwave your foods; just avoid frying. You can also eat things raw! The list of Fitz-approved options is pretty long. I've only put one cooking style on the "please don't" list. I bet that makes you do the big sigh of relief thing. Ahhhhh. That's better.

Try baking for crispy textures, roasting for deep flavors, broiling for quick, high-heat cooking, or air frying for a lighter crunch. If you barbecue, sauté, or microwave your foods without dumping too much salt, sugar, or unhealthy fats on it, you're good to go! Sautéing may require a small amount of oil or butter, but even with that, you could substitute a healthier option like broth. If you're creative, just about anything can be made deliciously healthy.

So Spicy!

Want to add bold flavor to your meals without extra calories, unhealthy fats, or junk? Say hello to your spice rack, it was built for your taste buds and to supercharge your health! Not only do herbs and spices make your food taste amazing, but they're also loaded with health benefits. Some, like turmeric and ginger, help fight inflammation, while others, like rosemary and cinnamon, may support memory and blood sugar balance. While some salt is okay, lower-sodium options include basil, cumin, turmeric, garlic, and chili flakes. Basically, your spice rack might double as your medicine cabinet.

You Devil

Sauces and dressings can make or break a meal, not just in taste but in nutrition. They can elevate your dish to gourmet levels or drown it in hidden sugars, salts, and unhealthy fats. Let's make sure yours enhances your dish in only positive ways. Sauces typically provide the featured flavor we're excited about, so make choices that truly bring out the best in the nutritious foods you're preparing, enhancing your meals, not sabotaging them. The best are made from whole, nutrient-packed ingredients like fresh herbs, nuts, and healthy oils. Think vinaigrettes, tahini, pesto, tomato sauces, and homemade salsa, all the flavor, none of the junk! Healthy homemade dressings make excellent marinades, too.

Bottled Up

There are plenty of yummy and healthy store-bought sauces, too, but you'll have to read labels because there are lots of "bads and uglies" you should avoid. Look out for high fructose corn syrups, which are frequently found in BBQ and teriyaki sauces. Soy sauce, teriyaki, and jarred marinara are often low in fat but may err on the too-high-sodium side. The US Food and Drug Administration says 5% Daily Value (DV) or less of sodium per serving is considered low, and 20% DV or more of sodium per serving is considered high. Pay close attention to serving sizes because the nutrition information on the Nutrition Facts label is usually based on one serving. Many sauces are packed with artificial additives and preservatives, things your body doesn't need and nature never intended. Consider corn syrup, soybean oil, "natural flavors," and large amounts of sugar as red flags when reading labels.

Even healthy sauces should be used in moderation. A 'light' dressing isn't so light if you drench your salad. Try dipping instead for more flavor and fewer calories! Overall, the healthiest dressings and sauces are made with a combination of whole foods, herbs, and spices. For easy, wholesome alternatives, try making your own sauces at home:

Salsa: A simple mix of fresh tomatoes, onions, jalapeños, and spices adds a kick to any dish.

Lemon Vinaigrette: Olive oil, lemon juice, and seasonings create a light, zesty dressing.

Tomato Sauce: Simmer tomatoes, garlic, oregano, salt, and pepper for a rich, flavorful base with no hidden junk!

You Sneaky Fox

Sneaking extra veggies isn't just about making food taste better; it's about boosting your nutrition and adding fiber, which can help with digestion, weight management, and overall health. Get creative in the kitchen; what veggies can you sneak into your next meal? Add some cauliflower to mashed potatoes, grate carrots into meatloaf, slide some spinach into lasagna, or toss zucchini into pasta sauce. If your kids refuse to eat certain veggies, this is a quality move, which falls perfectly under the Parental "Don't Ask, Don't Tell" policy. If you don't have kids to sneak veggies past, this trick also works for adults. Add extra greens to your meals for an almost invisible nutrition boost. It's a simple way to make every meal healthier without compromising taste!

Whole Grains are a Whole Lot Better

Trade white pasta, rice, and bread for whole-grain versions. Whole grains are rich in nutrients like B vitamins, iron, and magnesium, which help support your metabolism, promote heart health, and keep your body running at its best. They also contain more fiber, provide longer-lasting energy, and you'll experience less of a blood sugar rollercoaster. Switching to whole grains might take some time if you're used to white bread and pasta. Try gradually mixing whole-grain options into your meals; soon, you'll learn to love the extra flavor and texture!

Pitch the Processed Foods

By cutting out processed foods, you're doing your body a huge favor by helping reduce your risk of chronic diseases, improving digestion, and boosting your energy. Processed meats include hot dogs, bacon, and deli meats, which have been preserved by smoking, salting, curing, or adding chemical preservatives. Processed baked goods, frozen entrees, certain cereals, snacks, and chips are boxed, bagged, and canned and are often packed with sugar, salt, and chemicals. Instead of filling your pantry with the former, stock your fridge with unprocessed lean meats, produce, whole grains, and legumes. How do you know which chemicals to avoid? Look for ingredients you can't pronounce; those long, complicated words might be a red flag. It may not belong in your lunch if it sounds like it belongs in a lab. Do a little research on anything you don't immediately recognize as food before taking a bite.

Smarter Servings

Even with healthy foods, there can be too much of a good thing. Mindful eating is key to avoiding weight gain; slow down, savor your food, and tune in to your body's hunger cues. It's not just about what you eat, but how much you eat. To avoid overeating, use smaller plates, chew slowly, enjoy a tall glass of water while dining, and pay attention to when you feel full. You may also want to invest in a food scale to ensure you're not accidentally consuming more than you think. Remember that protein and fiber are the stars of satiety, so aim for a palm-sized portion of protein and fill half your plate with fiber-rich produce to keep you full and satisfied. Box leftovers for later, or share some healthy homemade cooking with your furry friend, Fido. If you find yourself reaching for food out of boredom or emotion, take a moment to pause and check in with yourself. Sometimes, a glass of water or a deep breath is all it takes to reset your cravings.

Meal Prepping Makes Sense

If you don't want to go through the process of cooking for each meal, make double or triple portions and freeze leftovers. Yes, it might take a little extra time to prepare, but the time you'll save on busy days is worth it. For variety, rotate your meals weekly or switch up your seasonings and sauces so you never feel like you're eating the same thing every day. That way, "future you" can grab a homemade meal instead of a super-sized order of regret from the drive-thru. Cooking at home is typically more affordable than restaurant meals, and this master move will benefit your body and bank account!

Savvy Snacking

There's a good chance you might get hungry or need a little boost between meals, and I encourage you to answer those calls. Frequent, balanced snacks may help manage energy and appetite, so spreading calorie consumption throughout your day is a good thing. Much better than the awkward "one big meal per day plan". Just choose healthy snacks! Enjoy quick peel-and-eat fruit, chopped veggies, trail mix, hummus, and whatever suits you instead of hitting a vending machine full of fried, processed, or sugary nonsense. Pro tip: Nuts make wonderful snacks, but they are high in fat and calories. Instead of tossing them down your throat like a madman, buy nuts in their shells. The process of opening each shell will slow you down and allow your stomach's satiety signals to sound off before you eat too much.

Eating shouldn't be too complicated. You don't need to count every macronutrient or deprive yourself of everything you love. Choose most of your meals and snacks from the list of healthy food items, purchase and prepare meals and snacks wisely, and spread your caloric intake throughout your day. This shouldn't drive you crazy. When you feel uncertain, yield to the Lil' Fitzy on your shoulder. She'll point you in the right direction, and when you do what she tells you to do ... prepare to feel that lil' smooch on your cheek!

Chapter 7

THE CASE AGAINST DIETS

Diets are short-term tactics that generate short-term results and are in no way a path toward supercharging anything! They tend to be based on restrictions that lead to suffering, frustration, and failure. Many people, maybe even you, have pursued diets with good intentions, but dieting does not equal eating wisely or achieving lasting results. In fact, you will not find the word "diet" in this book with a positive connotation attached, because I believe that dieting has been one of the most significant downfalls of healthy societies. Instead of people learning to eat the right amounts of the right foods, they've learned to eat with utter disregard for health and then try to undo the outcomes of their reckless behavior with a quick fix. Well, folks, quick fixes do not exist. Fad diets are crap! There, I said it, and boy, does that feel good. They are all absolute crap.

This is a reminder that the Exact Formula is NOT a diet. It's a sensible plan with structure and long-term sustainability. It has zero rigid exclusions and encourages you to make quality choices for nutrition and food satisfaction. That is something you can do for life. Don't hop on the next weight loss bandwagon; choose sustainable, long-lasting change instead. Think about it. Wouldn't getting to your favorite weight and staying there be phenomenal? Wouldn't it be nice to do so while still being able to have a slice of pizza, cake, or a beer once in a while? And wouldn't it be great to

Chapter 7 | The Case Against Diets

lose weight without having to fork over $300 per month to some snake-oil salesman promising you quick weight loss with their products?

Yeah. Let's get into that. Brace yourself, because I've just climbed onto my soapbox and I'm not holding anything back. I have utter disdain for the vultures in the fitness industry who have based their entire careers on scamming decent people who want a healthy body out of their hard-earned money. Nothing pisses me off more. It's vicious, and if I could tour the world popping each jerk who has sold a "weight loss supplement" in the mouth, I'd do it. Also, violence is bad. Don't punch people unless you're in a boxing ring.

Folks, other than the new string of medical-grade semaglutide injections (we'll get to that), nothing you buy at the supplement store will actually induce weight loss. No smoothies, bars, or pills with the term "weight loss" or "diet" on them are going to get you where you want to go. What works? Burning more calories than you consume. Period. Imagine if I tried to sell you an apple wrapped in "diet apple" packaging. Would you think I was a scammer? Of course! The same goes for bars, snacks, and smoothies wrapped in those words. Don't fall for it. You are not a sucker. At least, not anymore.

And another thing. I find it fascinating that most of these products are being sold by minimum-wage, part-time employees in a supplement store. Not scientists in any way. Why the hell would anyone take their suggestions on what chemicals to ingest? Really! I'm all down for taking quality advice from a physician or registered dietitian who has carefully reviewed your blood work, knows where you're deficient, and knows whether a certain supplement may work well with your other medications. But what makes "Bob," whose last job was selling tires, a wizard in weight loss and nutrition? Okay, what if Bob were a personal trainer? He likely earned some sort of certificate for teaching exercise online, and now he's your go-to for iron, magnesium, and potassium? NO! He's not. He's officially not.

The other cool place people score supplements, like they're shopping for crack, is in the trunk of their neighbor's car. You know, the neighbor who isn't even fit herself, yet is selling all sorts of solutions for you and your problems. Yep, she's also selling candles, kitchen stuff, weight loss supplements, and those sticky "weight loss wraps." I love the concept of wrapping your torso in some goo-filled plastic wrap with the notion that it's just going to melt your internal fat away, without melting your skin or organs. LOL! This craziness is actually for sale, these promises are actually made, and wonderful people actually pay money for it all.

Please stop being taken advantage of. Please stop taking advice from folks who have no legitimate expertise. Please stop looking for shortcuts that don't exist. Please stop wasting your money. I promise that if you adopt the Exact Formula and complement it with exercise and sleep, you will get where you want to go.

Supplements do have a place. Science is pretty cool, and there are definitely products to help us with our deficiencies. But you need to work with the right professionals to figure out which, if any, will serve you well. Don't just take the stuff your friend is taking or that you heard about on a podcast. If you invest in your lab work (may be covered by insurance if you have it) and a registered dietitian, you will only spend money on supplements that will actually be meaningful to you. This will help you save a fortune on all the products you genuinely do not need. Also, the Food and Drug Administration does not regulate supplements, so it is difficult to be sure if they contain the ingredients they claim to.

Quick story: many years ago, a popular publishing house hired me to write a book on boosting metabolism. I signed the contract

Chapter 7 | The Case Against Diets

and wrote the book. When I was done, they told me that they were going to include two chapters: one promoting "negative calorie foods," suggesting that you could burn more calories digesting certain foods than you consume, and the other promoting weight loss supplements. I responded reasonably, sharing that negative calorie foods do not exist and weight loss supplements were not only a farce but could be dangerous for readers who took certain medications. It was both unethical and dangerous to promote these concepts. Their response? "These topics sell books, so we're adding them!"

I was appalled. Unfortunately for me, I was listed in my contract as a freelance writer instead of the author, so I wouldn't get the final say on content. I dug my heels in and pulled out of the book. They kept my book, added a hack nutritionist's name to the title, and sold it. Hard lesson learned on the contract, but a perfect test of my commitment to your health and my reputation. I knew if I lied to you in those pages, nobody would ever trust me again. Know this: I've never sold out, nor will I.

The world has offered up an endless number of dumb diets. It's hard to imagine there have been so many bad ideas and even more people to fall for them. I know a woman in my town who has a "weight loss business." Gosh, outside of this, I like her. But she tells people not to eat fruit because it contains too much sugar. What? She actually advises people to stop eating raspberries, oranges, and apples. What the hell? It kills me. I've had friends go to her, banish fruit and many other things from their plates, and lose weight over a few months. Inevitably, everyone loses their minds from misery, quits, and regains all the weight they lost plus more. And that's precisely how diets work. Friends, if anyone ever tells you blueberries are bad for you (unless you're personally allergic), run. This is just one example of a dumb diet, and gosh, there are so many more. Let's cover a few of the most popular diets and why they're bad ideas.

Keto

Sure, keto can help with epilepsy, but for the average Joe, it's a nutritional dumpster fire. Slashing fruits, veggies, and grains? Hello, vitamin deficiencies and constipation. Guzzling saturated fat? Congrats on stressing your heart and kidneys. Plus, "keto flu" makes you feel like you've been hit by a truck, and obsessing over macros is about as fun as a root canal. "Keto crotch" and "keto breath" are two other experiences you may want to avoid. Sure, you might lose weight up front, but you could also lose muscle, sanity, and your will to live. This is not a recipe for long-term success.

Intermittent Fasting

Intermittent Fasting sounds edgy until you're hangry, lightheaded, and snapping at your grandma. Jamming all your nutrients into a tiny, arbitrary eating window is a recipe for brain fog, bad moods, and terrible food choices. It can wreck your social life, slow your metabolism, and mess with your hormones. Athletes? Good luck fueling or recovering properly. It's not magic, it's just skipping meals and hoping for the best. Long-term effects? Still a giant question mark. Also, if fasting is so important to you, congrats! You've been doing it your entire life. That's right. Humans have a natural fast built into each day called SLEEP. And when we wake up, we break that fast with, you guessed it, BREAKfast! Food is fuel. Eat it when you need it, not on the clock.

Cleanses

Cleanse diets are basically glorified starvation wrapped in a shiny label. Your liver and kidneys already detox your body just fine without the help of overpriced juices or cayenne pepper concoctions. These cleanses slash real food, protein, fats, and fiber, leaving you nutrient-deficient, weak, and hangry. Sure, you might lose a few pounds, but it's just water weight that'll boomerang back the second you eat a sandwich. Plus, they can wreck your digestion, dehydrate you, and foster a toxic mindset that your body needs constant punishment to be "clean." Instead of this ridiculous act of deprivation, keep your digestive system moving with lots of water and fiber, two things that promote real weight loss.

Sugar-Free

Gee. I'd really like to jump on board with this because refined sugar isn't helpful to our health. However, going sugar-free can be pretty difficult. You'd have to avoid all cookies, cakes, sodas, and juices. But you'd also need to avoid ketchup, barbecue sauces, most marinara sauces, cereals, protein bars, smoothies, and even many soups. This is a really rigid way to live. Instead, I encourage you to severely limit refined sugars, but be reasonable. It's nice to have a piece of cake at a birthday party or some marinara sauce on your chicken and veggies.

Low or No Carb

OMGosh. This one is ridiculous. Folks, carbohydrates are not the enemy. They literally give you ENERGY, which makes them more of a bestie. This is the impetus of the phrase, "Food is fuel." Carbs are the stars of that show. Healthy carbs include fruits, veggies, potatoes, whole grains, and beans. Not only do they give us the fuel to go, go, go, but they are also packed with fiber, which keeps our digestive system hopping, allowing us to go, go, go! Try driving anywhere without gas in your car or your electric battery charged up. Ain't happening! Of course, you can limit ultra-processed carbs with little nutritional value, but the good carbs? Keep them coming!

White Out

It's bizarre that avoiding all white foods is actually a thing. As I've said, limiting refined sugars and flours is good, but going cold turkey means you'll have a hard time enjoying a slice of pizza (which most people like to do on occasion). Potatoes often get targeted as an evil "white food," and nothing could be further from the truth. Did you know they are packed with vitamin C, potassium, vitamin B6, protein, iron, and fiber? They're also quite low in calories, considering the amount of satiety they provide. A five-ounce potato will only cost you 100 calories. FYI: I'm a lean woman who is a proud potato eater; I have one every day. Again, it's ideal to avoid refined flours and sugars, but you don't have to be radical about it.

GLP-1 Receptor Agonist /Semaglutide Injections

I'm going to address this, but start by reminding you that I am not in any way, shape, or form a medical professional. I'm not a doctor, nurse, pharmacist, etc. I've spent my entire career shouting, "Magic weight loss pills do not exist." And now they do, in the form of a shot. And it's not really magic; it is a prescription GLP-1 agonist with known, significant side effects and limitations, best used under medical supervision with lifestyle changes. I used to preach that if Oprah Winfrey hasn't found the magic weight loss drug, neither will you. She had all the money and resources, and was still overweight. But now these injections are on the market, and Oprah has slimmed down. So yes, it's obvious that these drugs, which I will not reference by brand name, can be effective. They were originally approved for those with type 2 diabetes, cardiovascular disease, and kidney disease, but are now often prescribed just for weight loss. I'm still on the fence as to whether I like them, because everything comes with a trade-off, right?

Chapter 7 | The Case Against Diets

I've read all the articles and spoken to many physicians, from cardiologists to primary care doctors, and the most common responses I receive on semaglutide for weight loss are positive. If an obese person uses them to achieve a healthy weight, they automatically diminish that individual's risks of heart disease, diabetes, stroke, and other nightmares, especially for folks in the morbidly obese category. I like that aspect a lot.

I've also heard stories of patients suffering from constant nausea, diarrhea, headaches, and dizziness. More serious risks include thyroid cancer, pancreatitis, gallbladder disease, and more. Through social media, I've heard people complain they've lost bone density and experienced other weird side effects. Again, I'm not a doctor, but you don't have to be one to know how to weigh risks.

What I can tell you is that obesity is terrifying. It puts people at risk for all of the super bad, life-altering stuff, with the worst being stroke, heart attacks, and sudden death. When a lean person dies of cardiac arrest, we're shocked. When it happens to an obese person, we think, "Damn shame, but it was bound to happen!" You don't want to be in the "of course you died of heart disease" category. My wish is for everyone to achieve their ideal weight and true health through the guidance I've provided here in this book. Healthy habits do not require a warning label like these shots. If you are obese, please don't take advice from friends; instead, have a discussion with your doctor. Just know that even with shots, you'll eventually have to adopt healthy habits to maintain a healthy weight and achieve fitness. If you do not, you will regain the weight you lost and feel worse than ever.

Health, fitness, and an ideal weight are absolutely within your reach, and you don't need scams, schemes, or starvation to get there. You need real food, real movement, real sleep, and a relentless commitment to yourself. Stay the course. Fight for your future. Build the body and life you deserve, one wise choice at a time. Your power isn't sold in a bottle or hidden in a fad. It's already in you. Get to work!

Chapter 8

FOUR PILLARS OF FITNESS & THE F.I.T.T. PRINCIPLE

Being truly fit isn't just about how far you can run or how much weight you can lift. It's about mastering all Four Pillars: Strength, Cardiorespiratory Endurance, Flexibility, and Balance, to move confidently, powerfully, and pain-free in everyday life and adventure. True fitness means being able to move for long periods, at different intensities and in different ways, without pain or instability. That's right. You must be proficient in all four areas to qualify as FIT. Even elite athletes can fall short of true fitness if they neglect any of these Four Pillars.

Though many people who exclusively focus on cycling or walking, for example, believe they are fit, most fail to meet the mark. Having a passion for a particular type of exercise is fantastic and one of the keys to keeping you going; however, if you only do that one particular exercise, you may be cheating your body. If you exercise in a way that targets each pillar, though, you move into an entirely different category of human. This training will make you more likely to feel great, look fabulous, exude energy, and think clearly while avoiding unnecessary aches and pains.

Fitness isn't as simple as "going for a walk," but it's also not as complicated as counting carbs and competing in triathlons. To qualify as physically fit, you must put in some effort and see results in four categories: strength, cardiorespiratory endurance,

Chapter 8 | Four Pillars of Fitness & The F.I.T.T. Principle

flexibility, and balance. I call them the Four Pillars of Fitness because each is a vital component, and without even one element, the roof could cave in.

Now, let's put this idea to the test. Do these people qualify as FIT?

1. A marathon runner who doesn't have the strength to do five push-ups or carry his luggage.

2. A bodybuilding champion who can't touch her toes or reach behind her to scratch her own back.

3. A yoga instructor who becomes breathless after climbing two flights of stairs.

4. A competitive swimmer who can't stand on one foot for 30 seconds without falling.

The answer to all four examples is NO. None meet the criteria to qualify as fit. This is important to understand because too many people laser-focus on one or maybe two areas of fitness and completely neglect the others. I am deeply embedded in the running community as a race announcer. I host many of the largest and most iconic road races in America, many of which are marathons. One would think that all marathon runners would qualify as FIT. But that prediction would be wrong. And it makes me sad. Sad because I know how much time and effort go into preparing for and conquering the 26.2-mile distance. Surely, that would pay off with an undeniable certificate of fitness, right? Nope. The reason is that many runners tend to only run. This isn't true across the board, but it is for a large chunk of that population. So many of my favorite athletes tend to overlook the power of training for strength, flexibility, or balance. Their cardio-respiratory endurance is off the charts, and that's fantastic, but that doesn't compensate for the tightness and weakness that leave them susceptible to all sorts of painful runner burdens like IT

Band Syndrome and Plantar Fasciitis. Ouch! If only they knew that modest efforts in strength, flexibility, and balance would help them run further, faster, and pain-free. If only they knew how much better their body would look, feel, and perform overall if they did. Commit to all Four Pillars if you want to be truly FIT and not just good at one thing. Your body will thank you.

Four Pillars of Fitness

Muscular Strength

Muscular strength allows you to lift, push, pull, press, and move powerfully against gravity and other forces of resistance. It helps you carry groceries, open that obnoxiously-heavy door, and keep up with life's physical demands. Body weight exercises such as squats, lunges, push-ups, calf raises, crunches, and bridges are great choices because they require zero equipment and utilize gravity to make you stronger. Using tools such as free weights, bands, cables, kettlebells, plyo-boxes, and medicine balls will add variety and challenges to your training.

Cardio Respiratory Endurance

When your heart and lungs are in top form, they can effortlessly pump blood throughout your body and process oxygen. The stronger these organs are, the easier breathing will be at rest and work. You can enhance cardiorespiratory endurance by performing aerobic exercises that make you huff and puff. Running, cycling, swimming, dancing, jumping, cross-country skiing, and boxing are great examples. Aerobic activity is done at a pace where you huff and puff but can keep going for an extended period. For example, running at a moderate pace is preferable to sprinting a short distance and then stopping.

Flexibility

This is your body's ability to bend, reach, and twist through a wide range of motions comfortably and without injury. You should target all the muscles in your body for this benefit. Increased flexibility will allow you to extend your body parts in various directions without risking sprains, strains, and tears. It will also help you avoid the aches and pains that stem from stiffness. Have you ever heard anyone enthusiastically proclaim that their back was stiff with a smile? Not a chance. Flexibility promotes mobility and makes everyday movement easier and safer, whether you're reaching for something on a high shelf or twisting to look behind you. Prioritize stretching multiple times daily and pursue workouts like yoga and tai chi. Stretch in bed, at your office, at the airport, or anywhere else. Even tiny bits here and there can make a positive impact.

Balance

Do this, and you'll be less likely to fall. That's a simple explanation, right? Sure, you've probably gone your whole adult life without face-planting like a drunken sailor. I got it. But many people do fall, and doing so as a grownup is way more jarring and painful than it was when we were kids. I assure you, you no longer bounce!

Putting time into this pillar of fitness will enhance something called proprioception. That's your body's natural ability to respond to an imbalance without purposely thinking about it. If, for example, you step off the sidewalk and onto the squishy grass while walking, with quality proprioception, your brain will instantly tell your ankle not to roll, it will hold its position, and you won't fall. But without that practiced skill, you may go boom. Balance training can be done anywhere at any time. One of my favorite go-to moves is to stand on one foot while brushing my teeth or waiting in line at the grocery store. Simple, yet impactful.

Commit to all Four Pillars if you want to stay strong, energized, and injury-free. Train smart, move often, and keep your body performing at its best.

The F.I.T.T. Principle

Want to get fitter, faster, and stronger without second-guessing your workouts? The F.I.T.T. principle, Frequency, Intensity, Time, and Type, gives the structure you need to make every session count. Let's break it down so you can train smarter, not just harder.

Frequency – How often should you exercise?

For a healthy individual, I'd suggest exercising most days of the week. After all, your body was designed for movement. Whether doing structured exercise, sports, gardening, working, child rearing, or staying active throughout the day, you were not built to sit on the couch for hours on end. Instead, aim to exercise deliberately four to seven days a week, and when that's not possible, find ways to stay active. Every bit of movement adds up! For those days when you can't intentionally exercise, being active will go a long way. Every ounce of effort counts.

Intensity – How hard should you exercise?

Intensity is the difference between a workout that maintains your fitness and one that actually improves it. Pay attention to these signs of effort as we break this down, pillar by pillar. Focus on the keywords grunt, huff and puff, wince, and wobble.

Cardio

Huff and Puff! If you can walk and talk forever, you're likely not working hard enough. If you are sprinting and can't squeak out, "Gee, this sucks." you're working too hard. If you're huffing and puffing like the Big Bad Wolf but can keep going for 10 minutes or more, you're in the zone!

Strength

Go for the grunt! No, you don't have to shout like that pumped-up dude slamming barbells in the weight room. But, to become stronger, you should challenge your muscles with added resistance or repetitions that make you grunt from exertion, working to a point where you can no longer lift, press, push, or pull.

Flexibility

Wincing is a sure sign you're making progress. That "Wooooh, I feel that!" moment is your sweet spot. Pushing past that point could lead to injury, so don't become overzealous.

Balance

Wobble, baby! Balance training usually entails standing on one foot, or standing on squishy objects. If an exercise makes you wobble, it means you're challenging your balance and improving. Wobbling doesn't mean that you're "bad" at the exercise, it means you're working to become better. If you're super-still, you're not making progress.

Remember to work at intensities that make you huff, puff, grunt, wince, and wobble! Progress only comes when you push past your present capabilities.

Time – How long should you exercise?

Thirty minutes or more of any type of exercise daily is the gold standard because it allows you to get your heart rate up and work on various body parts in various ways. In most circumstances, the more you do, the more significant your progress will be, but don't stress if you can't fit in a long workout session every day. Even five minutes of movement, jumping rope, lunges, or stretching can be beneficial. Just start where you are, gradually increasing time and effort. If you can manage five minutes today, know it is significantly better than doing nothing. Aim to do more next time, and progress will come.

Type - What kind of exercise?

Besides incorporating the Four Pillars of Fitness, it's a wise idea to vary your choices for exercise within each pillar. When you change up the type of exercise you do, your body has to adjust to the new challenge and will grow more capable because of it. If you only walk, for example, don't expect to be great at swimming or cycling. Think about how your body moves with these three exercises and which muscles are utilized. There is a tremendous difference! If you mix up your routines, your body will benefit from the struggle to succeed.

Keep the F.I.T.T. Principle in mind when designing your workouts. Structure your training around Frequency, Intensity, Time, and Type; trust the process, and watch your fitness levels rise

Chapter 9

EVERYTHING EXERCISE

You. Supercharged!

This supercharged chapter is your guide to building a smart, effective exercise strategy that covers every pillar of fitness. No matter the day or the place, with equipment or without, you'll always have a way to move, improve, and make your body better.

Strength Training - What You Should Know

Strength training is the fountain of youth! It's the ticket to power, resilience, strong bones, a faster metabolism, sexy curves, and more. If you'd like your body to look and feel younger, this pillar of fitness can't be beat. I have a question for those who have previously shied away from strength training. On any given day, doing any given thing, would you rather be stronger or weaker? Can you come up with one instance when weakness is superior to strength? I'm confident you'll conclude that strength is always preferred. If you believed that strength training would automatically make you bulky, you were wrong. Even for men, bulky muscles typically require intense training and aggressive fueling. Women often fear that strength training will make them "big," which is quite sad because, for the most part, women do not produce enough testosterone to generate excessive muscle mass. Certainly not muscles that would be considered "bulky." You might be surprised to know that strength training can actually make you smaller because it boosts your metabolism, helping you shed fat faster.

Chapter 9 | Everything Exercise

Besides knowing how to perform particular exercises, strength training has some guidelines based on research. Stick with the following parameters to make the most progress.

Total Body Training. When plotting out your strength training workouts, remember that all muscles matter. That's right. All of them! Strength training isn't just about big biceps and flat abdominal muscles. Strength training is about having the ability to move your body in various ways, with the power to pull, push, lift, and press against resistance. It's about being able to hoist yourself off the ground, as well as carry groceries into your home without struggling. Strength is required to open that jar of pickles, slam your car's trunk shut, and hold your grandchild. Even the most mundane tasks regularly challenge your back, lats, shoulders, and glutes, so it would be unacceptable to ignore them when exercising.

Many people tend to work what I call "vanity muscles" and neglect the others. Strong, curvy biceps, abs, and glutes are always popular, but if you only train the muscles that excite you in the mirror, you'll suffer from imbalances or risk injuries without garnering the benefits of a well-rounded plan. Train wisely, train everything, and the results will speak for themselves

The 48-Hour Rule. Studies show that to reap the benefits of strength training, your muscles need approximately 48 hours to rest, recover, and rebuild between workouts. Effective strength training causes tiny tears in your muscle fibers. These tears are the reason your muscles feel so sore and weak after a workout, but they are good tears that your body will remedy with its fancy response team. However, if you do not allow a 48-hour window for repairs, then your muscles remain in a constant state of breakdown. So, if you work your biceps on Monday morning, just wait until Wednesday morning to train them again. This rule applies to all of your muscles, including your abs. It is also exclusive to strength training. Cardio, flexibility, and balance training do not require this 48-hour rest period.

Opposing Muscle Groups. Opposing muscles are those that work against each other. Ideally, these muscles will possess equal strength. Your biceps, for example, are responsible for bending your arms, while your triceps do the work of extending your arms. If your biceps are significantly stronger than your triceps, you risk injury to the weaker triceps and your elbow joint. I advise putting an equal amount of effort into training both. If you can lift 15 pounds doing a biceps curl, you should be able to press 15 pounds for a triceps extension.

Other opposing muscle groups are the back (traps) and chest (pecs), shoulders (deltoids) and lats, biceps and triceps, quadriceps and hamstrings, calves and anterior tibialis, abductors and adductors, abdominals and lower back (erector spinae), and iliopsoas and glutes.

Train larger muscles first. Do this to avoid potential performance issues caused by fatigue. We usually need our smaller accessory muscles to help activate and work our larger muscles, but we do not necessarily need our larger muscles to engage our smaller muscles. If, for example, you did some killer exercises that fatigued your biceps and triceps, those smaller muscles would not likely be able to perform well enough to do chest-focused exercises such as the bench press or push-ups. You need your arms to work your chest. However, you do not need to activate your chest muscles to work your arms. So, split your body in half, top and bottom, and train the largest muscles first. Pro tip: Your larger muscles are closest to your belly button. Start close to it and work your way out toward your fingers and toes. For example, work your glutes before your calves.

Sample order for an upper body strength training session:
chest, back, shoulders. lats, biceps, triceps, and forearms

Sample order for a lower body strength training session:
glutes, hip flexors, quadriceps, hamstrings, adductors, abductors, anterior tibialis, and calves

Core training comes last! Your abdominal and lower back muscles must be strong to help maintain proper form for most exercises. If you train them before exercises like push-ups or military presses, your form could suffer, putting you at risk for pain or injury. Save crunches and bridges for the end of your workout.

How to choose the perfect amount of resistance. Your priority is to find a resistance that challenges you without hurting you. Whether you are utilizing dumbbells, kettlebells, machines, bands, body weight, or any other strength training tool, figuring out how much will only come via trial and error. Always start with a choice you believe will be easy and advance in small increments as you acclimate. Choose a resistance that forces you to grunt by the eighth repetition. If you can't do at least six repetitions of an exercise, you should reduce the resistance. If you can easily do more than 10 repetitions, you should try a heavier option. If you struggle to lift your arms and legs or stand up without any additional tools, that's okay too. Sometimes, gravity is all the resistance you need. If this is true for you, consider your limbs your dumbbells, and get serious about lifting them in all directions to get stronger. Every exercise I recommend with equipment can be done without. Stay consistent, and you'll be working with resistance tools soon enough. Remember, the point is not to debilitate your body with soreness, instead, be smart and progress with baby steps.

How many repetitions should you do? It depends on your goals. If you're just getting started, aim to do 10 repetitions of a weight that feels mildly challenging. Work your way up to three sets of 10 repetitions over time. Your goal should be to choose enough resistance that reps 8-10 always feel like a struggle and make you grunt. If you are working toward serious size and strength, choose the type of resistance that will exhaust your muscles in 6-8 reps. More weight + fewer reps + protein = bigger, stronger muscles.

"What if I only want to tone?" That's a common question, and here's my honest answer. There is no such thing as toning. Either you are working to grow stronger, or you aren't. "Toning" is often the wish of women who fear bulkiness. Remember, unless you're using steroids, going crazy with protein or making massive efforts to grow large muscles, you won't. I'm looking you in the eyes right now. Strength training will only make you better. Do not skip this pillar!

Cool Strength Training Tools:

Gravity! Your body vs gravity is a match made in fitness heaven. Gravity is free, always with you, and can make lifting your body parts a real challenge. Push-ups, pull-ups, squats, lunges, crunches, and leg lifts are just a handful of the exercises you can do with this cool tool.

Dumbbells are the most popular strength training tool; they come in many different sizes and can be used sitting, standing, or lying down.

Resistance Bands are inexpensive and can be used to work most muscle groups. They're gentle yet challenging and are often a preferred choice for physical therapists and bodybuilders alike. They are lightweight and easy to travel with.

Chapter 9 | Everything Exercise

Cable Machines allow you to do similar exercises as you do with bands, with the ability to add resistance.

Kettlebells are relatively small equipment that work your muscles in a wide range of motions and are fun to use.

Machines are most commonly found at fitness centers. They are large and provide a stable choice for working one muscle at a time, often without utilizing your core for stability. Machines make it easy to adjust resistance and usually come with instructions posted on them. If you'd like to keep more of your body engaged while exercising, choose other options.

Scheduling Strength Training: Train each muscle group every other day for the best results. If you can't make that happen, train every third day. Training once weekly will not likely lead to progress, only maintenance. Feel free to work your entire body in each workout, or break up your workouts into sections, upper and lower body on various days of the week.

Cardio - What You Should Know

Cardiovascular exercise, also known as cardiorespiratory exercise, will increase the capacity and strength of your heart and lungs. The more powerful your heart is, the more easily it will pump oxygen-rich blood through your body. This lowers your heart rate and blood pressure, which are symbolic of good health and fitness. Increasing your lung capacity strengthens your breathing muscles, making delivering oxygen to your body and brain easier. The more powerful your heart and lungs are, the more comfortable vigorous exercise will be, and the longer it will take your body to exhaust or "poop out."

On a mission to burn a bunch of calories? Vigorous cardio gets it done, especially if you're working hard and/or for a long time. Strength training increases your metabolism for the long haul, but cardio burns up calories now! Any exercise that makes you huff and puff for an extended period counts as cardio: swimming, cycling, dancing, running, boxing, hiking challenging routes, and cross-country skiing are popular options.

Picking your pace. This is very personal, so do not compare yourself to anyone else. Your goal should be to exercise at a pace that makes you huff and puff, but not hyperventilate. You should be able to say "Gee, this is hard!", but not carry on a conversation without struggling. I recommend performing somewhere between a level of 6-to-8 on a scale of 1-to-10, with 10 being the hardest. Find the sweet spot of challenging yourself without going overboard. If you do too much, you'll eventually be forced to stop exercising, which defeats the goal of doing an extended cardio session.

Today's efforts should make tomorrow's easier, and consistency will eventually make today's struggles look like child's play. Progress will reveal itself when you can comfortably do things that previously wore you down. This is what stamina and endurance look like. Stay the course to turn fatigue into fitness and, eventually, athleticism.

The gold standard for cardio is 30-60 minutes daily. But you can do much less if necessary; and, if you have time for two to three hours of cardio, even better yet! You may think exercising for more than an hour sounds bonkers, but think about all of the youth, collegiate, and professional athletes who train for hours on end. The million plus people who run full marathons yearly, and senior citizens spending entire mornings playing pickleball. Know that it is safe and ideal to extend your sweat sessions when you can.

Chapter 9 | Everything Exercise

If you're starting out or bouncing back from illness or injury, skip the gold standard and stick with YOUR standard! Start with one minute of walking, wiggling, swimming, or dancing once or a few times daily. Tack on time and intensity whenever you can. You've got to start somewhere, and right now, you can only start where you are.

Cardio - Moves to Make You Huff and Puff. Examples include cycling, walking, hiking, running, group dance classes, swimming, water walking, martial arts, canoeing, stand-up paddleboarding, snow shoeing, basketball, soccer, lacrosse, and ultimate frisbee

Stretching - What You Should Know

Mobility stems from stretching. Keeping your muscles flexible is one of the most significant things you can do to avoid pain and genuinely feel good. Have you ever heard someone say "My back is so stiff" with a positive connotation? Never. Mobility is your freedom to bend, twist, extend, and reach without pain or injury. Pliable muscles feel good and allow us to move in all directions.

Your joints will benefit too. Your shoulder should be able to move your arms through an enormous circular range of motion. To maintain that range, you should perform that motion daily. The same goes for your hips and spine. Humans were not built to move only in a linear forward motion (walking, sitting, lying flat). Instead, we were designed to rotate, twist, move laterally, and bend. Stretching is the perfect time to put your joints and muscles through their complete ranges of motion. As the old saying goes, "If you don't use it, you lose it." And just like strength training, you should stretch all of your muscles, not just your hamstrings.

You should stretch throughout each day. But there are times when particular stretches will benefit you more than others.

Twist and Shout: Extending and twisting in bed before your feet hit the floor is almost instinctive for many, and often comes with a weird little yawn and yell. Fun! Spend some time tossing yourself around before you get up - it's good for you!

Rise and Shine: Once you're up and before the day begins, dedicate at least three minutes to moving and stretching your body in all directions. Your upper and lower body, plus your torso.

Stretch Breaks: Build in as many short or long stretch breaks throughout your day as you can. Schedule them in or do them at random. If you work at a desk, set a reminder to stretch every 30-60 minutes.

Connectivity: Attach stretching to other activities you do daily. For example, every time I let my dogs into the backyard to go potty, I stretch my hips.

Reach for More! Stretching at the end of a workout session is the ideal time to improve flexibility. Once your core temperature has increased and your body has been through the paces, your muscles are ripe for progress, so push each stretch until you wince. Hold for 10-20 seconds. Relax for a few moments, and repeat.

Yoga and Tai Chi: An entire class dedicated to stretching and mobility? Seems like a win. Look for free online classes, or find a studio nearby to take part in a group or do personal training. If you don't like the weird words your instructor uses, just ignore them like I do.

Chapter 9 | Everything Exercise

Sleepy Time: Bookend your beautiful morning stretches by reaching and twisting before or after you get in bed. You can also stretch in bed when you're stuck there and not feeling so good.

It's Gumby Damn it! The more you do, the better you'll be, so stretch like your name is Gumby. In the shower, in the airport, on the plane, at your aunt's house, at your job, at the dog park, and in the exam room while you wait for your doctor. This is clearly a case of more being more!

Balance Training - What You Should Know

If you don't like falling, this should be high on your list of priorities. Remember that even the most impressive athletes sometimes take a tumble, and without exception, they wish they hadn't. To make progress in balance training, you should constantly be testing it. And by testing it, I mean that you should do things that make you wobble, adjust, and look like you are off-balance. You are not making progress if you are standing on one foot motionless. If you are standing on one foot, flailing your arms around like a drunk, you are doing the right thing. As with the other three Pillars of Fitness, struggle leads to progress.

Balance training will usually require you to stand on one foot, stand on something squishy, or both. If you're unsteady, try standing on one foot while holding on to a wall, countertop, friend, or another stationary object. Do this for five to thirty seconds. Once you've conquered that skill, try standing on one foot without holding on to anything. And then do so while moving your arms in a variety of ways. Advanced challenges include playing catch, shaking your booty, and lifting weights while standing on one foot. You can also try standing on official balance training tools like the BOSU or balance disk, or test your balance by standing on a couch cushion. When standing on squishy objects, start on both feet and eventually move on to single-leg challenges.

The key is to do things that make your feet, ankles, knees, and hips adjust to keep you upright. Done regularly, these exercises will improve your proprioception (your instinctive response to being thrown off balance) and decrease your chances of falling.

Circuit Training is a clever way to add variety and save time while exercising. It is done by doing short bursts of different exercises without resting. This is wise if you'd like to squeeze a quality workout into a condensed period. Design your circuit workout by choosing four to 10 different exercises. Commit to doing a predetermined amount of time or reps of each exercise, as well as a certain number of rounds. Mix and match any sort of exercises to challenge your body and keep yourself entertained. If you alternate between cardiovascular exercises and strength training exercises without resting in between, you'll reap the benefits of an elevated heart rate that comes with cardio, even while you're strength training.

Interval Training is done by alternating short bursts of high-intensity exercise with longer segments of less intense exercise. This is a fantastic way to increase cardiovascular endurance. If you went to a track, for example, and ran as fast as you could for as long as you could, you might collapse before you completed one lap. Sprinting is anaerobic, which means you're not using oxygen as an energy source. So when you run out of oxygen, you're done! Alternating longer periods of slow running with short bursts of fast running will help increase your speed and endurance while strengthening your heart and lungs. This model of training can be done with any sort of aerobic exercise. Swim slowly for 60 seconds, then swim fast for 15 seconds. Cycle slowly for two minutes, then spin fast for 30 seconds. Choose shorter, intense intervals as you begin, and increase them as you become fitter. If you're just returning to fitness, begin with one minute of low intensity and five seconds of higher intensity. Baby steps!

Chapter 9 | Everything Exercise

Beast Mode sounds good to you? Hell yeah! You can turn your body into a high-caliber machine by being aggressive and consistent with your workouts. Take my huff, puff, grunt, wince, and wobble recommendations seriously and challenge yourself often. Aim to finish your workouts with rosy cheeks and a stinky body. Train in a manner that makes you want to sprawl out on the floor in a puddle of sweat like a starfish when you're done. Be consistent, because half the battle is showing up. If your workouts are challenging and you train almost daily, your body will have no choice but to respond. When your homies start complimenting you on your obvious physical upgrades, tell them you're supercharged!

Sporty Spice, that's you! It doesn't matter how old you are or what kind of shape you're in, sports are for everyone. Going beyond the standard gym workouts or fitness classes will have unique and special benefits for your body and mind. Whether you play a sport you've enjoyed your whole life or try something new, joining a team and competing at a high or low level is important. Sports make us move our bodies in unique ways, challenge our coordination, incentivize us to improve, bring social opportunities, and provide the adrenaline rush that only comes from missing or scoring points. Also, they can be really freaking fun.

It makes me cranky that so many people give up on sports after leaving high school. The benefits grown-ups enjoy from playing sports are the same as those children experience: physical fitness, intellectual stimulation, stress relief, learning to lead, follow, win, and lose with grace, encouragement to do your best, and the excitement that comes from competition. Please pick a sport and join in. Racquetball, triathlon, swimming, kickball, ping pong, cross-country skiing, sailing, ballroom dancing, running, golf, disc golf, ultimate frisbee, T-ball, soccer, etc. Revisit something you used to love and try something new. It will add enjoyment to your days, give you something to look forward to, and positively impact your body. Whether playing to win championships or simply to have fun, sports are a particularly powerful tool for supercharging your life.

Warm-Ups and Cool Downs

These essential steps are meant to ease your body into and out of your workouts without injury. Cars can go from 0-to-60 without tearing a hammy. You and I cannot, probably.

Warm-Ups

Before you get into the hard stuff, spend five to 10 minutes preparing your muscles to go through the motions they'll be doing at top speed. During this time, your heart rate should gradually increase, your core temperature should rise, a drop of sweat may form above your eyebrow, and your body should go from stiff to supple. Gradually increasing your range of motion for the muscles you'll be training will limit the likelihood you'll experience sprains, strains, or tears. Blending low-level cardio movement with dynamic (active) stretching is ideal. Knee lifts, reaching, twisting, arm circles, jumping jacks, running slowly, and other moves that make sense for your planned workout will suffice.

Cool Downs

Instead of slamming on the brakes once you've completed the most intense portion of your workout, ease back out of it. Stopping abruptly can lead to dizziness and nausea, but a gradual end to your workout can feel great and reduce recovery time. Slow your pace, breathe deeply, and do some static (stationary) stretching once your heart rate has returned to normal.

Chapter 9 | Everything Exercise

Fitz's Five Star Exercises

These are my favorite strength training moves for quick results. To make your muscles harder and stronger in a hurry, do them all, or a variety of them, every other day. They incorporate multiple muscle groups and are quite challenging. You can modify each to make them easier as you get started or add resistance, time or repetitions to increase difficulty. Do them all during the same workout or sprinkle them in.

Push-ups, pull-ups, squat jumps, lunges, burpees, angry-ups, lateral gait, mountain climbers, planks, and Supermans

Exercise Instructions

- Mix and match any of these exercises: standing, seated, or horizontal.
- Use bands, dumbbells, ankle weights, or your own bodyweight.
- Keep your knees soft when standing, and avoid locking out your knees and elbows throughout each exercise.
- Maintain good posture throughout every movement.
- Affix bands to stable objects that will not budge when you pull on them.
- Start small when choosing resistance and progress slowly.
- Aim for 6-10 reps of each strength move (or fewer if needed).
- Hold each stretch or balance exercise for 10-30 seconds.
- Don't forget to breathe naturally.

STRETCH AND STRENGTH TRAIN ANYWHERE

In this section, you'll learn how to strengthen and stretch each body part. You can perform these exercises with any equipment and in any location you choose. My hope is that you will commit much of this information to memory, so you will never miss workouts by claiming you didn't know how. I've said it before, but when you know better, you should do better. When you know how to train all muscle groups, you should be able to exercise in the fanciest gym in the world or in the desert. You can also take this book with you wherever you go!

CHEST

Bench Press with Dumbbells

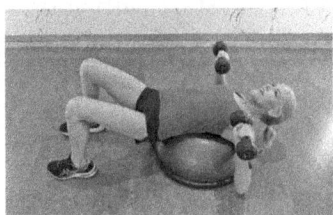 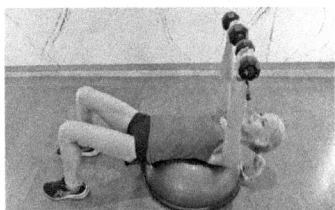

Lie on your back on an elevated surface. Start with your hands near your chest and push forward until your arms are almost straight and your hands are over your shoulders.

Flies with Dumbbells

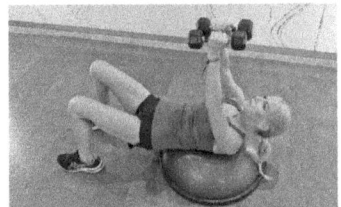 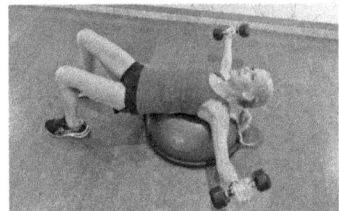

Lie on your back on an elevated surface. Start with your arms almost straight, hands facing each other and over your shoulders. Slowly lower your weights out to the side until your hands line up with your shoulders. Keep elbows soft.

Bench Press with Band

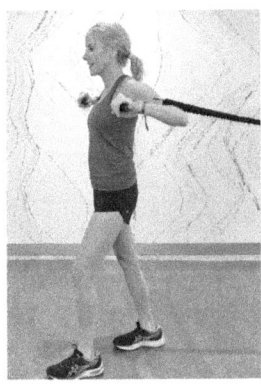 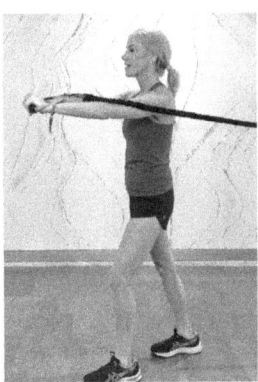

With your bands affixed behind you, stand with soft knees. Start with your hands near your chest and push forward until your arms are almost straight and your hands are in front of your shoulders.

Flies with Band

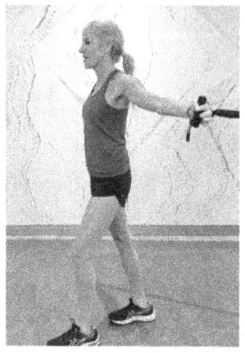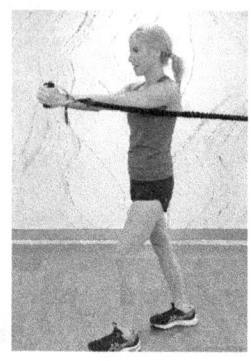

With your bands affixed behind you, stand with soft knees. Start with your arms almost straight, hands facing each other, and chest height in front of you. Slowly bring your arms to the side until your hands line up with your shoulders. Keep elbows soft.

Push-ups

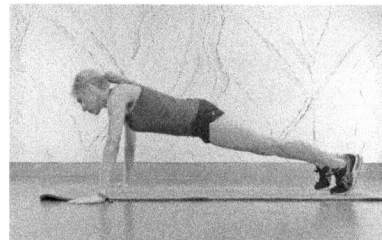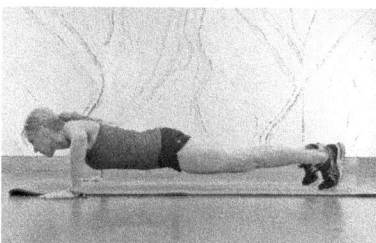

Start in a plank position with hands under your shoulders and a flat back. Lower your body toward the ground and return to starting position.

Flat Back Push-ups on Knees

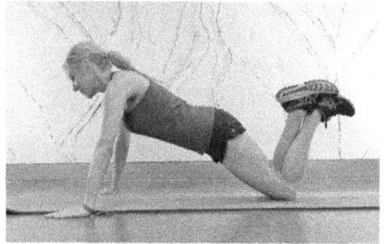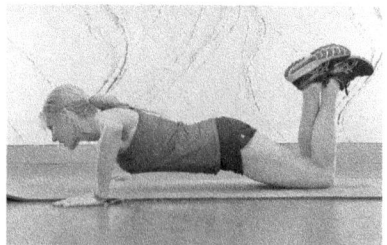

Start on your knees with hands under your shoulders and a flat back. Lower your body toward the ground and return to starting position.

Chapter 9 | Everything Exercise

Torso Push-ups on Knees

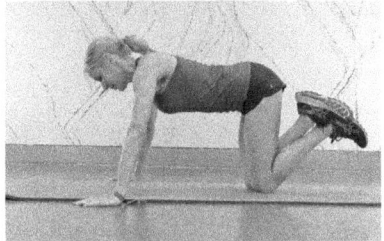 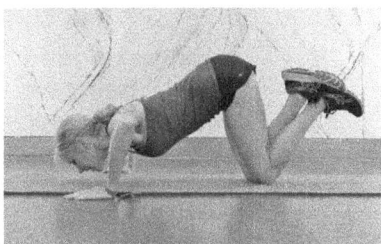

Start with your hips over your knees with hands under your shoulders. Lower your shoulders and chest toward the ground and slowly return to starting position.

Wall Push-ups

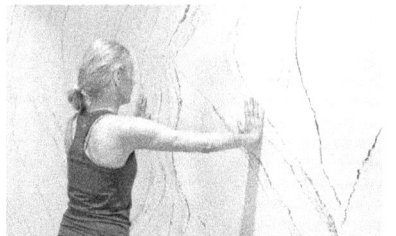 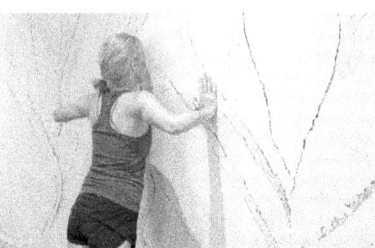

Stand with your hands pressed against a wall at shoulder height with arms only slightly bent. Slowly bring your chest closer to the wall and then push away before you kiss the wall.

Seated Chest and Biceps Stretch

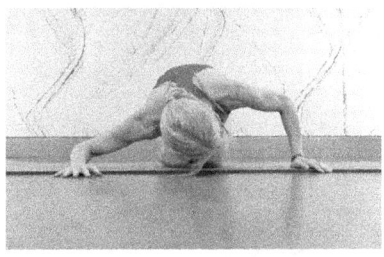 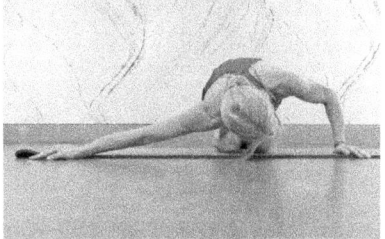

Sit on your knees, with your tush resting on your heels. Extend your left arm to one side, palm on the floor. Press your left shoulder into the floor while rotating your torso to the right. Repeat the same stretch with your left arm bent and elbow touching the floor.

Standing Chest and Biceps Stretch

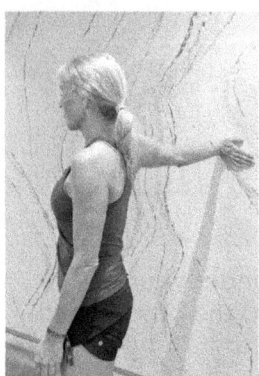

Stand with your right arm extended to the side, palm pressed against a wall, fingers pointing behind you. Rotate your torso to your left.

BACK

Rows with Dumbbells

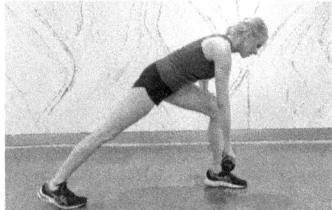 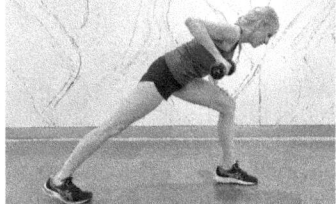

Stand in a lunge position with your left arm resting on your left thigh, flat back. Start with your right arm extended toward the ground. Slowly raise your right hand to your right shoulder.

Reverse Flies with Dumbbells

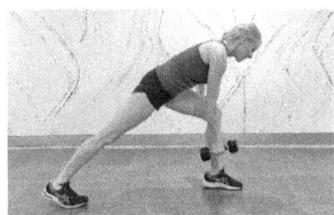 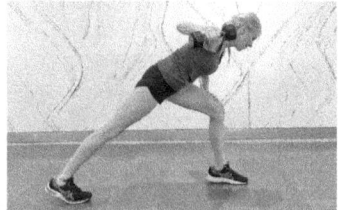

Stand in a lunge position with your left arm resting on your left thigh, flat back. Start with your right arm extended toward the ground and slowly lift it out to the side of your body, ending at shoulder height.

Rows with Band

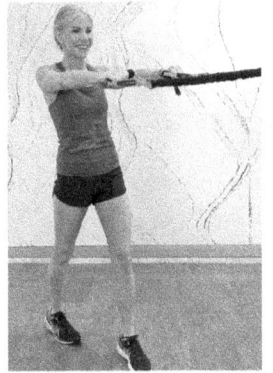 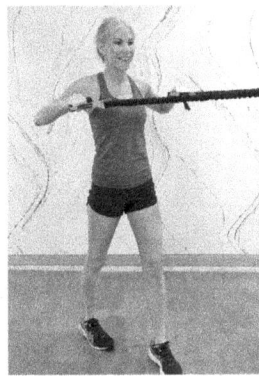

With your band affixed in front of you, stand with soft knees. Start with both arms extended at shoulder height. Slowly pull the band to your shoulders.

Reverse Flies with Band

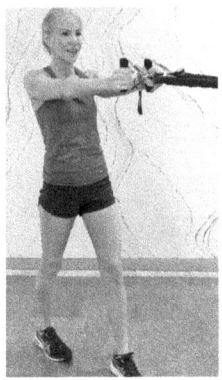 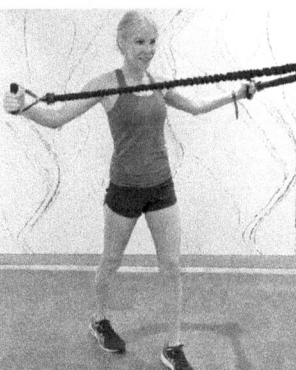

With your band affixed in front of you, stand with soft knees. Start with both arms extended at shoulder height. Slowly pull the band to your sides until they are level with your shoulders. Keep your elbows soft but not fully bent.

Back Stretch

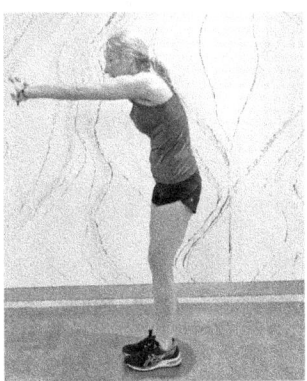

Stand with soft knees and hands clasped together. Reach your hands far out in front of you while arching your back.

LATS

Lat Pull with Dumbbells

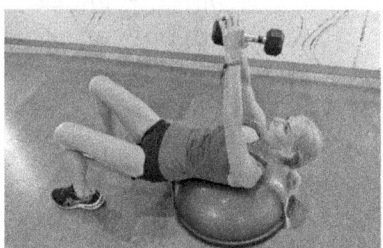 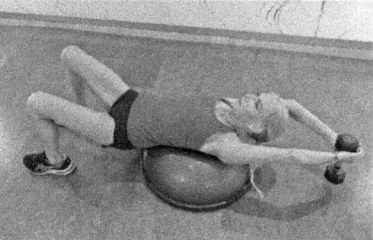

Lie on your back on an elevated surface. Hold one dumbbell with two hands. Start with your arms straight over your chest. Extend your arms behind your head until you can not reach any further.

Lat Pull with Band

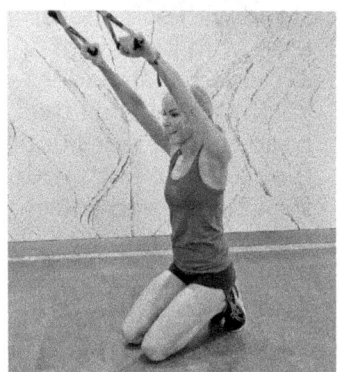 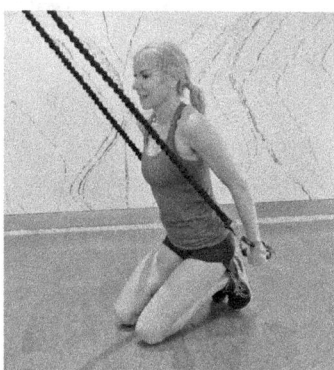

Begin on your knees with your band affixed above you, holding both handles with your arms extended overhead. Slowly pull your arms toward the ground. Keep your elbows soft but not fully bent throughout the entire motion.

DELTOIDS

Military Press with Dumbbells

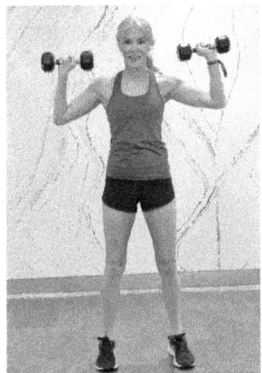 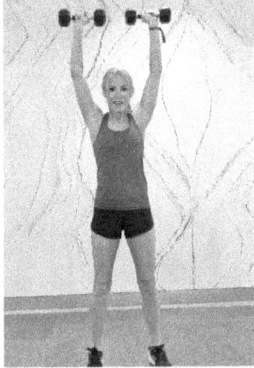

Stand with knees soft and arms up as shown. Press weights toward the ceiling.

Lateral Raise with Dumbbells

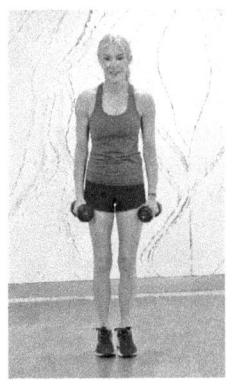 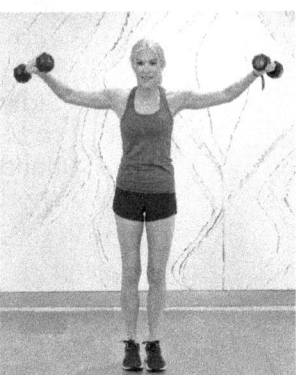

Stand with your knees soft and arms extended, hands facing the sides of your thighs. Slowly raise both arms to the side until your hands are level with your shoulders.

Front Raise with Dumbbells

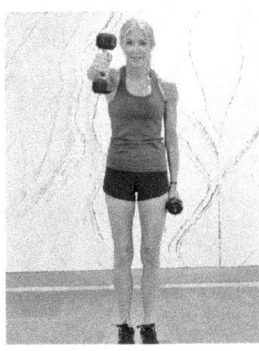 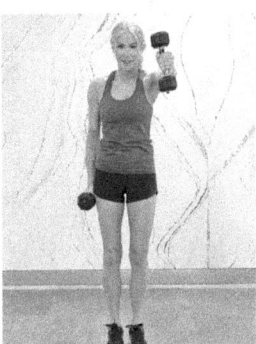

Stand with knees soft and arms extended with hands facing the top of your thighs Slowly raise one arm in front of you until your hand is level with your shoulder.

Military Press with Band

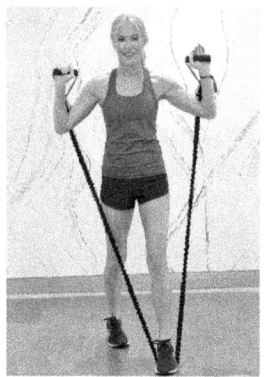 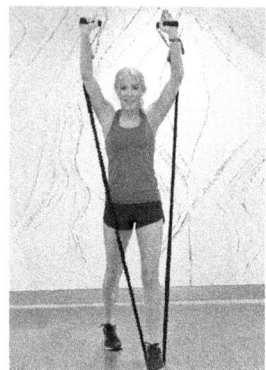

Stand on the center of your band with knees soft and arms up as shown. Extend hands toward the ceiling.

Lateral Raise with Band

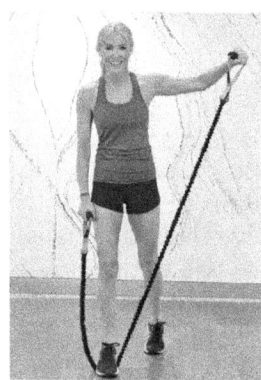 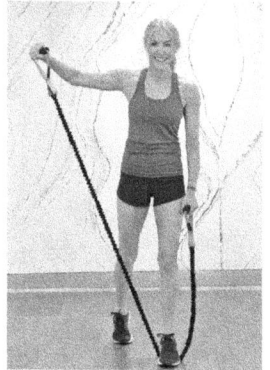

Stand on the center of your band with knees soft and arms extended with hands facing the sides of your thighs. Slowly raise one arm to the side until your hand is level with your shoulder.

Front Raise with Band

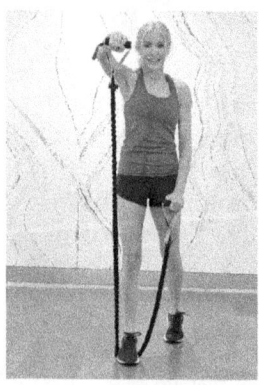 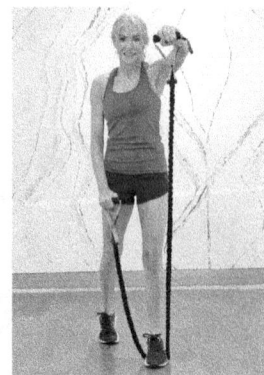

Stand on the center of your band with knees soft and arms extended with hands facing the top of your thighs. Slowly raise one arm in front of you until your hand is level with your shoulder.

Chicken Wing Stretch

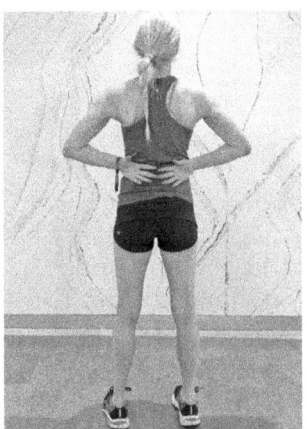

Place the back of both hands onto your low back and bring both elbows toward the front of your body.

Cross Chest Stretch

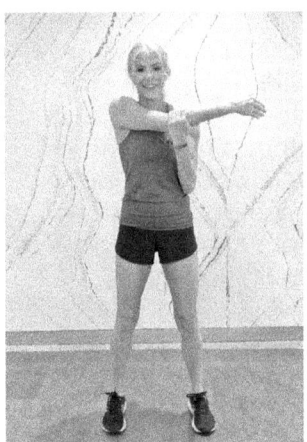

Bring one extended arm across your chest. Use the opposite hand to pull your extended arm even further across your chest.

BICEPS

Single-arm Biceps Curl with Dumbbells

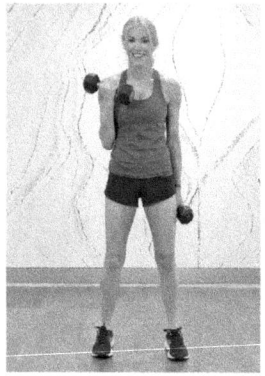 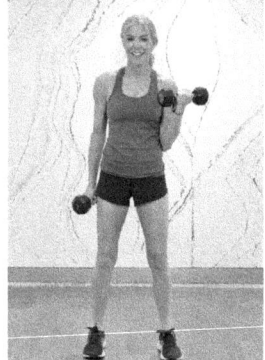

Stand with soft knees with hands at your sides. Keep your elbows pinned tight to your body and slowly bend one arm until your hand is close to your shoulder.

Biceps Curl with Dumbbells

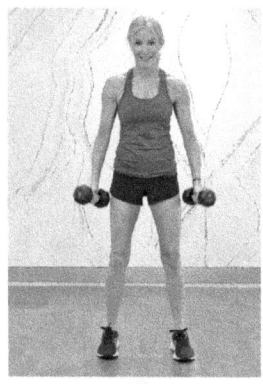 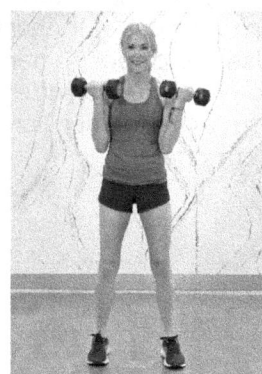

Stand with soft knees with hands at your sides. Keep your elbows pinned tight to your body and slowly bend both arms until your hands are close to your shoulders.

Biceps Curl with Band

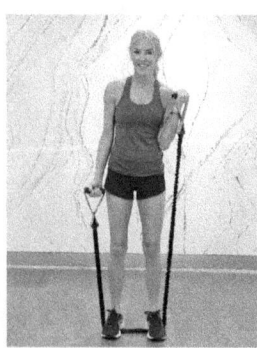 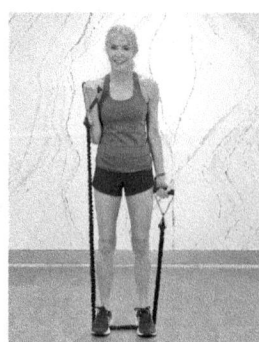

Stand on the center of your band with soft knees and hands at your sides. Keep your elbows pinned tight to your body and slowly bend one arm until your hand is close to your shoulder.

Biceps Stretch

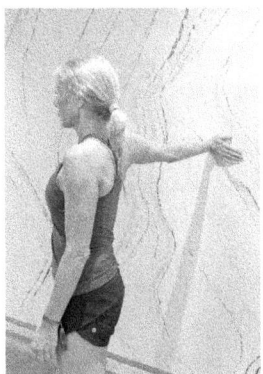

Place one palm against the wall with your fingers pointing behind you. Extend that arm and rotate your body away from the wall.

TRICEPS

Triceps Extension with Dumbbells

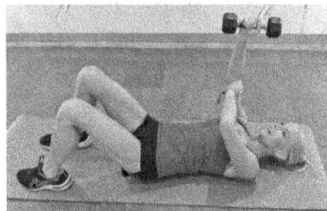 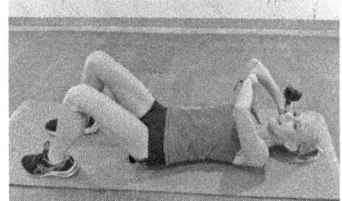

Lie flat on your back with your knees bent. Hold the weight in your right hand with your arm extended straight above your right shoulder. Support your right arm with your left hand to prevent wobbling. Slowly lower the weight toward your right shoulder.

Criss-Cross Triceps Extension with Dumbbells

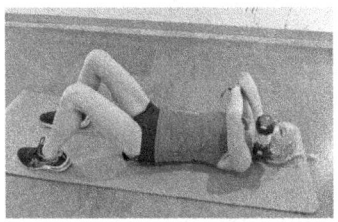 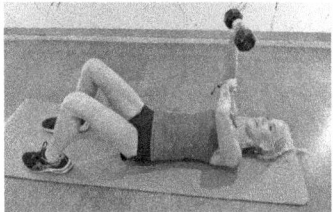

Lie flat on your back with your knees bent. Hold the weight in your right hand with your arm extended straight above your right shoulder. Support your right arm with your left hand to prevent wobbling. Slowly lower the weight toward your left shoulder.

Triceps Extension with Band

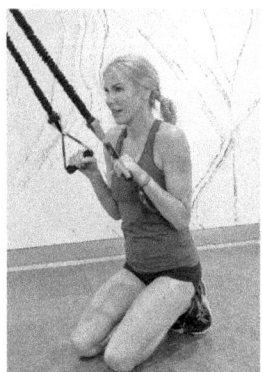 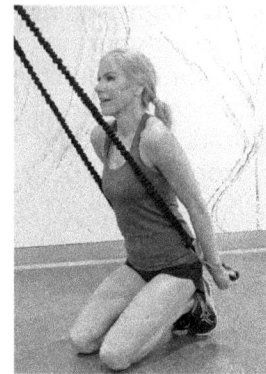

Begin on your knees with your band affixed above you. Holding both handles with your elbows pinned tight at your sides and your hands near your chin, slowly extend your arms toward the ground.

Single-Arm Triceps Extension with Band

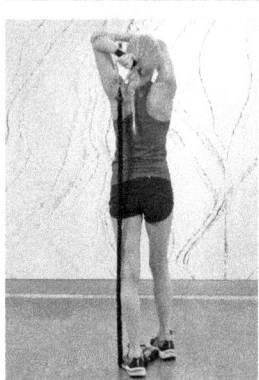 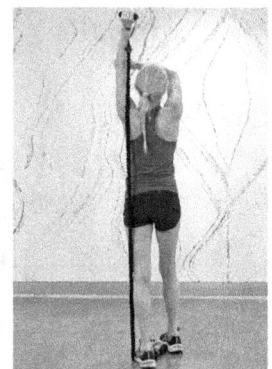

Stand on a band with soft knees. With your left arm bent and your elbow above your head, hold a band handle behind your shoulder. Slowly extend your arm to the ceiling as shown.

Single-Arm Triceps Extension with Dumbbells

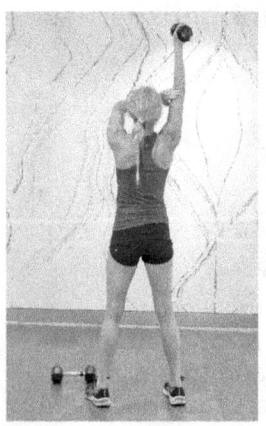 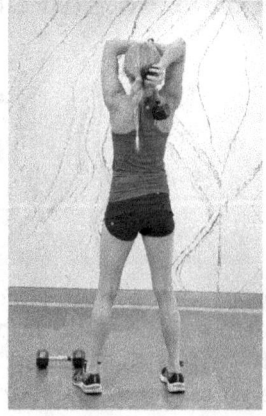

Stand with soft knees. Hold a weight in your left hand with your arm extended straight, reaching up to the sky. Support your left arm with your right hand to keep it stable. Bend your left arm, so the dumbbell drops behind your head. Slowly return to starting position.

Dips on the Floor

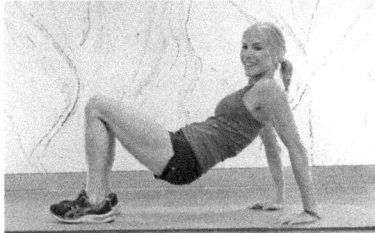 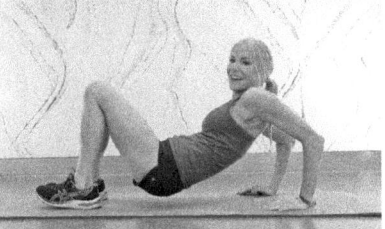

Sit on the ground with your legs in front of you and your knees bent. Begin with your hands on the floor behind you, fingers pointed towards your tush, and arms extended. Slowly bend your arms and extend them to return to the starting position.

Triceps Stretch

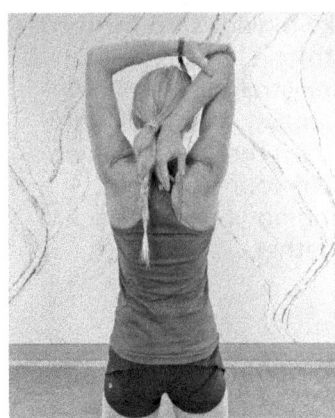

Place your right hand behind your neck with your elbow high. Grab your right elbow with your left hand and gently pull your right arm back. Simultaneously press down on your right forearm with your left thumb to enhance the stretch.

GLUTES & QUADRICEPS

Squats

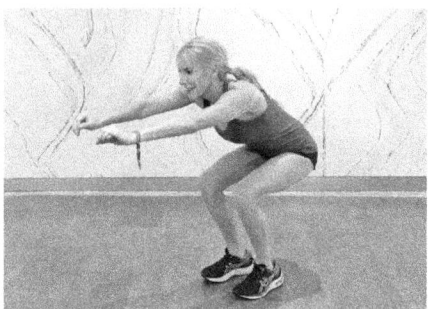

Sit back until your thighs are parallel to the ground. Do not allow your knees to jet forward over your toes.

Lunges

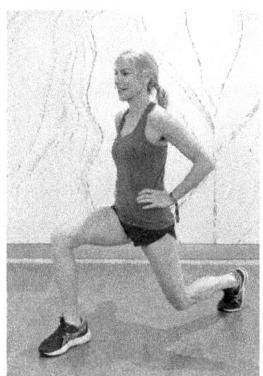
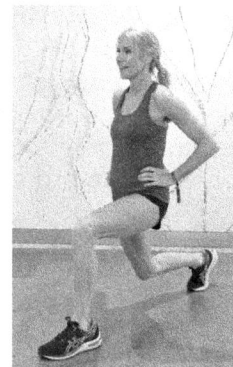

Take a giant step forward with one leg. Keep your back straight while dropping your back knee toward the ground. Push off of your front foot, bringing your feet back together.

Single Leg Squat

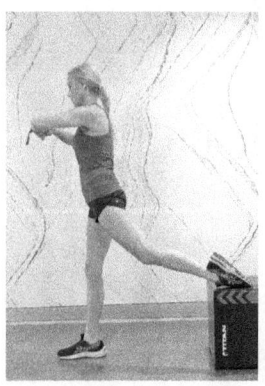
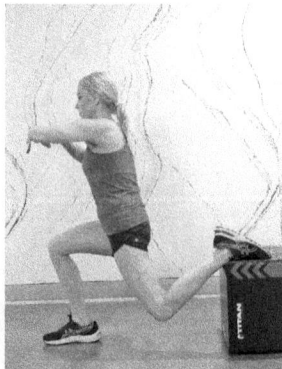

Stand on one foot with your other foot resting on a chair or plyo box. Slowly lower the knee of your back leg towards the ground and return to starting position. Do not allow your front knee to jut forward past your front foot.

Chapter 9 | Everything Exercise

Walking Lunges

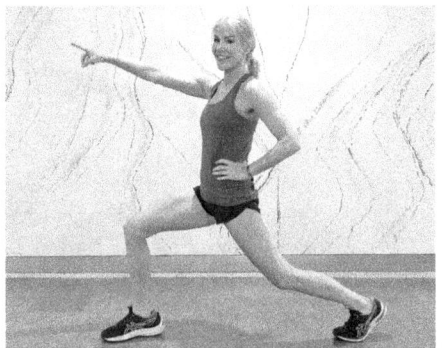

Begin with both feet together. Take a giant step forward with one leg dropping your back knee toward the ground. Bring your back foot up to your front foot. Continue forward, alternating legs.

Squat Jump

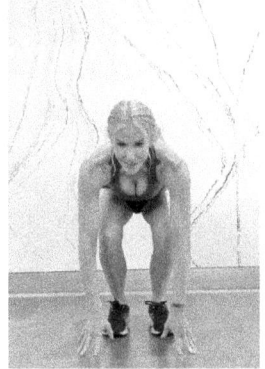 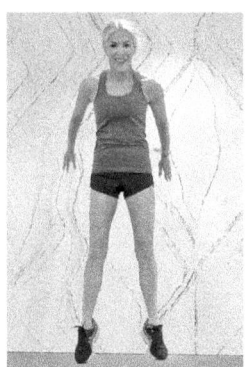

Stand with feet shoulder width apart. Squat down low and jump up high.

Hip Thrusts

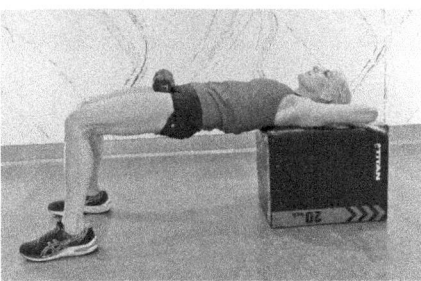 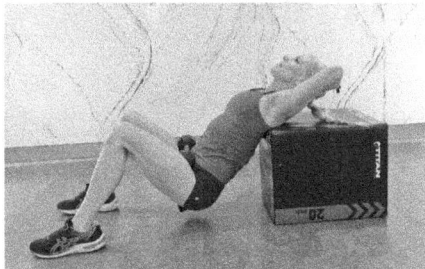

Rest your shoulders on a bench or plyobox with your feet flat on the floor. Place a weight on your lap. Begin with your hips folded and glutes close to the ground. Slowly lift your hips so they're parallel to your knees and shoulders. Drop your hips slowly and repeat.

Kick Backs with Band

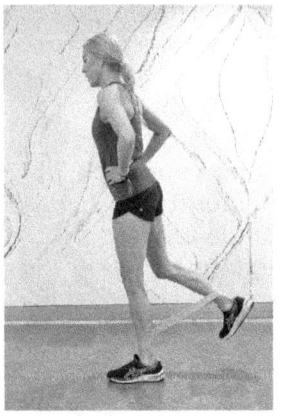 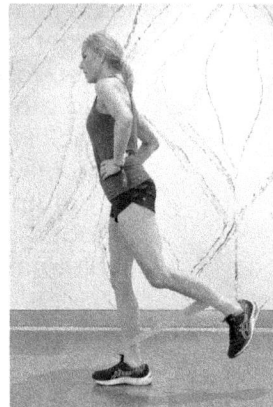

Stand with soft knees and a band looped around your ankles. Keeping toes on both feet pointed forward and knees almost straight, extend one leg backward as far as you can.

Prone Donkey Kicks

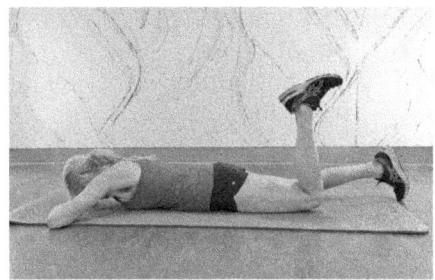 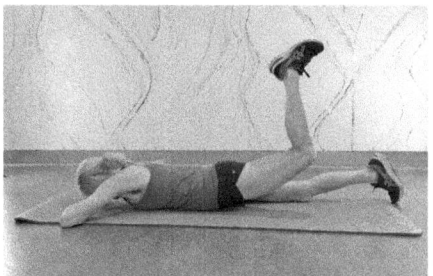

Lie face down with your forehead resting on your hands. Bend one leg and lift your heel to the ceiling. Pulse that foot up and down.

Quad Stretch

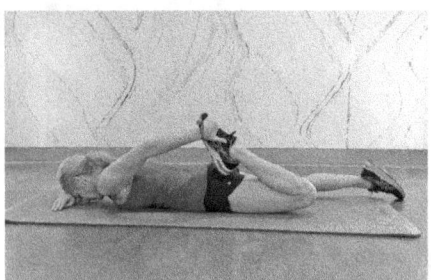

Lay face down on the ground. Grab your left foot with your left hand and bring your foot as close to your tush as possible.

Single Leg Folded Glute Stretch

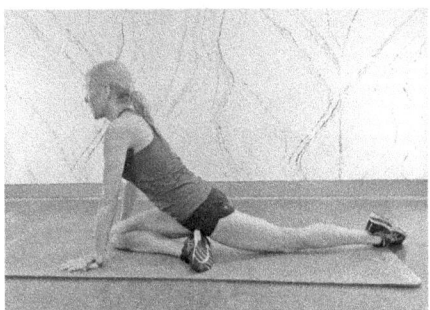 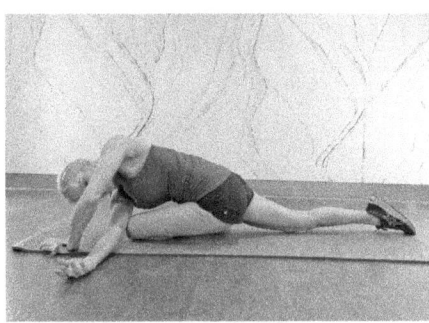

Lean forward over your left knee with that leg bent across your body, and extend your right leg behind you. Increase the intensity by twisting your right arm across your body, pressing your shoulder to the ground.

Single Leg Seated Glute Stretch

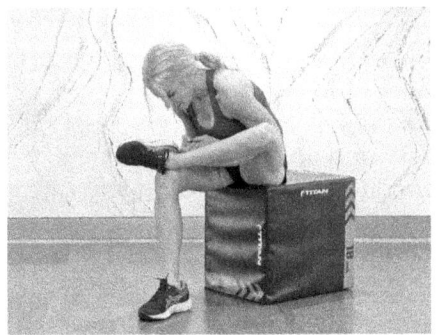 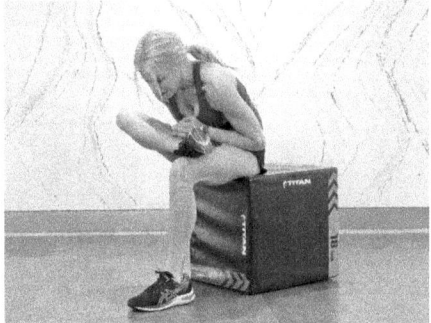

Sit on a plyobox or bench. Lean forward over one knee with that leg bent across your body, and your foot resting on your other knee.

HIP FLEXORS

Knee Lifts with Band

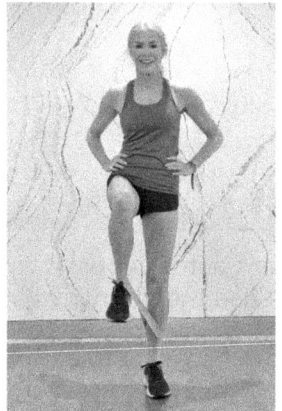 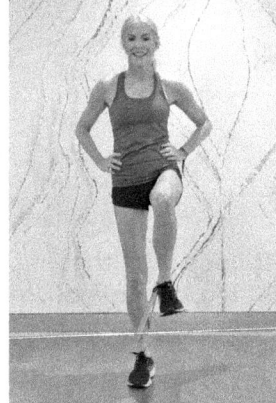

Stand with soft knees and a band looped around your ankles. Keeping toes on both feet pointed forward, alternate lifting your knees as high as possible. Keep your back straight.

Double-Leg V-Up

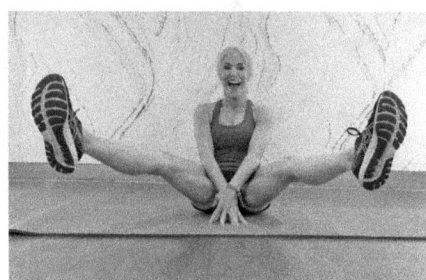

Sit on the ground with both legs in front of you in a "V" shape. Place both hands on the floor between your legs for balance. Simultaneously lift both straight legs off the ground and hold as long as you can.

Single Straight Leg Lifts

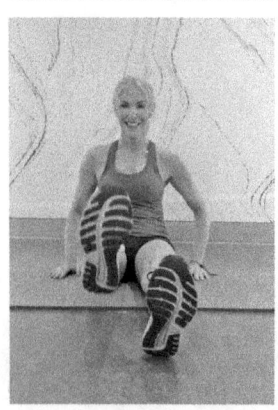 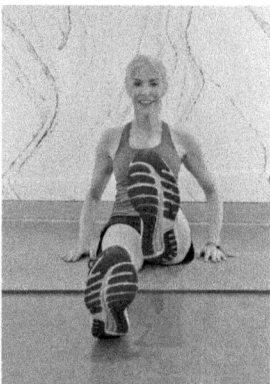

Sit on the ground with both legs extended in front of you. Alternate lifting one straight leg off the ground and holding as long as you can.

Kneeling Hip Flexor Stretch

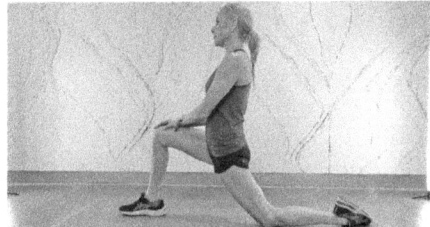

Start in a forward lunge position with your back knee on the ground. Lean your back hip all the way forward.

Kneeling Hip Flexor Stretch Level #2

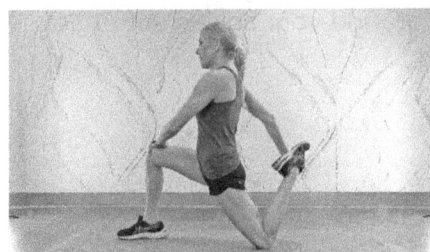

Start in a forward lunge position with your back knee on the ground. Grab your back foot with the opposite hand and lean your back hip forward.

Kneeling Hip Flexor Stretch Level #3

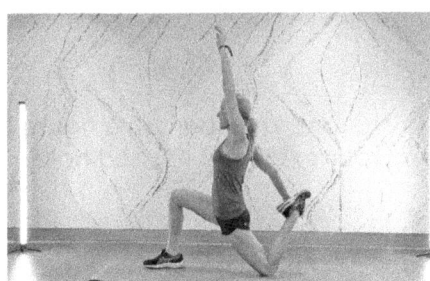

Start in a forward lunge position with your back knee on the ground. Grab your back foot with the opposite hand, reach your other hand to the ceiling and lean your back hip all the way forward.

Standing Hip Flexor Stretch

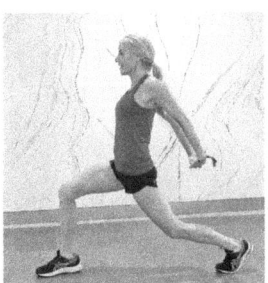 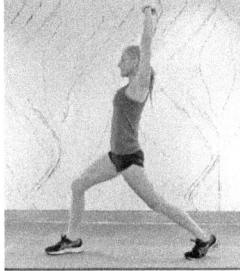

Start in a forward lunge position. Lean your back hip all the way forward. Extend both hands towards the sky.

HAMSTRINGS

Prone Hammy Curls with Band

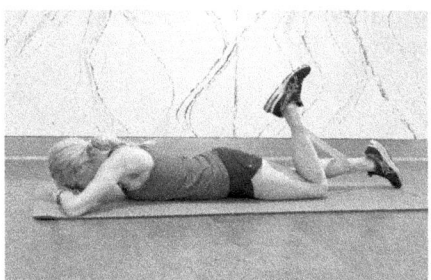 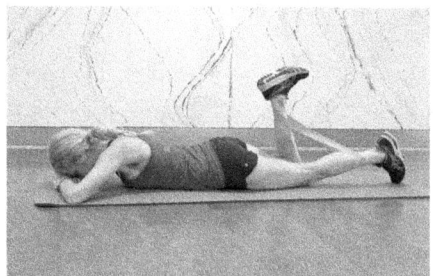

Lie face down with the band looped around your ankles. Alternate bending your legs to kick your tush.

Hammy Stretch

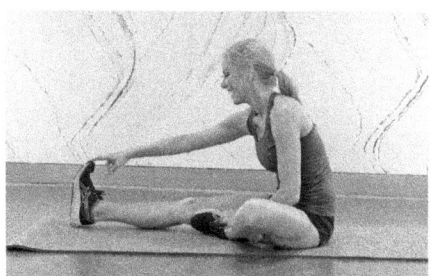

Sit on the floor with one leg extended and one knee bent in a figure-four position. Lower your chest toward your extended leg and hold.

Advanced Hammy Stretch

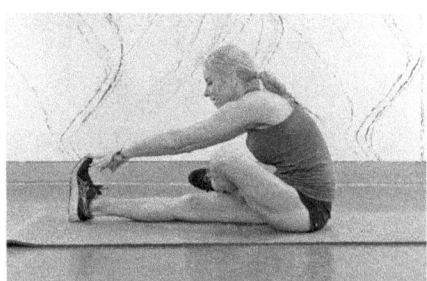

Sit on the floor with one leg extended and one knee bent on top of the extended leg. Lower your chest toward your extended leg and hold.

GLUTE MEDIUS/ABDUCTORS

Lateral Gait with Band

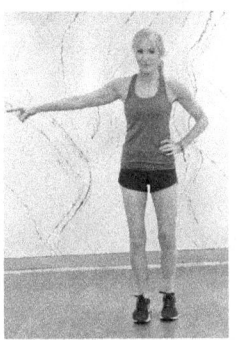 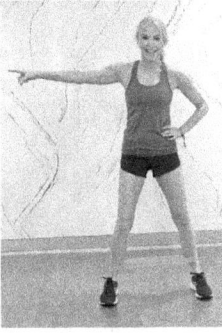

Stand with soft knees and a band looped around your ankles. Take a giant step to the right and bring your left foot in so your feet are together. Take several more giant steps to the right side, and then take several giant steps to your left. Keep your toes pointed forward throughout the exercise.

Clam Shells with Band

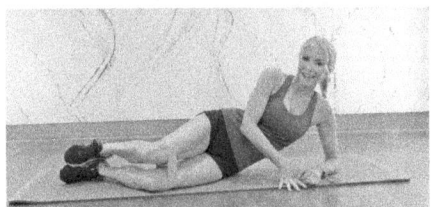 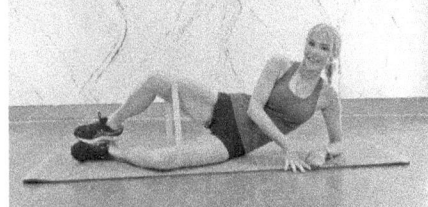

Rest on your side with your knees bent, legs stacked on top of each other, with a band around your thighs, just above your knees. Keeping your feet together, slowly lift your top knee towards the ceiling like you're opening a clam shell.

Lying Lateral Leg Lifts with Band

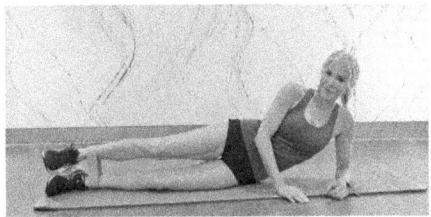 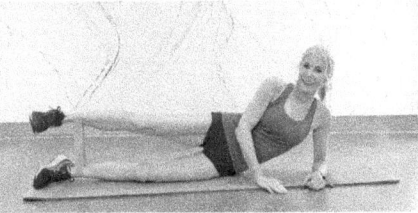

Rest on your side with your legs straight and stacked on top of each other, with a band around your ankles. Keep your legs almost straight with your toes pointed forward, and slowly lift your top leg towards the ceiling.

Booty Bridges

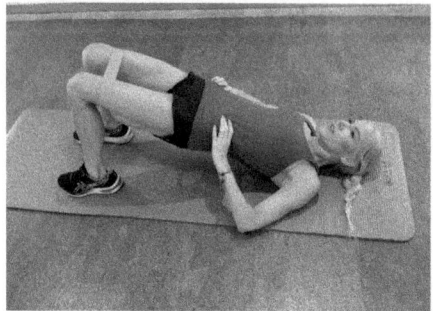 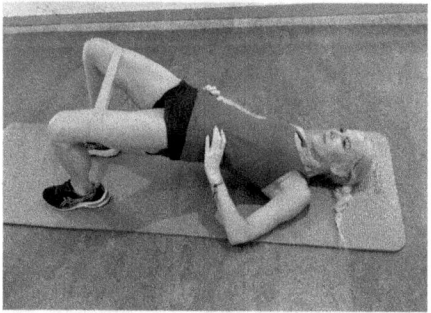

Lie face up with your shoulders and feet touching the ground, and a band around your thighs. Lift your hips so your body forms a straight line between your knees and shoulders. Keeping your hips high, bring your knees apart and slowly back together.

Criss Cross Applesauce Glute Stretch

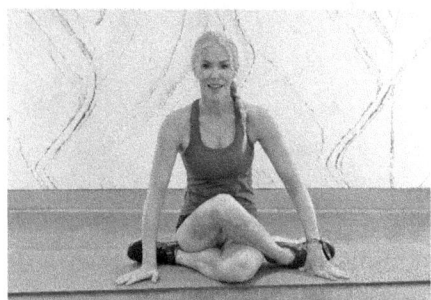 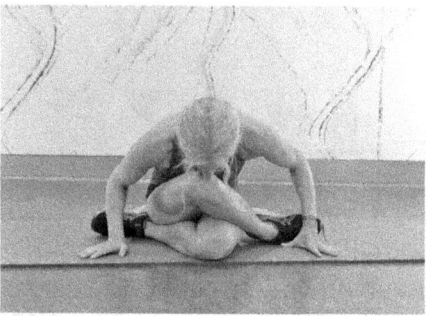

Bend and cross one leg on top of the other. Try to stack your knees on each other (or come close). Lower your chest to your thighs and hold.

ADDUCTORS

Squeezes

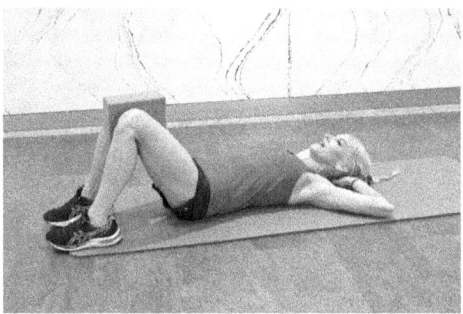

Lie on your back with your knees bent and a pillow, yoga block, or rubber ball between them. Either squeeze your pillow hard for 10-30 seconds or squeeze and release in a pulsing motion.

Squeezes with Bridge

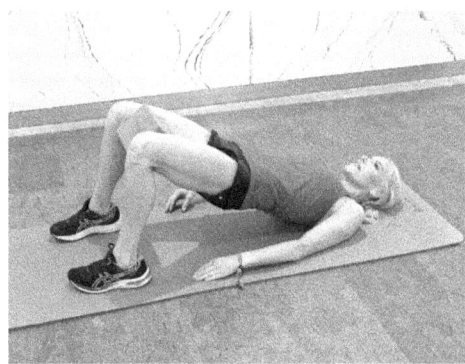

Begin in bridge position with a pillow, yoga block, or rubber ball between your knees. Either squeeze your pillow hard for 10- 30 seconds or squeeze and release in a pulsing motion.

Standing Adductor Stretch

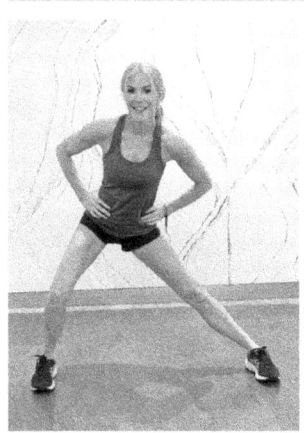 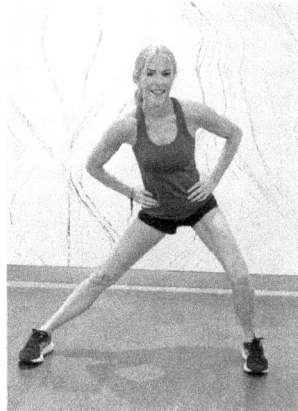

Stand with feet very far apart with toes pointing forward. Bend one knee and shift your weight over to that side.

Army Crawl Stretch

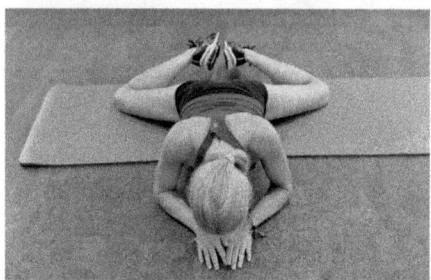 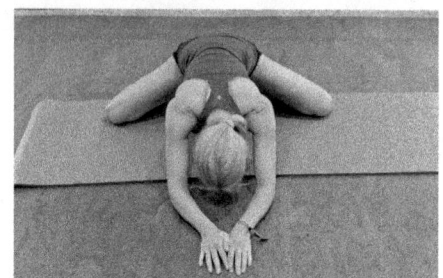

Get on the ground with your knees spread apart, feet together, and your tush seated back on your heels. Lower your hips and chest as much as possible with your arms extended over your head. Keep your hips and chest near the ground and drive your hips forward. Hold both positions for 10-30 seconds.

Adductor Stretch with Band

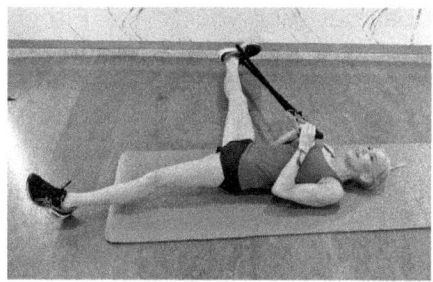

Lie on your back with a band wrapped around one foot, holding the handles at your chest. Gently pull the banded foot out to the side until you feel a good stretch.

Chapter 9 | Everything Exercise

ABDOMINALS

Plank

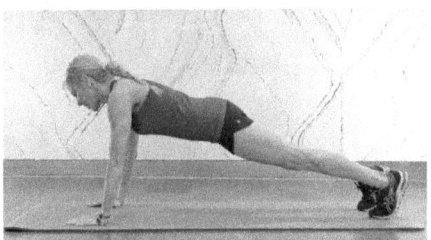

Lie face down on the ground with only your toes and hands touching the floor. Keep your hands directly below your shoulders, and remain still with your body forming a straight line between your heels and shoulders.

Forearm Plank

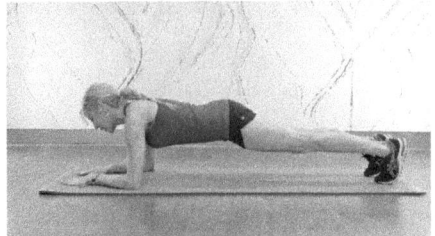

Lie face down on the ground with only your toes and forearms touching the floor. Remain still with your body forming a straight line between your heels and shoulders.

Planks with Arm-Lifts

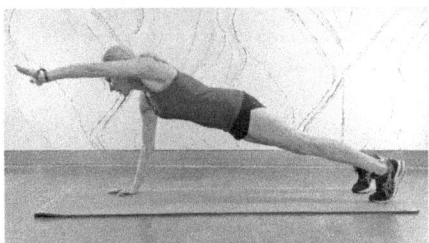 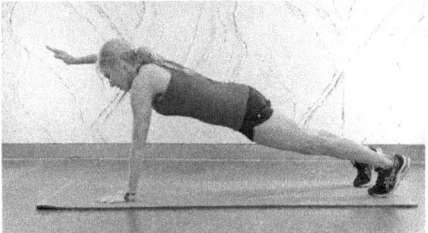

Begin in either plank position and alternate lifting your arms until they're parallel to the ground.

Planks with Leg-Lifts

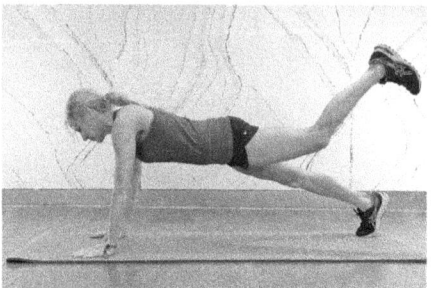 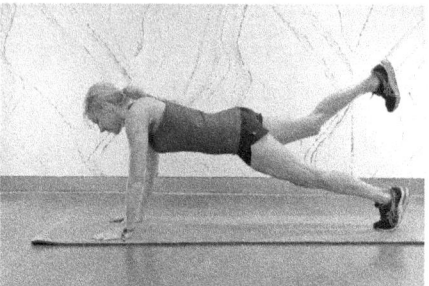

Begin in either plank position and alternate lifting your legs to the ceiling.

Side Plank

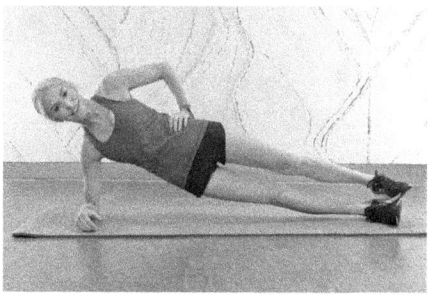

Hold your body up on one elbow (or hand) and the side of one foot. Remain motionless without allowing your lower hip to drop toward the floor.

Side Plank Leg-Lifts

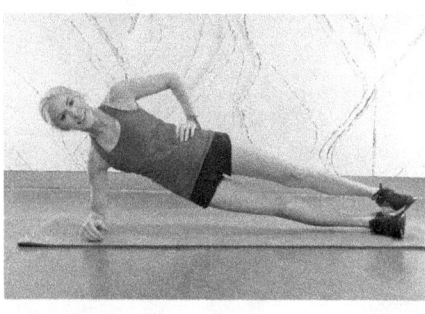 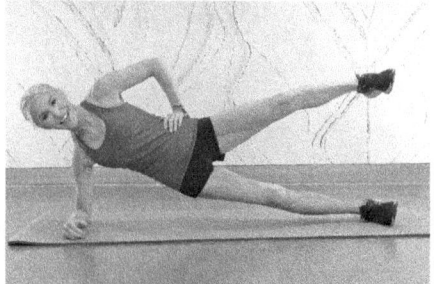

Begin in the side plank position and slowly lift and lower your top leg.

Side Plank Leg-Lifts with Band

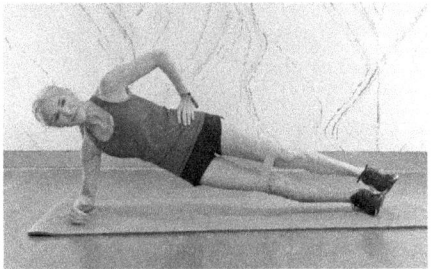 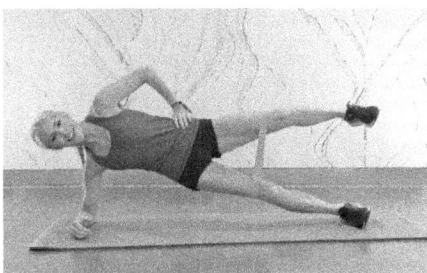

Begin in the side plank position with a band around your ankles and slowly lift and lower your top leg.

Side Plank Knee to Elbow

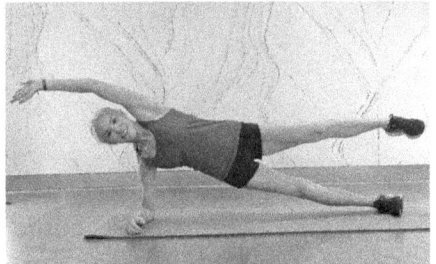 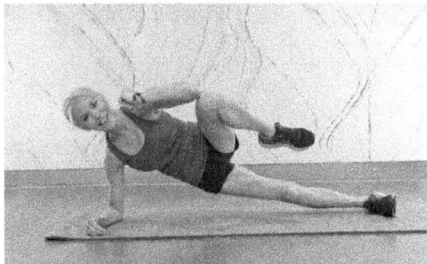

Begin in the side plank position with the top arm extended over your head. Slowly bring your top elbow and knee together and return to the extended position.

Crunches

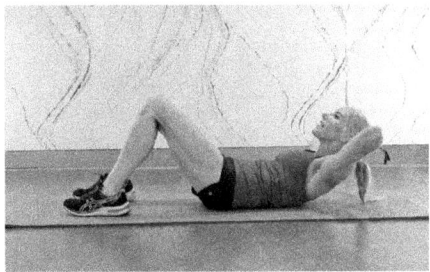

Lie on your back with your knees bent and feet flat on the floor. With your chin high, slowly lift your shoulders off the ground and return to starting position.

Oblique Crunches

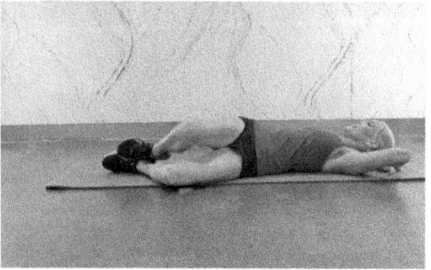 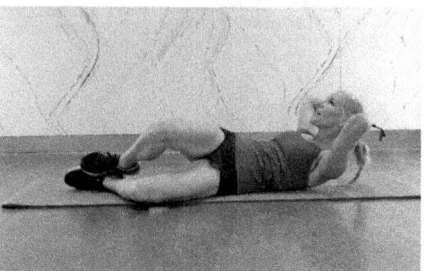

Lie on your back with your knees bent and twisted to the side. With your chin high, slowly lift your shoulders off the ground and return to starting position.

Full Oblique Sit-Ups

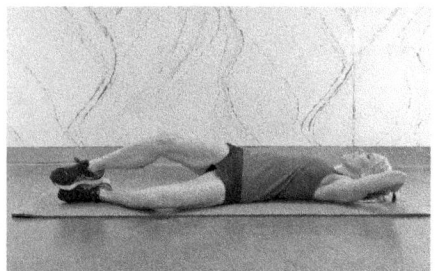 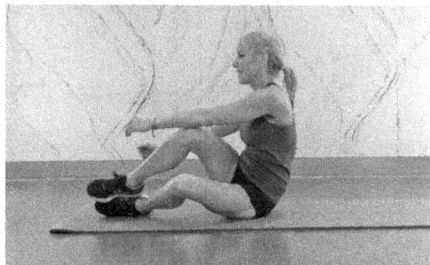

Lie on your back with your knees bent and twisted to the side. With your chin high, slowly lift your shoulders off the ground until your torso is upright, and return to starting position.

Full Extension Crunch

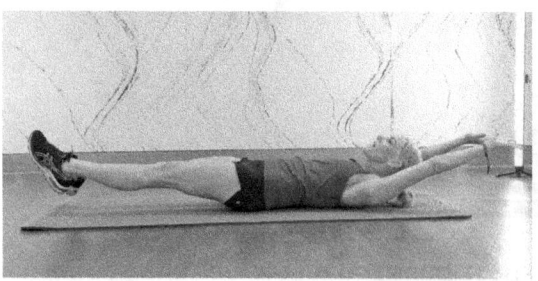 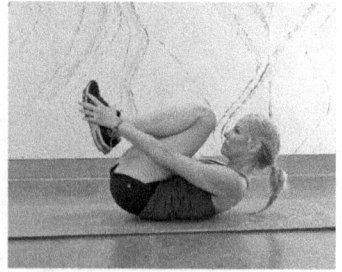

Lie on your back with your arms and legs extended, hovering over the floor. Slowly tuck your knees and grab your toes with your hands. Return to full extension.

Straight Leg Criss-Cross Crunches

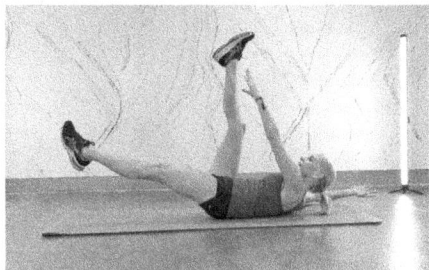 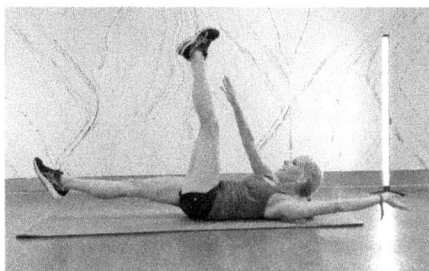

Lie on your back with your legs extended. Keeping your chin high, lift at the shoulder and rotate your right hand toward your left foot. Twist and lift your left hand toward your right foot.

BOSU Crunches

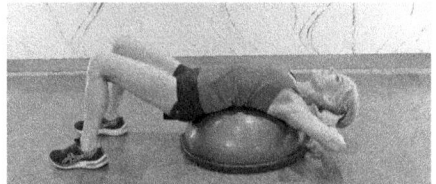 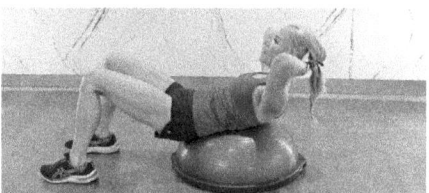

Lie with your back arched resting on the dome side of a BOSU with your knees bent and feet flat on the floor. With your chin high, slowly lift your shoulders off the BOSU and return to starting position.

Standing Rainbow Stretch

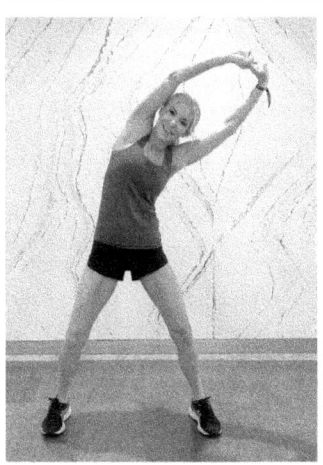 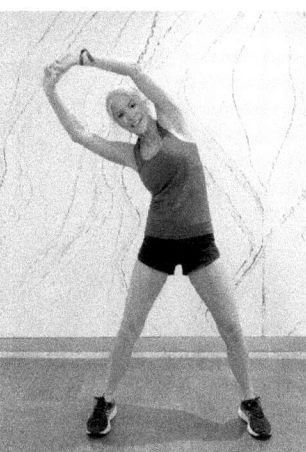

Clasp hands and reach to the ceiling. Lean to one side while reaching high and then the other.

Upward-Facing Dog

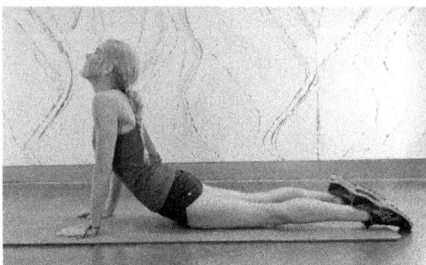

Lie face down with your hands below your shoulders. Lift your torso off the ground by extending your arms. Look up towards the ceiling.

ERECTOR SPINAE/LOW BACK

Supermans

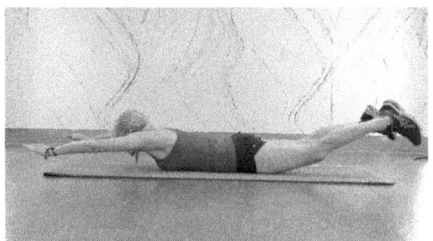

Lie face down with arms and legs extended. Lift both arms and legs off the ground and hold that position for 10-30 seconds.

Superman Swim

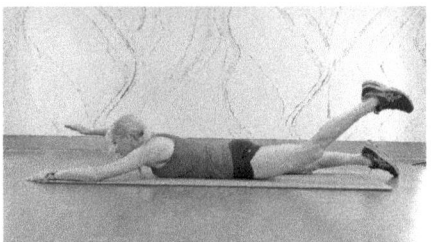 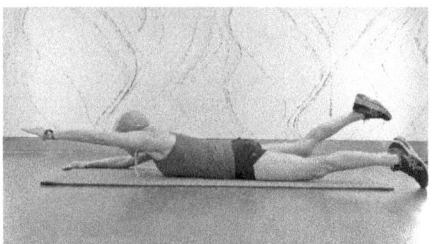

Lie face down with arms and legs extended. Alternate lifting opposing arms and legs as if you are swimming.

Superman Leg Lift

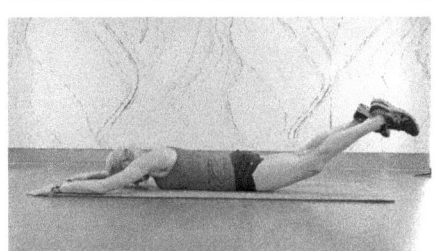

Lie face down with legs extended. Lift both legs off the ground. Hold, or lift and lower in a pulsing motion.

Superman Chest Lift

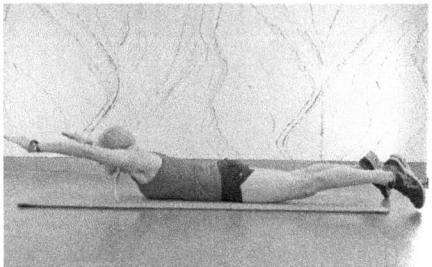

Lift your chest, shoulders, and arms off the ground. Hold, or lift and lower in a pulsing motion.

Bridge

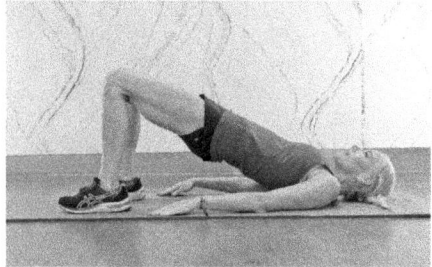

Lay face up with your shoulders and feet touching the ground. Lift your hips so that your body forms a straight line between your knees and shoulders. Hold, or lift and lower in a pulsing motion.

Single-Leg Bridge

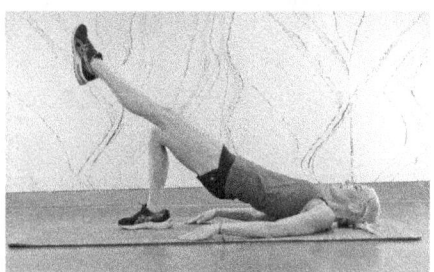 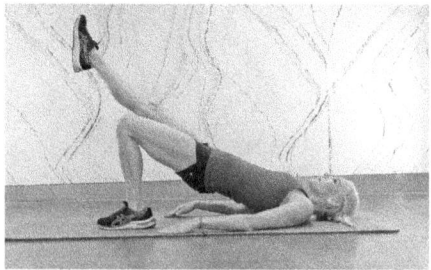

Begin in the basic bridge position and lift one leg so that your body forms a straight line between your foot and your shoulders.

Bridge Thrusts

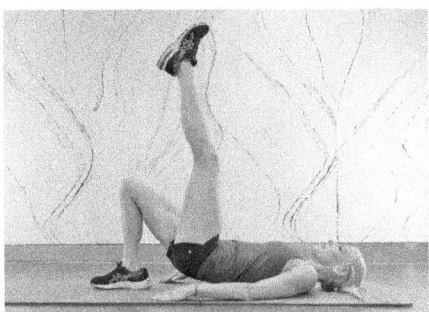 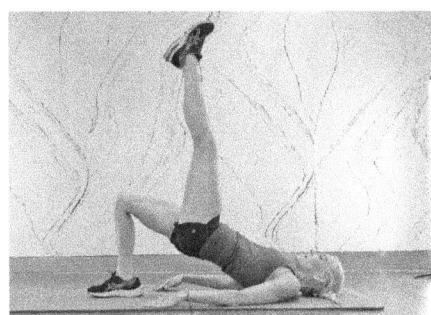

Begin in the basic bridge position with one leg straight up in the air. Slowly lower and lift your hips in a pulsing motion.

Marching Bridges

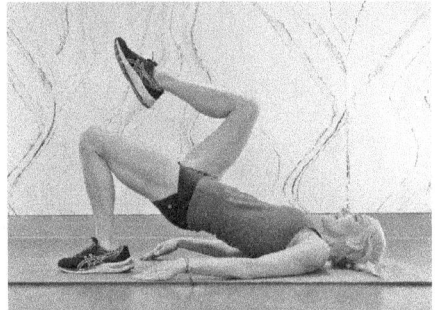 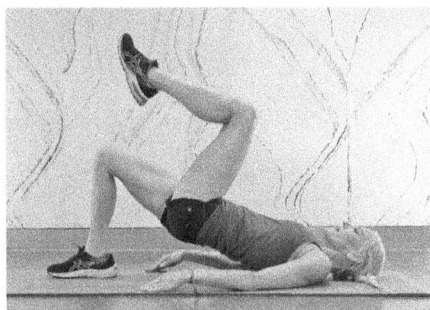

Begin in the basic bridge position and slowly alternate lifting knees in a marching motion.

Angry Cat

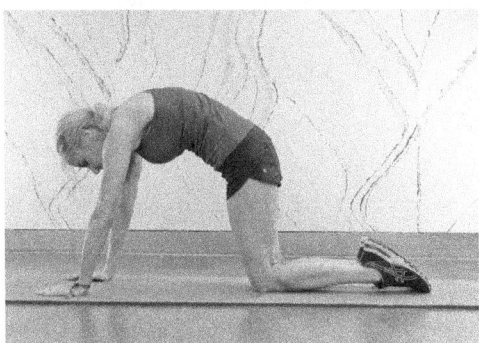

Begin on your hands and knees, and arch your back.

Child's Pose

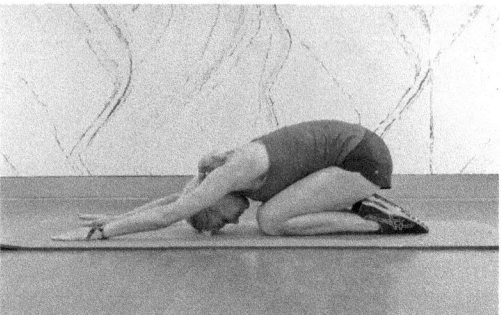

Start on your hands and knees. Sit your tush back on your heels with your arms extended out in front of you.

Army Crawl Rainbow Stretch

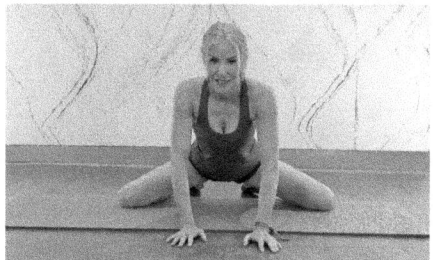

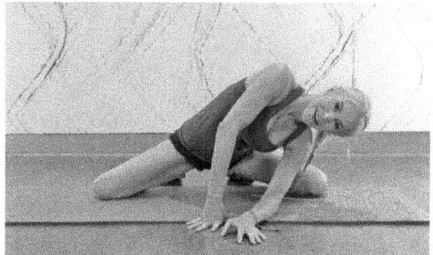

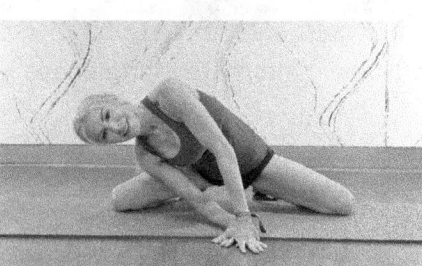

Begin on the ground with your knees spread apart, feet together, and your tush seated back on your heels. Lean your torso as far as you can from one side to the other. Hold for 10 to 15 seconds on each side.

CALVES

Calf Raises

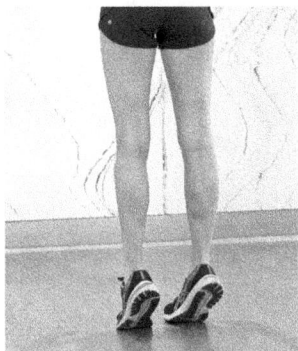

Stand with feet shoulder-width apart and knees soft. Lift your heels off the ground, rising onto your toes. Hold, or lift and lower in a pulsing motion.

Single-leg Calf Raises

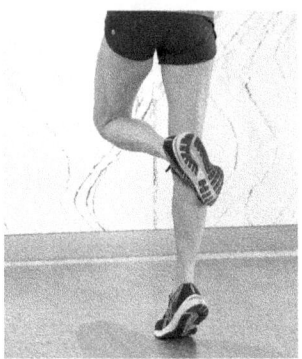

Stand on one foot with your knee soft. Lift your heel off the ground, rising onto your toes. Hold, or lift and lower in a pulsing motion.

Calf Stretch

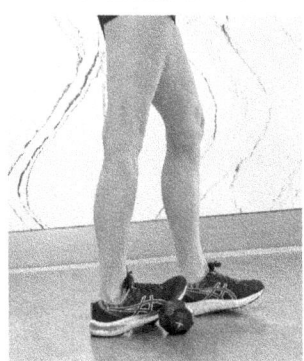

Stand with one foot in front of the other with the forefoot of your front leg elevated onto a dumbbell (or similar height object).

ANTERIOR TIBIALIS

Toe Taps

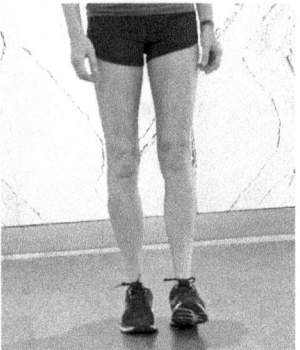

Stand with feet shoulder-width apart and knees soft. Alternate lifting your toes off the ground.

Weirdo Walk

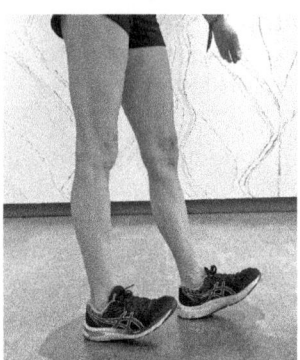

Walk 10-100 steps with your toes lifted, only your heels touching the ground.

Chapter 9 | Everything Exercise

COMPOUND EXERCISES

Angry Ups

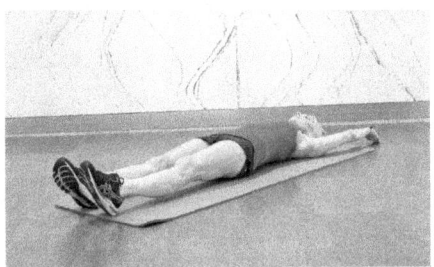

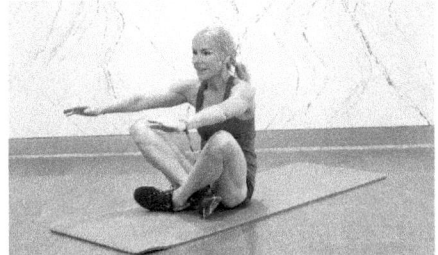

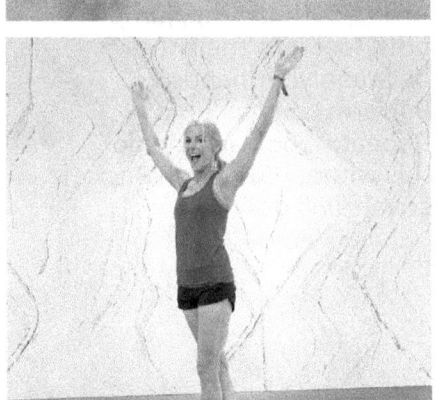

Begin lying flat on your back with your arms extended above your head. Lift your arms to the ceiling (do not touch the ground), cross your ankles, and use your lower body and abdominal strength to rise to a standing position. With arms still high, lower your body back into the starting position.

Mountain Climbers

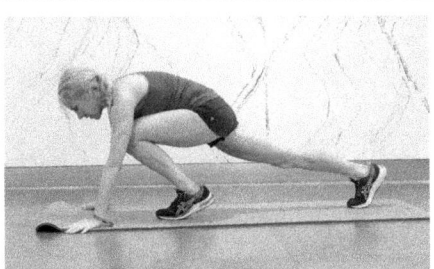

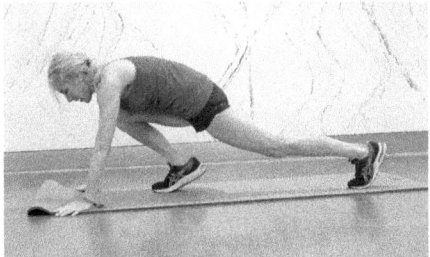

Begin in plank position with your right knee bent to your chest. Quickly extend your right leg while bringing your left knee to your chest. Repeat in a rhythmic motion for up to a minute.

You. Supercharged!

Burpees

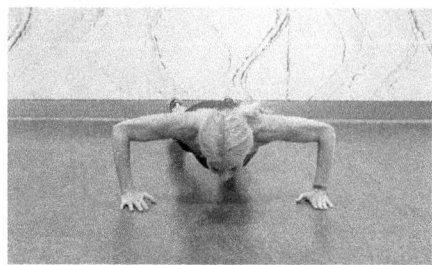

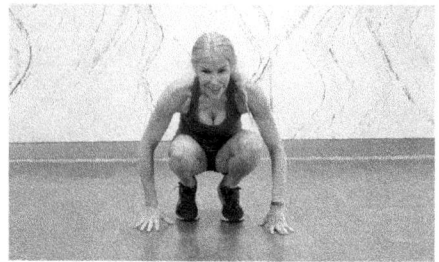

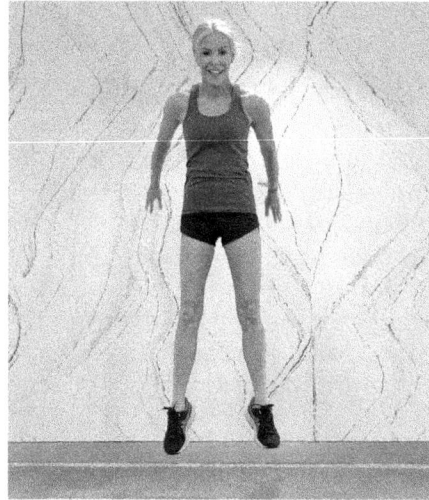

Begin with a push-up. After your push-up, jump both feet into the space between your hands. Perform a squat jump. Repeat! *You can also do this without jumping. Basic squats will do!

Chapter 9 | Everything Exercise

CHAIR EXERCISES

If exercising standing up doesn't feel good at any point, you can accomplish a whole lot in a seated position or with the support of a chair. You can do these exercises at home, the office, a fitness center, and anywhere else. Choose comfortable and sturdy chairs, and prioritize movement when doing mundane activities like watching TV. Don't be too shy to do these exercises while sitting in waiting and exam rooms. Have confidence that you can make tremendous progress with the help of a chair.

Chair fitness classes are growing in popularity at fitness centers everywhere. They cater to a wide variety of people who cannot exercise standing or simply prefer not to do so. They're often really fun and a superb way to socialize. Leave your ego at the door, and get to work!

Flies with Band

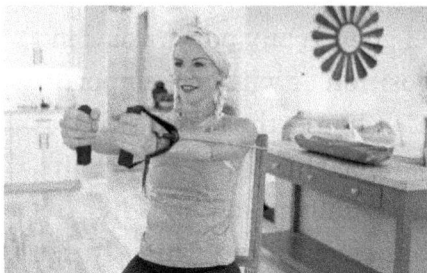 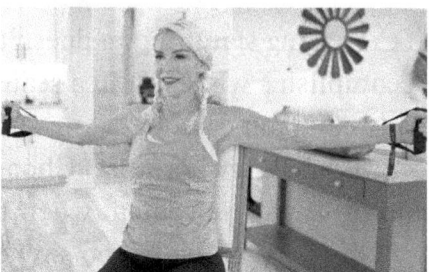

With the band affixed behind you, start with your arms almost straight, hands facing each other, and chest height in front of you. Slowly bring your arms to the side until your hands line up with your shoulders. Return to starting position.

Bench Press with Band

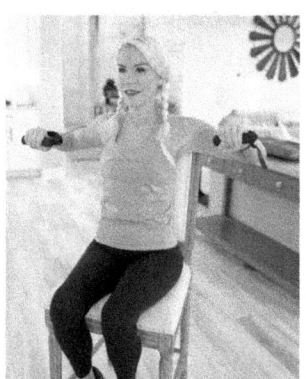 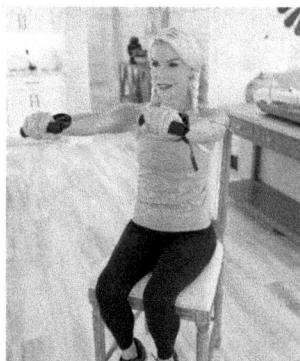

With your band affixed behind you, start with your hands near your shoulders and push forward until your arms are almost straight at shoulder level.

Military Press with Dumbbells

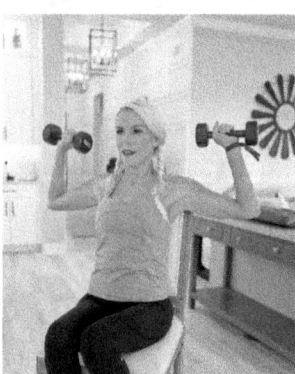 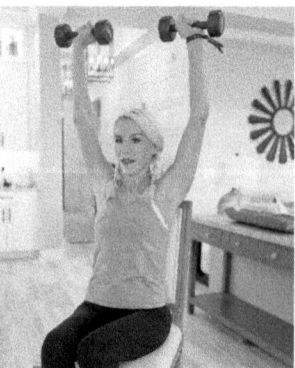

Start with arms wide, elbows bent, and hands facing forward. Press weights toward the ceiling and slowly return to starting position.

Lateral Raise with Dumbbells

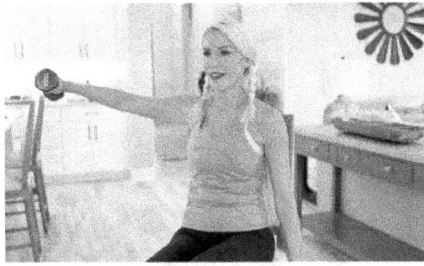
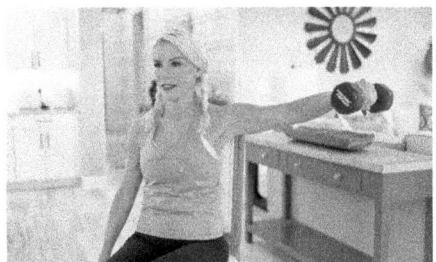

Start with arms extended toward the ground. Alternate each arm to the side until your hand is level with your shoulder.

Straight Leg Lift

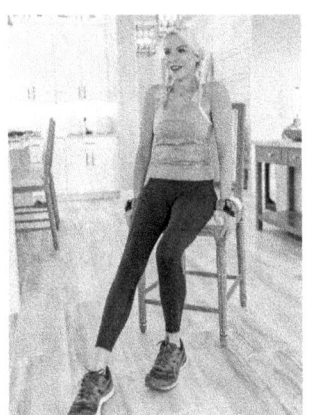
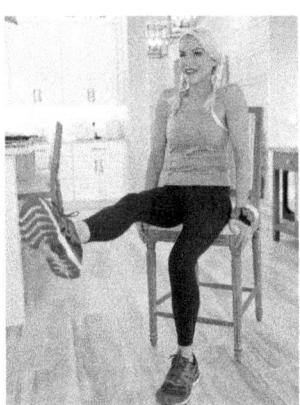

Sit forward on your chair with one leg extended. Slowly lift that leg straight up and down multiple times.

Straight Leg Lateral Lift

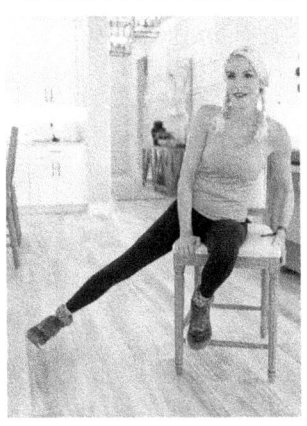
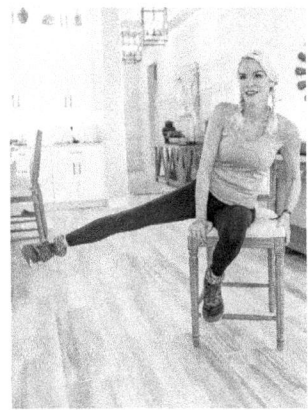

Sit towards the right side of your chair with your right leg extended. Keep your toes pointed forward and slowly lift that straight leg up and down multiple times.

Cardio Flap

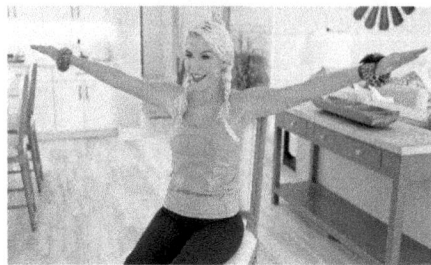 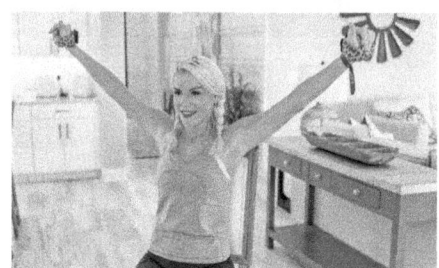

Bring your arms straight out to the side with or without weights and flap your arms up and down like a bird.

Kick Twist

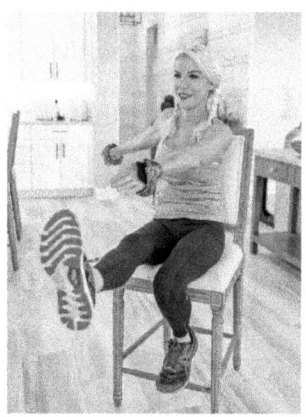 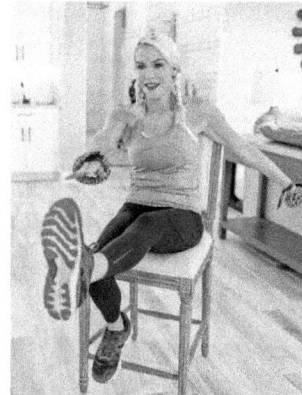

Simultaneously kick one foot while twisting and reaching for it with your opposite hand. Kick, twist, and reach!

March

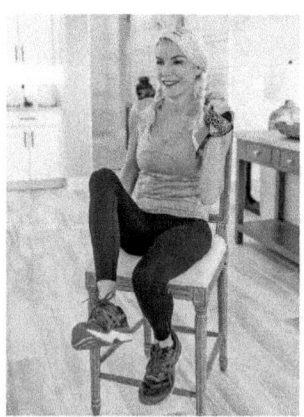 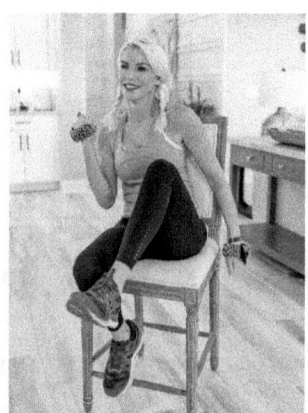

March in your chair by lifting your knees and pumping your arms.

Chapter 9 | Everything Exercise

Boxing

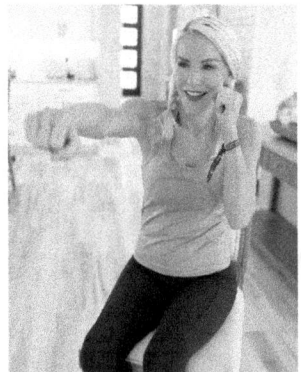 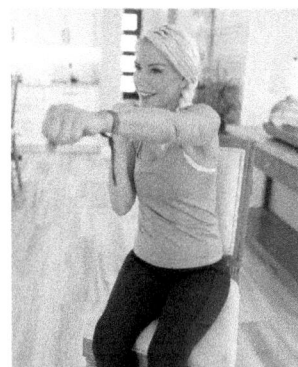

Start with your fists near your face and elbows pinned close to your body. Do a variety of punches on both arms until you've had enough.

Rainbow Stretch

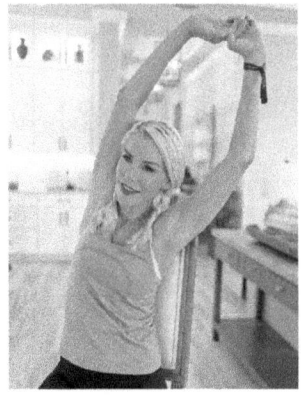 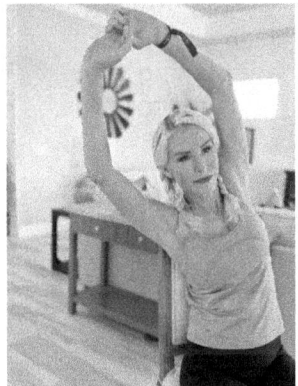

Clasp hands and reach to the ceiling with them. Lean toward each side, making a rainbow with your hands.

Lat Stretch

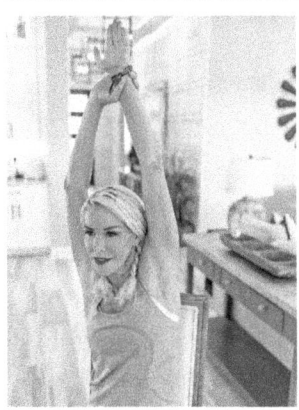 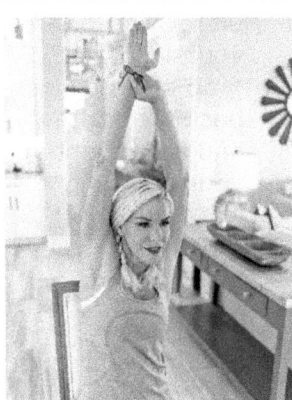

Reach one arm up high overhead. Grab that wrist with your opposite hand and gently pull your extended arm higher.

Shoulder Stretch

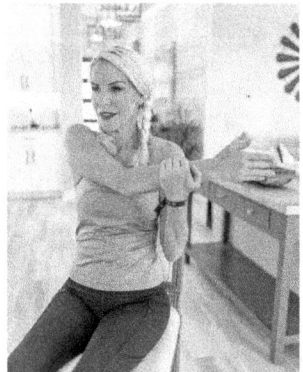 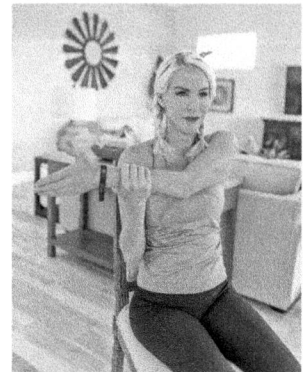

Bring one extended arm across your chest. Use the opposite hand to pull your extended arm even further.

Low Back Stretch

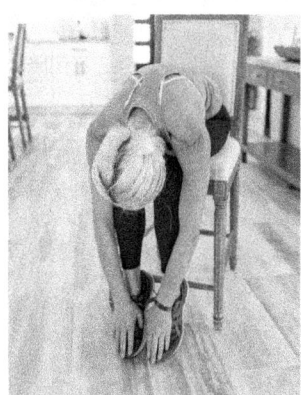

Fold forward in your chair, reaching your hands towards your toes.

Open Chest Stretch

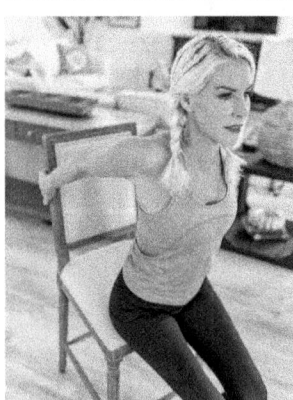

Sit forward on your chair and grab the chair back with both hands. Straighten your arms and lean your chest forward.

Twisty Back Stretch

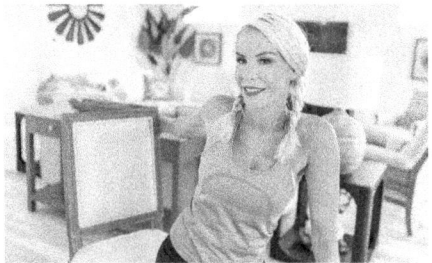 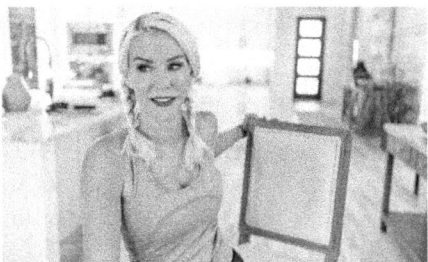

Sit forward in your chair, twist backward, grabbing the left side of your chair back with your right hand. Hold and then switch sides.

Lengthening Stretch

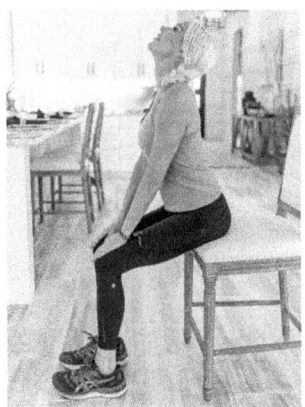

Sit forward on your chair with both feet flat on the floor. Push your chest forward, arch your back and look up.

Angry Cat

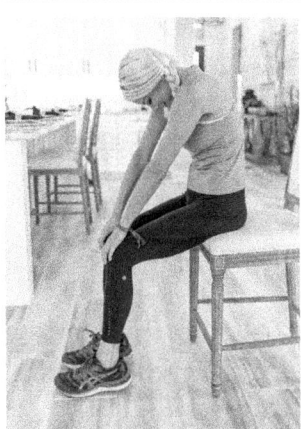

Sit forward on your chair with both feet flat on the floor. Drop your chin and lift your upper back towards the sky.

Hamstring Stretch

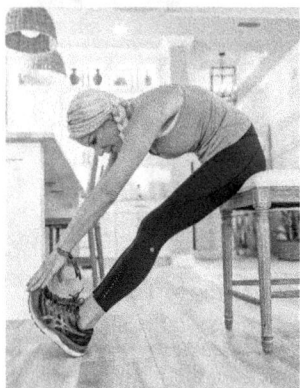

Sit forward in your chair with both legs extended in front of you. Reach towards your toes with both hands.

Piriformis/ Glute Stretch

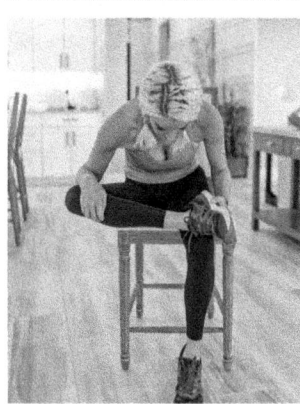

Cross one foot over the opposite knee. Fold your chest forward.

Cardio Lower-Body Twist

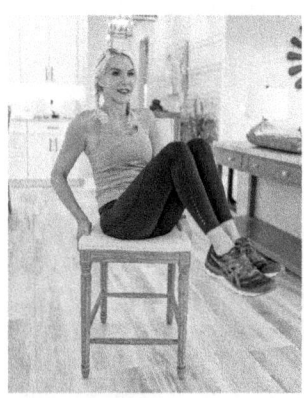 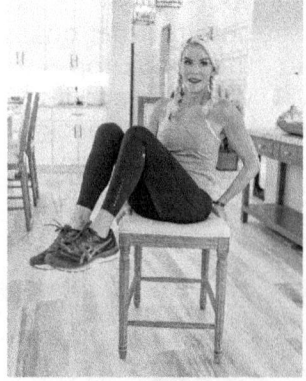

Start seated with both feet on the floor, holding onto the sides of your seat. Lift both knees up and to one side. Put both feet back on the floor. Lift both knees in the opposite direction and repeat.

Chapter 9 | Everything Exercise

Chair Squats

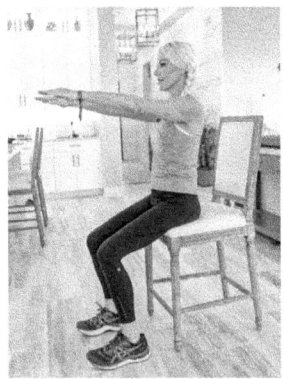 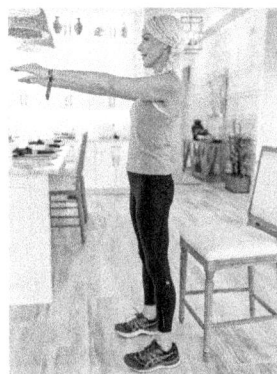

Begin seated normally in your chair. Stand up. Sit back down. Repeat.

Triceps Stretch

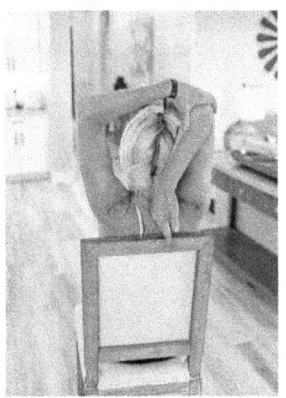 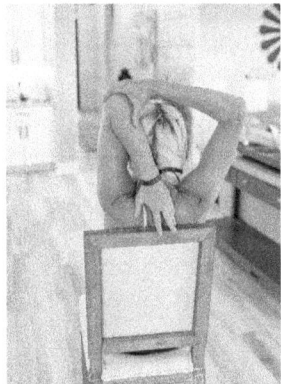

Place your right hand behind your neck with your elbow high. Grab your right elbow with your left hand and gently pull your right arm back. Simultaneously, press down on your right forearm with your left thumb to enhance the stretch.

Lateral Leg Lifts

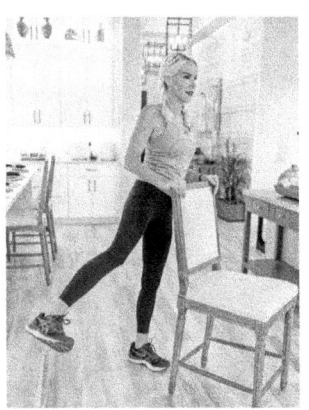

Stand with soft knees using your chair for balance. Keeping all your toes pointed forward, slowly lift one leg to the side and lower it.

Forward Leg Lifts

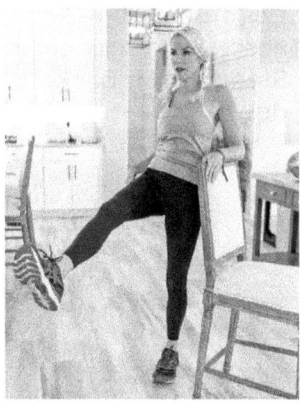

Stand with soft knees while holding onto your chair for balance. Keeping all your toes pointed forward, slowly lift one leg in front of you and lower it.

Kick Backs

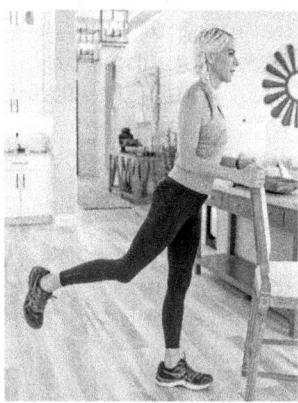

Stand with soft knees while holding onto your chair for balance. Keeping all of your toes pointed forward, slowly lift one leg behind you and lower it.

"No" Neck Stretch

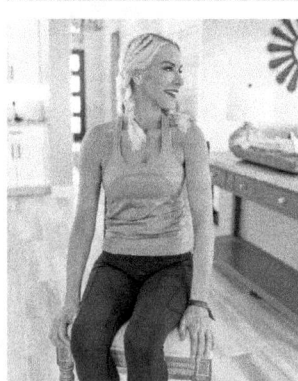

Sit up straight. Keep your chin level (don't look up or down). Slowly look over one shoulder and hold.

Assisted Neck Stretch

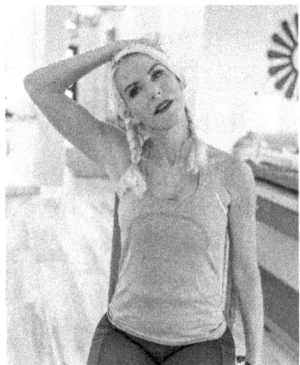

Sit up straight. Keep your chin level (don't look up or down). Place one hand on your head and gently press down, bringing your ear closer to your shoulder.

Abductions with Bands

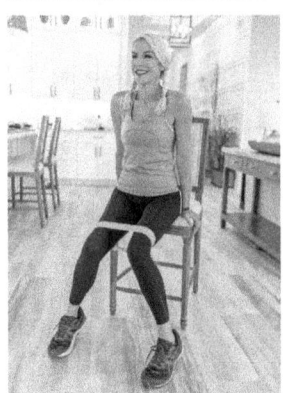 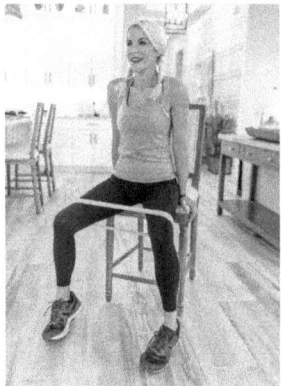

Sit forward on your chair with both feet on the floor and a band wrapped around your thighs (just above your knees). Pull both knees apart and then return to starting position.

Balance with Support

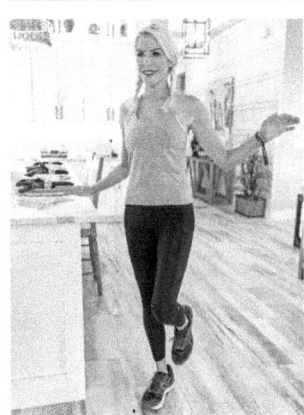

Stand on one foot while holding onto a stable chair, a countertop, a wall, or a friend. If you feel ready for progress, let go of support. Incorporate other balance training exercises near support until you're stable enough to train without it.

BED EXERCISES

Whether you are in bed due to illness or injury, or just want to start and end each day with some feel-good movements, your bed can be a productive place to exercise. I exercised in bed regularly during cancer care, which was incredibly beneficial, and still do so when watching TV or reading a book. At home, in a hotel, or in a hospital, when you can't stand or even sit in a chair, these exercises may help you maintain strength, flexibility, and mobility, while preventing stiffness. Always do what you can, when you can. This is the epitome of the "no excuses" lifestyle.

Taller Stretch

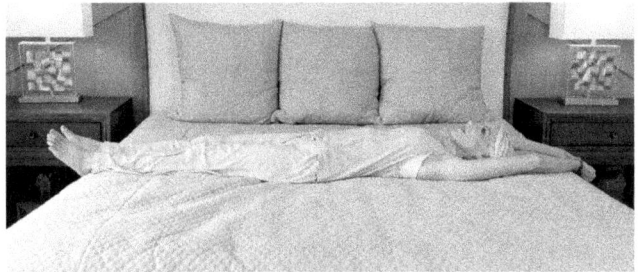

Lie flat on your back with legs straight, and arms extended overhead. Reach in both directions as if you're trying to make yourself taller.

Taller Pillow Stretch

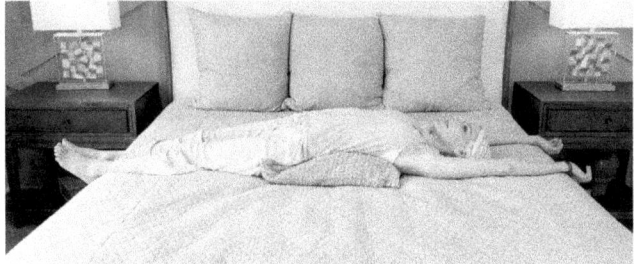

Lie flat with a pillow under your back, legs straight, and arms extended overhead.

Pillow Side Stretch

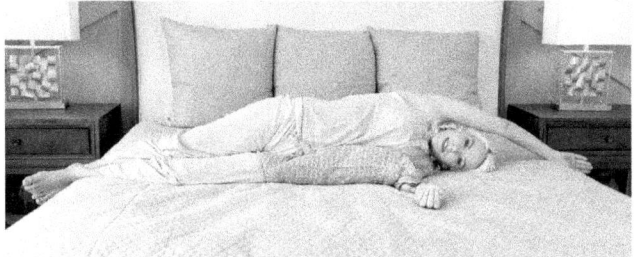

Lie on your side with a pillow under your hips and torso, with legs straight and arms extended overhead.

Prone Pillow Stretch

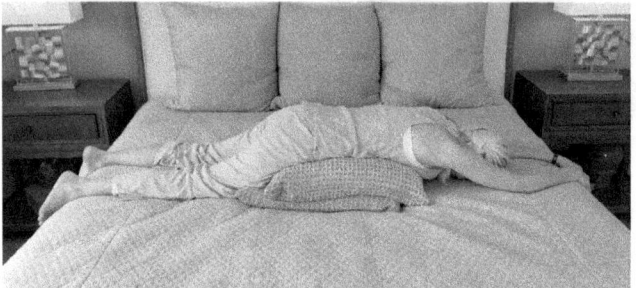

Lie face down with a pillow under your tummy, legs straight, and arms extended overhead. Relax.

Knees to Chest

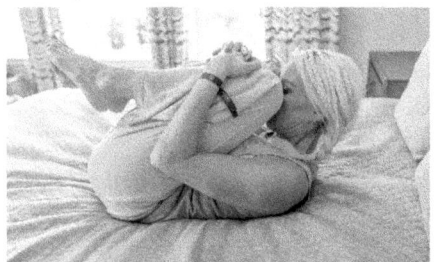

Lie on your back and bring your knees into your chest. Hug your knees tight while tucking your chin into your knees.

Army Crawl Stretch

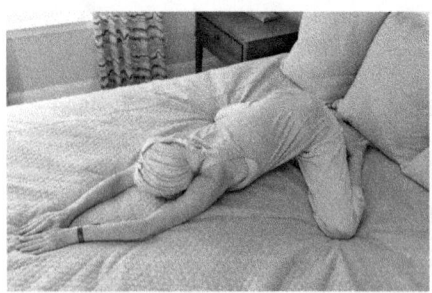 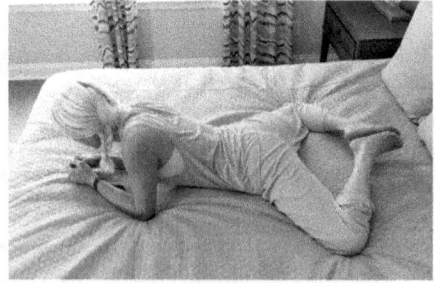

Get on the bed with your knees spread apart, feet together, and your tush seated back on your heels. Lower your hips and chest as much as possible with your arms extended over your head and hold. Keep your hips and chest low and drive your hips forward, and hold.

Chapter 9 | Everything Exercise

Angry Cat Stretch

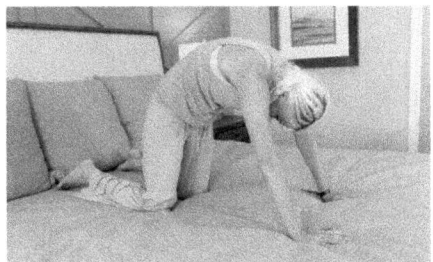

Begin on your hands and knees, and arch your back high.

Upward Facing Dog

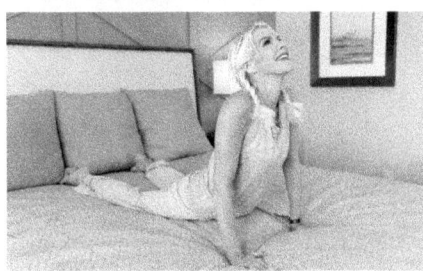

Lie face down with hands below your shoulders. Lift your torso high off the bed by extending your arms. Look up towards the ceiling.

Quad Stretch

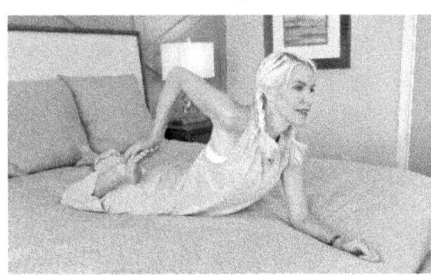

Begin in a prone position with hands below your shoulders. Bend your right leg and grab your right foot with your right hand.

Adductor Stretch

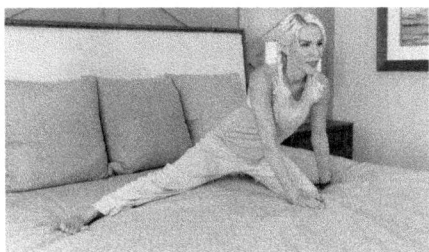

Begin on your left knee with your right leg extended to the side. Shift your upper body weight to your left knee.

Chest and Biceps Stretch

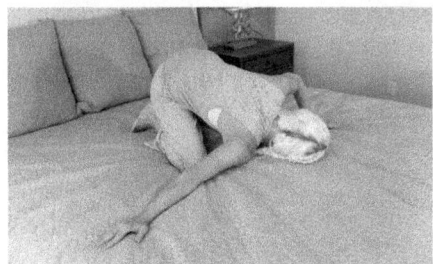 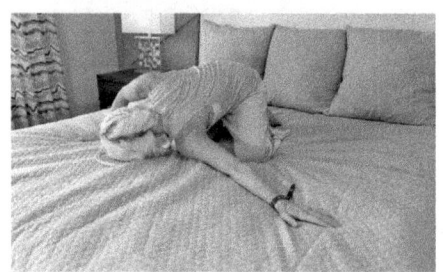

Sit on your knees with your tush resting on your heels. Extend your left arm to one side with your palm on the bed. Press your left shoulder into the bed while rotating your torso in the opposite direction.

Hip Flexor Stretch

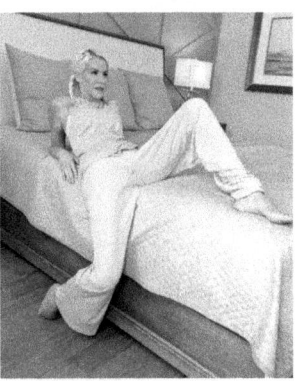

Begin near the edge of your bed with your left leg on the bed and your right leg off the side. Bend your right knee, placing the top of your right foot on the ground.

Low Back Stretch

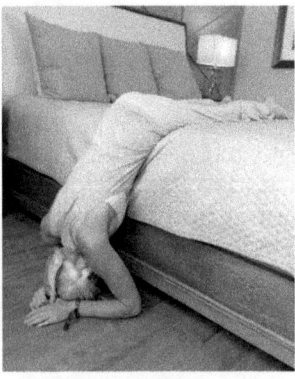

Fold your torso over the edge of the bed, resting your forearms on the ground. Relax.

Side Stretch

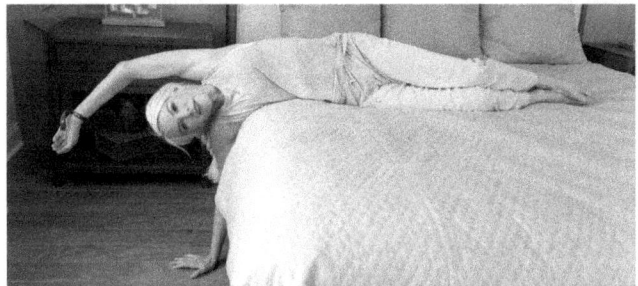

Begin in a side-lying position with your right armpit on the edge of the bed and your right hand on the ground. Reach your left arm up overhead and lean into the stretch.

Extended Twisting Stretch

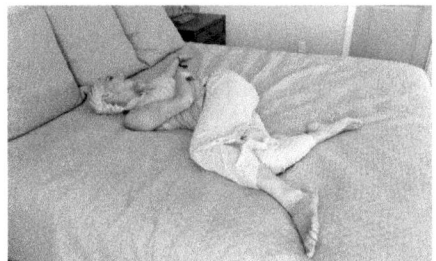

Lie on your back. Cross your left leg over the right side of your body. Twist your torso in the opposite direction, looking over your left shoulder.

CrissCross Applesauce Stretch

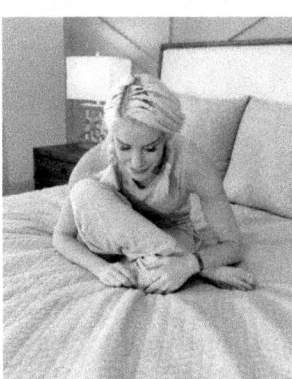

Bend and cross one leg on top of the other. Try to stack your knees on each other (or come close). Lower your chest and hold.

Headboard Stretch

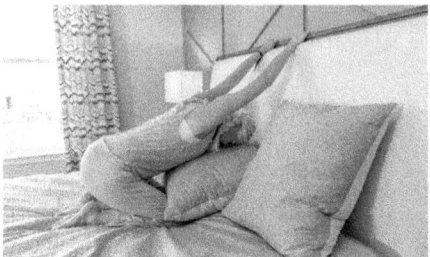

Kneel facing your headboard. Grab the top of your headboard or the wall near your bed. Sit back on your heels and drop your chest towards the bed.

Hamstring Stretch with Bathrobe Belt

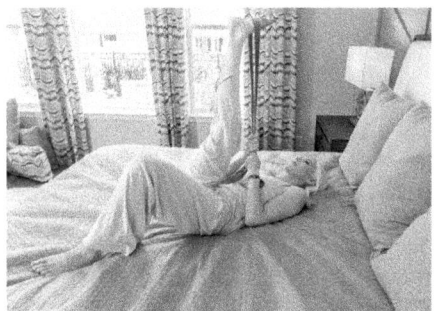

Lie on your back with your left leg bent and your right leg in the air. Wrap the center of your bathrobe belt around your right foot, extend your leg, and gently pull the right leg toward your chest

Adductor Stretch with Bathrobe Belt

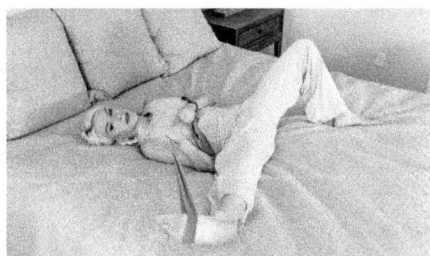

Lie on your back with your left leg bent and your right leg in the air. Wrap the center of your bathrobe belt around your right foot, extend your leg, and gently pull the right leg out to the side.

Chest Stretch with Bathrobe Belt

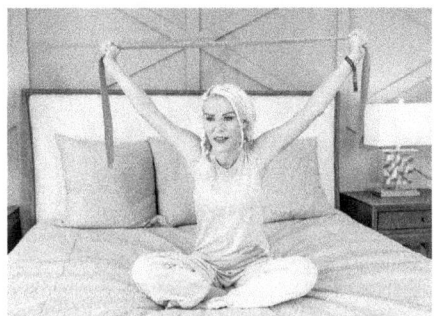 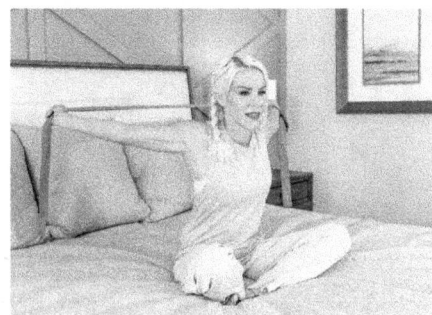

Sit straight up on your bed. Hold a bathrobe belt taut above your head with extended arms. Slowly lower your arms behind you. Loosen your grip on the belt as necessary to complete the motion.

Lateral Leg Lifts

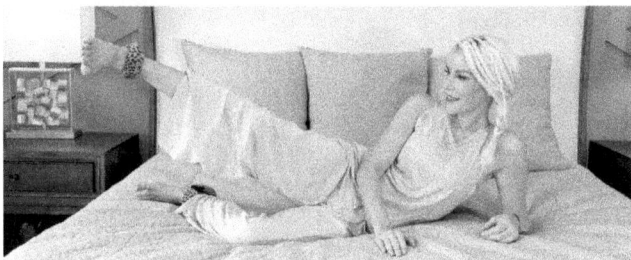

Rest on your side with your legs straight and stacked on top of each other. Keep your top leg almost straight with your toes pointed forward, and slowly lift it towards the ceiling.

Bent-Knee Lateral Leg Lifts

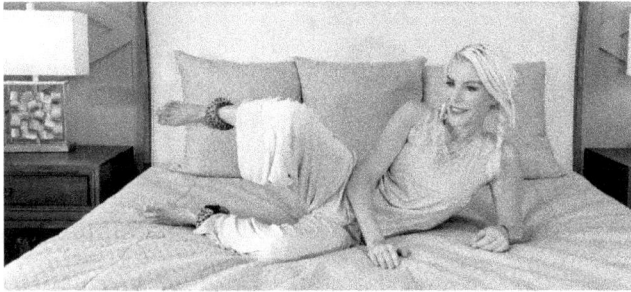

Rest on your side with your legs bent and stacked on each other. Slowly lift it towards the ceiling.

Straight Leg Lifts

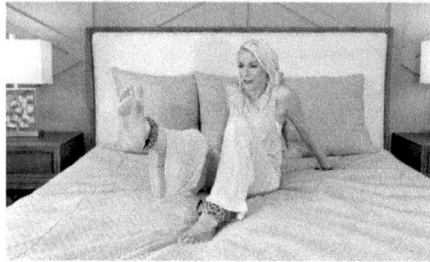 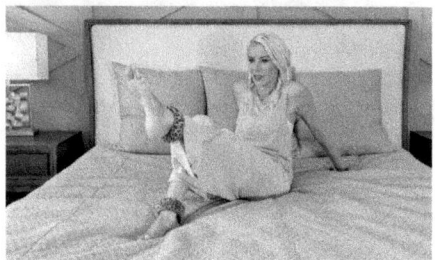

Begin in a reclined seated position with your arms supporting your upper body. Extend one leg in front of you, lifting it up and down.

Crunches

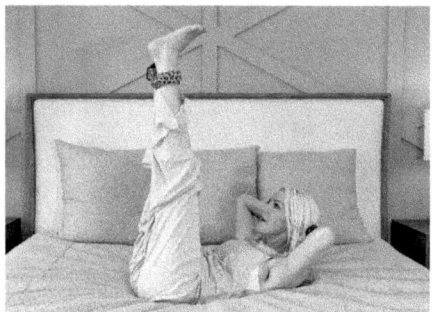

Lie flat with your knees bent or your feet high in the air. Lift your shoulders and lower them.

Lying Triceps Extension

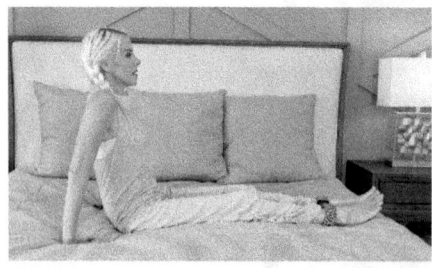 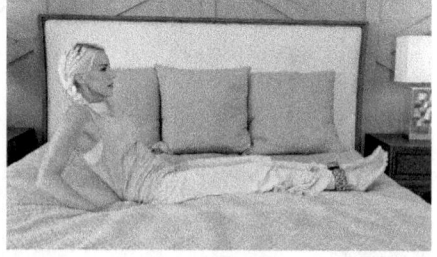

Begin in a seated position with your legs extended. Your straight arms should support your upper body, and your fingers should point toward your tush. Slowly lower your back about 50% of the way toward the bed. Using your triceps and abs, rise back up into starting position.

Chapter 9 | Everything Exercise

Bridge

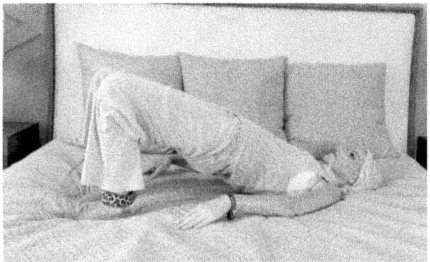

Lie face up with only your shoulders and feet touching the bed. Lift your hips so your body forms a straight line between your knees and shoulders. Hold, or lift and lower in a pulsing motion.

Marching Bridges

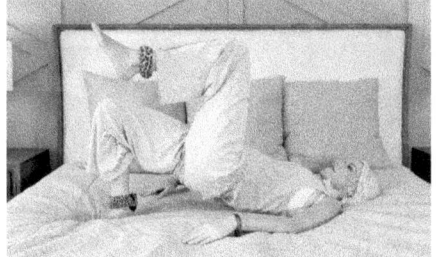 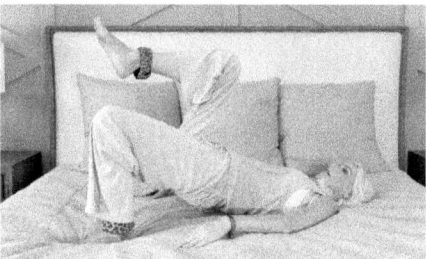

Begin in the basic bridge position and slowly alternate lifting knees in a marching motion.

Single-Leg Bridge

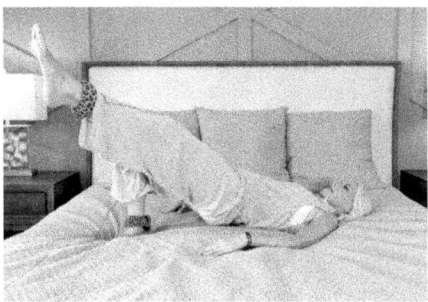

Begin in the basic bridge position and lift one leg so that your body forms a straight line between your extended leg and your shoulders.

Superman Swim

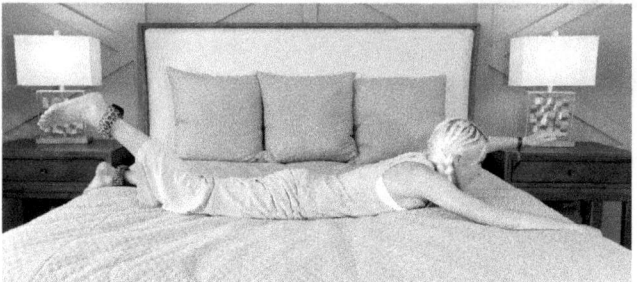

Lie face down with arms and legs extended. Alternate lifting opposing arms and legs as if you are swimming.

Superman Leg Lifts

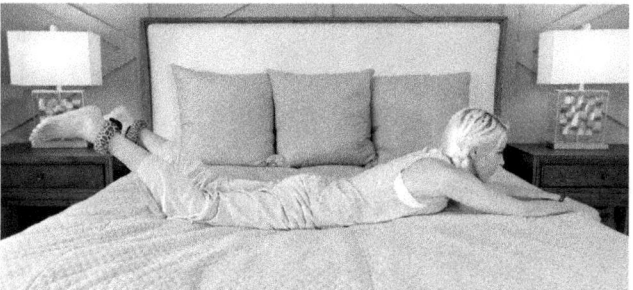

Lie face down with legs extended. Lift both legs off the bed. Hold or lift and lower in a pulsing motion.

Superman Chest Lift

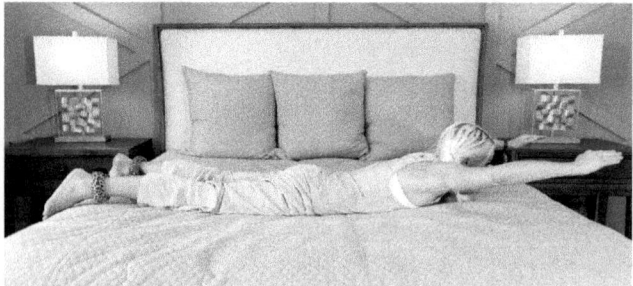

Lie face down with arms and legs extended. Lift your chest, shoulders, and arms off the bed. Hold or lift and lower in a pulsing motion.

Plank

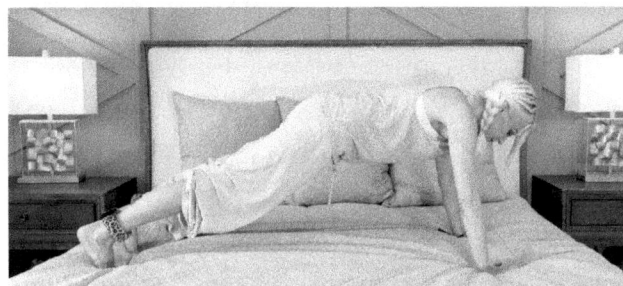

Lie face down with only your toes, hands, or forearms touching the bed. Keep your hands directly below your shoulders, and remain still with your body forming a straight line between your heels and shoulders.

Side Plank

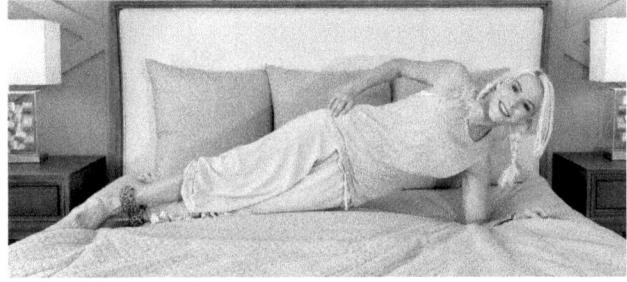

Hold your body up on one elbow (or hand) and the side of one foot. Remain motionless without allowing your lower hip to drop toward the bed.

Donkey Kicks

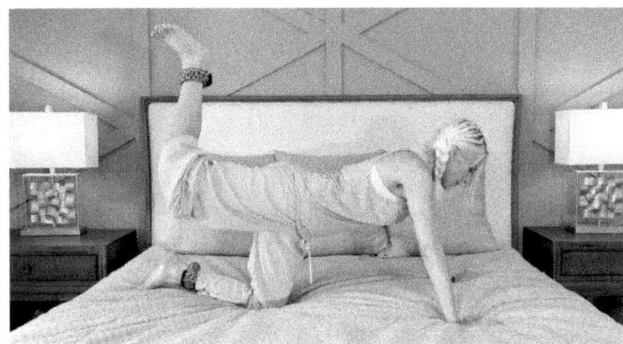

Begin on hands and knees. Lift one bent leg towards the ceiling as if you were trying to kick backward, and return to starting position.

Upper Body Motions

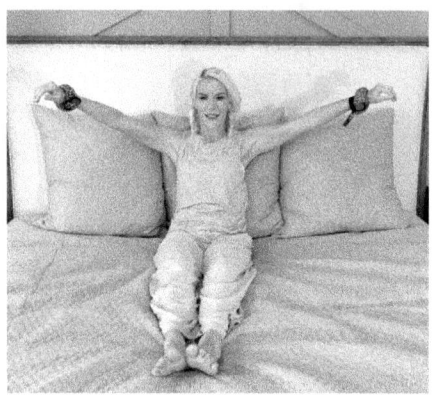
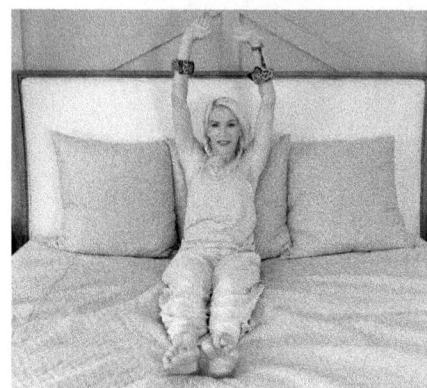

Recline back on some pillows and lift your straight arms up and down in various directions.

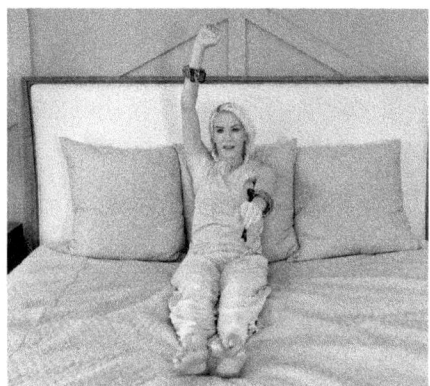
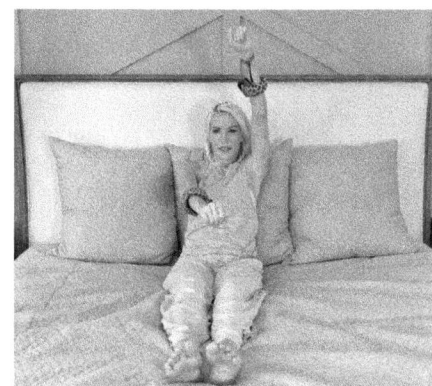

Recline back on some pillows and lift your straight arms up and down in various directions.

Chapter 9 | Everything Exercise

SHOWER STRETCHES

Stretching in the shower can feel magical. With warm water pouring over your body, it's a wise way to increase mobility while preparing your body for a big day or gently wind down for quality sleep. The shower is a wonderful place to stretch and relax, but you must show prudence and be cautious not to move quickly or do anything that would result in a fall. Only stretch if the shower floor is a textured non-slip surface, and you feel stable. Safety first! Play music, move slowly, breathe deeply, and enjoy these gentle movements.

Soggy Taller Stretch

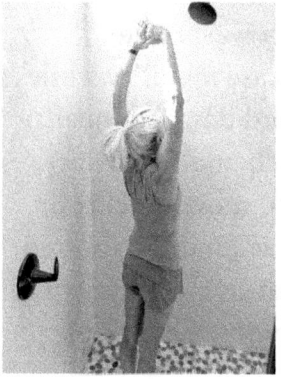

Clasp hands and reach to the ceiling.

Soggy Wall Stretch

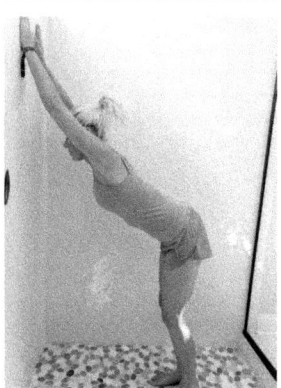

With arms extended, place the palms of your hands against the shower wall and lean forward.

Soggy Side Stretch

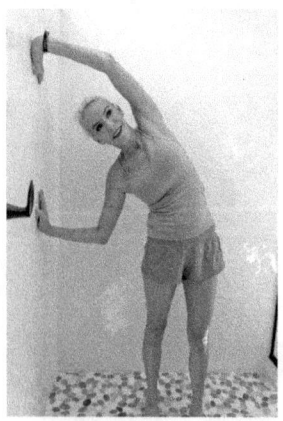

With one side to the wall, place the palms of your hands on the wall - one low and one high. Arch your torso toward the wall.

Chapter 9 | Everything Exercise

Soggy Adductor Stretch

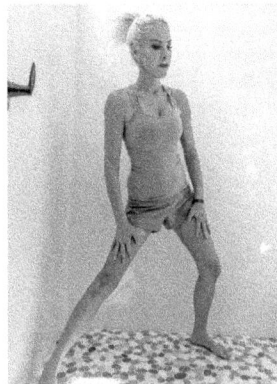

Stand with feet fairly far apart and shift your weight to one side, bending one knee. Stand with feet far apart. Reach up to the sky and over your head.

Soggy Chicken Wing Stretch

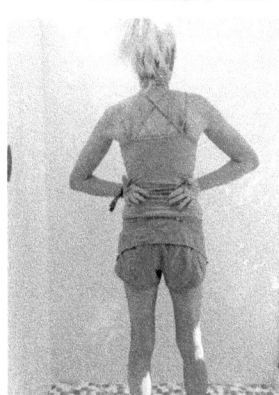

Place the back of both hands onto your low back and bring both elbows toward the front of your body.

Soggy Tricep Stretch

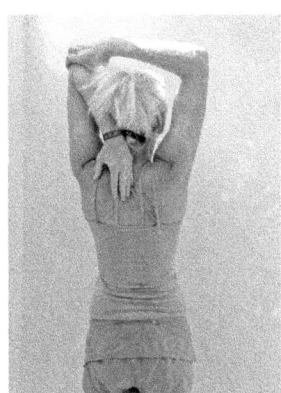

Place your right hand behind your neck with your elbow high. Grab your right elbow with your left hand and gently pull your right arm back. Simultaneously, press down on your right forearm with your left thumb to enhance the stretch.

Soggy Angry Cat

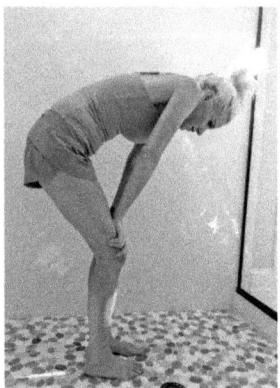

Stand with feet together and knees slightly bent. Place your hands on your thighs and arch your back toward the sky.

Soggy Standing Chest Stretch

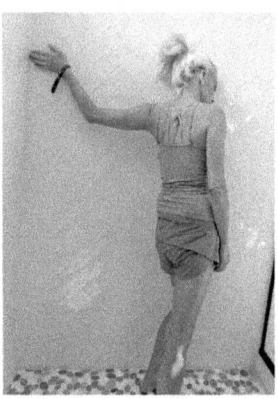

Stand close to a wall with your right arm extended to the side and your right palm pressed against it. Press your right shoulder against the wall and rotate to your left.

Soggy Calf Stretch

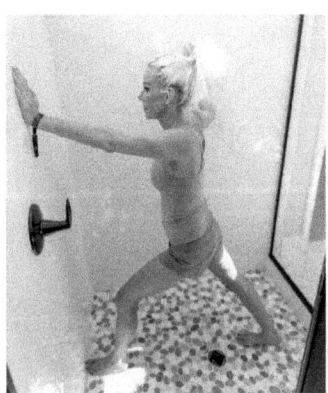

Stand facing a wall in a lunge position with your back leg almost straight, pressing that rear heel to the ground.

Chapter 9 | Everything Exercise

Stretch Soggy Up and Over Stretch

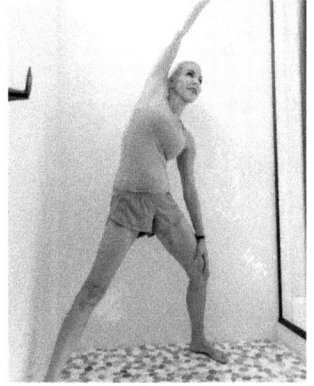

With a wide stance, reach as far up and over as you can.

Soggy Rainbow

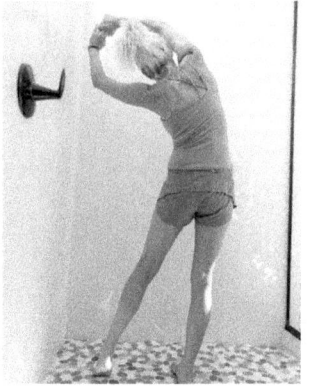

Clench your hands overhead and lean your body from side to side.

Soggy Standing Biceps

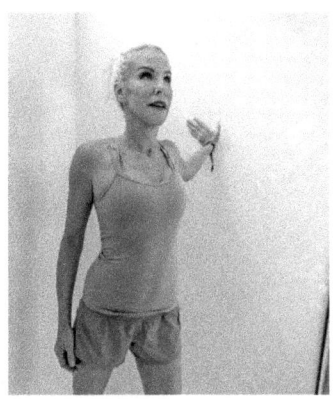

Place one palm against the wall with your fingers pointing behind you. Extend that arm and rotate your body away from the wall.

Soggy Standing Hamstring Stretch

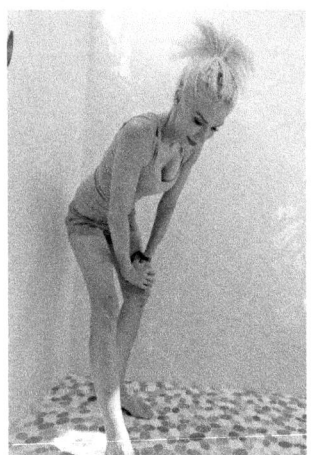

Extend one heel before you, and shift most of your weight onto your base leg. Sit back and lean forward slightly toward the extended leg. Remain mostly upright to avoid tipping over.

BALANCE TRAINING

Until you're super steady, stand near a wall or another robust and stable object for support. Aim to hold each challenge for 10-30 seconds, but start small. Don't get frustrated if you wobble; wobbling leads to progress!

Flamingo

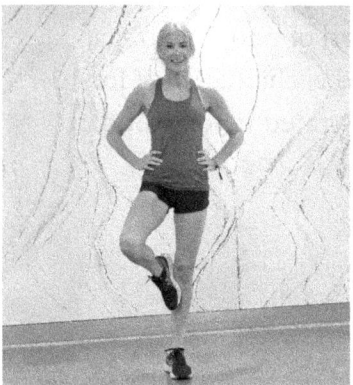

Stand on one foot.

Blind Flamingo

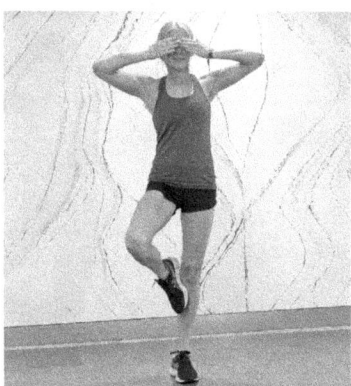

Stand on one foot with your eyes closed.

Flappy Flamingo

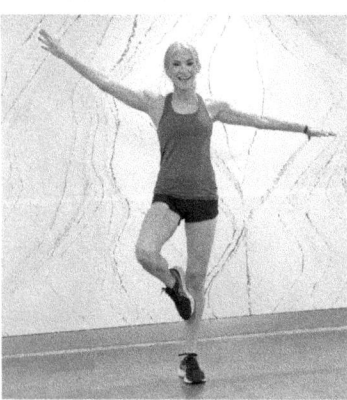

Stand on one foot and move your arms in various ways.

Chapter 9 | Everything Exercise

Kicky Flamingo

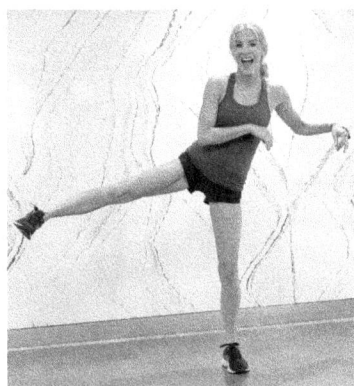

Stand on one foot and kick your free leg around in various directions.

Firm Flamingo on a Bubble

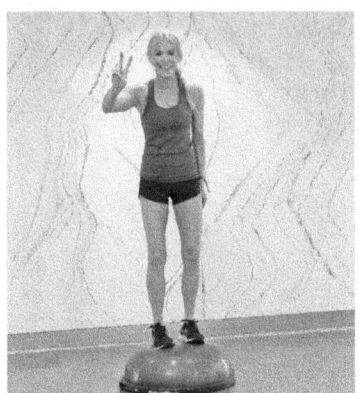

Stand on BOSU with the dome side up on two feet.

Flamingo on a Bubble

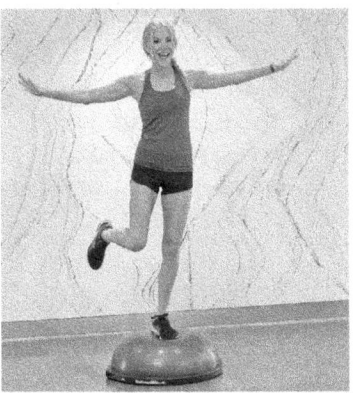

Stand on BOSU with the dome side up on one foot. This is advanced!

Flamingo Plays Catch

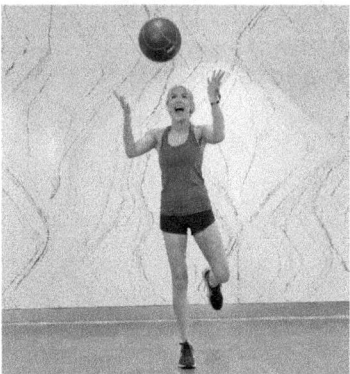

Stand on one foot while throwing and catching a ball. Do this with a partner or alone, with a bouncy ball or medicine ball.

Buff Flamingo

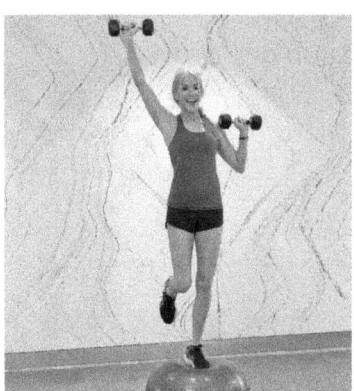

Stand on BOSU with the dome side up on one foot. Perform any of your favorite dumbbell exercises.

Flamingo Jump Squats

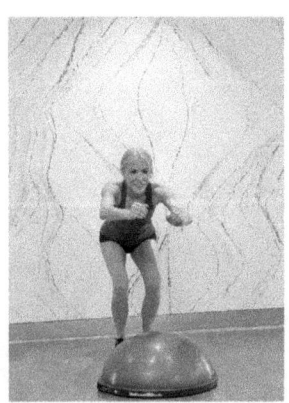 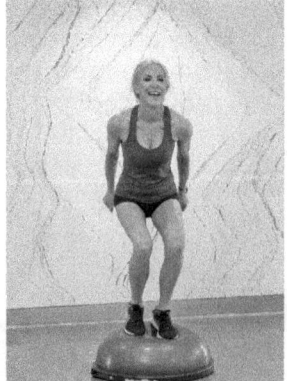

Squat down behind a BOSU with the dome side up. Jump onto the BOSU and stick the landing. This is advanced!

Chapter 10

SLEEP LIKE AN ANGEL

Few things can have such an immediate impact on the way you feel, look, and perform as quality sleep. Sleep is essential for supercharged health because it allows the body to repair, boosts immune function, and supports brain health, enhancing memory, mood, and overall well-being. After a solid slumber, we wake up feeling refreshed, revitalized, and ready for the day. Poor sleep causes us to feel bad, function on a very low level, and put ourselves and others at risk for accidents and mistakes.

Not much strikes more fear into our hearts than an early wake-up call. Panic sets in when you're booked on a 5:30 am flight, and the clock strikes 9:00 pm. Doing the negative math is agonizing. "If I hit the hay right now, I would only get six hours of sleep!" That's because you know that getting too little sleep is torturous. Your eyes will burn, your brain will be foggy, and you will be cranky. Feeling this way on a special occasion, for a trip, or an early morning event, is hard enough. Feeling this way daily because you fail to prioritize quality sleep can make your life miserable!

Sleepy people are rarely successful and happy. They often skip workouts, make lazy nutrition choices, drink too much alcohol, and fail to think clearly, creatively, or quickly. They can be snippy,

Chapter 10 | Sleep Like an Angel

downright rude, and impossible to work or live with. Low energy, overweight, and unhappy are also descriptions that fit the bill. I find it confusing when adults brag about how little sleep they get. It happens to all of us occasionally, but some folks make it a lifestyle and try to impress us with it. Know this: your lack of quality sleep shows. You don't have to tell us. We see it in your face, hear it in your voice, and experience it with your mistakes. Do us all a favor, get some sleep! We prefer you to be refreshed and energized at your best. Rest is part of the preparation for excellence.

Revitalizing sleep is rarely accidental. Much like exercise and nutrition, you should put some thought and effort into making it the best it can be. Adults are generally recommended to get 7-to-9 hours of sleep per night for optimal health and well-being, but like everything else, whether it be more or less, you should choose the right amount for you.

Stick to a regular sleep schedule.

Go to bed and wake up at the same time every day, even on weekends, if possible. In the same way parents sleep-train babies, you can train yourself. Even if you struggle to fall asleep at your desired bedtime, enjoy the peaceful rest you get until you fall asleep. Know that, eventually, your body will fall in line and do what you're telling it to do.

Create a bedtime routine.

Wind down with relaxing activities like reading or taking a warm bath to signal your body it's time to sleep. Try out a few techniques to see what works best. Chill activities like knitting and cuddling your cats should be calming. Arguing with your spouse will not. Choose wisely as bedtime approaches.

Limit screen time.

Avoid phones, computers, and TVs at least 30 minutes before bed, as blue light can interfere with melatonin production. If you want to get serious about this, remove the television from your room and leave your phone and computers outside before you turn in. Another great option is to turn the ringer and notifications off on your tech devices so a phone call, text, or email can't wake you up.

Optimize your sleep environment.

Make it dreamy by keeping your bedroom cool, dark, and quiet, and invest in a comfortable mattress and pillows. Think COZY!

Avoid caffeine and large meals before bed.

Stimulants and heavy foods can disrupt sleep.

Get regular exercise.

Physical activity can promote better sleep, but avoid vigorous exercise close to bedtime.

Sleepy Sounds.

If sweet silence won't work, invest in an app or machine to provide some sort of white noise. The sounds of rain, thunder, the ocean, or static might be the secret to calming your mind, while drowning out noisy neighbors, barking dogs or snoring spouses.

Manage stress and anxiety.

Calm your mind with relaxation techniques such as deep breathing, meditation, or journaling.

Chapter 10 | Sleep Like an Angel

Super-Recharge with Cat Naps

The ability to grab 20 refreshing minutes of Zzzz's is a gift. Some folks poo-poo napping as if they're too good for it. Rubbish! Nobody is above napping. If you need or want a little shut-eye, you shouldn't have any emotional hang-ups about it. You don't judge your cell phone when the battery gets low; you plug it in! A nap works the same way. Meow!

I recommend finding a quiet, comfy, and safe place. My go-to is the couch swing in my backyard. I adjust the pillows, cover up with a blanket, and pass out. Works every time. If my mind is racing, I'll put on a boring podcast. Without revealing which one helps me nod off quickly, I'll share that the hosts have monotone voices and speak slowly. I set the alarm on my phone if I have somewhere to be or something to do. Don't be ashamed to try napping in the back of your car (in a safe lot), on a plane, or in your bed. If you're willing to take naps when needed, you'll benefit by having more gusto to get through the rest of your day. On the days when your efforts fall short and you can't get to sleep, you'll at least benefit from a short amount of rest with your eyes closed.

Shut-eye is essential to supercharged health. It's the downtime your body needs to relax and recover from all of the demands you put on it each day. Getting yourself a great night's sleep or a hearty nap is something you should be proud of, and feel the benefits of immediately. While your peers are roaming around like zombies, enjoy the perks that come from snoozing like a baby in its mama's arms.

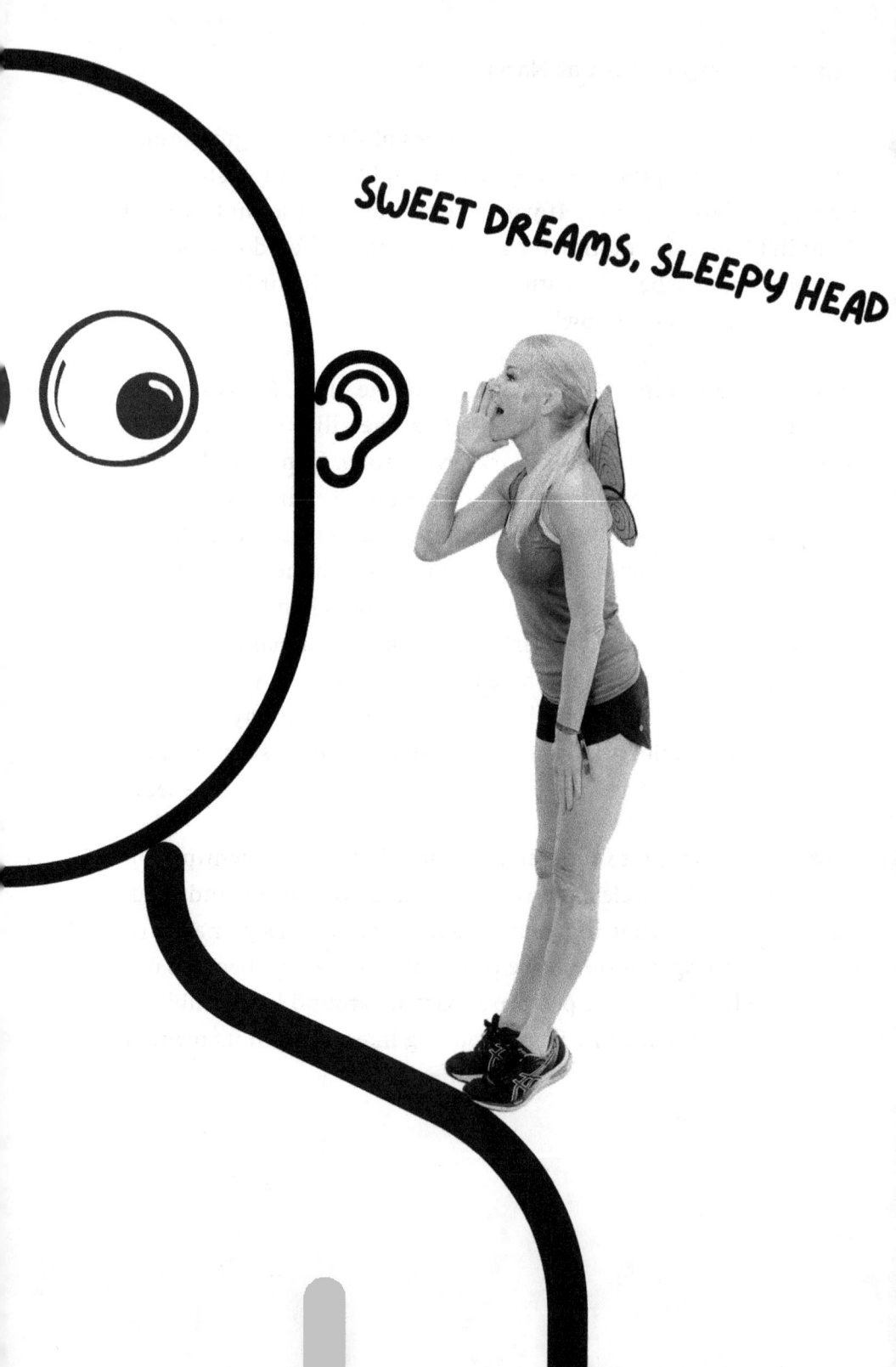

Chapter 11

MOTIVATION VS DISCIPLINE

You. Supercharged!

By this point, I hope you're pumped full of knowledge and excitement, ready to launch your mission for fitness, health, weight loss, and, of course, endless happiness. As a wise scholar once said, "Let's F'ing Goooooo!" Unfortunately, that scholar was found three weeks later, passed out on his couch, pants unbuttoned, buried in pizza boxes. Why? He had all the motivation in the world, but zero discipline. And discipline, also known as the Big D, is your secret weapon for long-term success.

Motivation is great. When you're excited about something, it's fun and feels easy to charge forward. But in a head-to-head battle for what matters most, let me be crystal clear: **discipline beats motivation every single time.** And it's not even close.

Motivation is a fleeting feeling. It's a spark, a powerful quote, a killer workout, an inspiring story. But it fizzles fast. Discipline, though? That's your commitment to doing the right thing no matter what. When it comes to chasing big goals, motivation is practically irrelevant.

Do I want to pay my property taxes every year? Nope. But I do it. Not because I'm jazzed about writing checks, but because I'm disciplined. Just like brushing your teeth, nobody's thrilled about it, but you do it anyway. That's discipline. You don't have to love

Chapter 11 | Motivation vs Discipline

your 6 a.m. workout, skipping the junk food, or going to bed early. You do those things because they're in your best interest. That consistent follow-through? That's where the magic lives.

I've seen folks get fired up, shout their goals from the rooftops, "Hey, everyone! I'm going to lose 50 pounds!" only to post pictures of themselves chugging cocktails the very next day. That's not discipline. That's a dopamine high followed by a margarita face-plant. Discipline is waking up and doing what needs to be done, especially when you don't feel like it. That's what separates dreamers from doers. So what gets you through those "blah" days? Not motivation. **Choices. Perspective. Action.**

When you're in a funk, don't spiral. Don't reach for a drink or sabotage yourself in other ways. Instead, remind yourself: "Life may not be perfect right now, but I can make it better". For me, it starts with fresh air. Stepping outside shifts everything. Hugging my dog calms me. Music heals. Exercise clears the gunk. I'll punch a heavy bag, go for a swim, or lift weights, whatever it takes to sweat out the sadness. Sometimes, I even pick up my guitar. I don't wait for motivation. I pursue things known to lift my spirits. And I *never* let other people's opinions steer my ship. If someone hates my guts? That's their problem. You don't have to accept every insult tossed your way. Build a force field around you and move along, happy and free.

Sticking with your plan is vital when you've got something big to achieve. About a year after I finished chemo, I was invited to run the iconic Boston Marathon. Once I said yes, I knew I'd have to train aggressively and smart. I faced tons of obstacles: constant travel to announce races, Florida's nasty heat and humidity, and, oh yeah, lingering weakness from cancer treatments. But I didn't fail myself. I ran in every town I visited, swapped outdoor runs for treadmill workouts at home, and refused to let my limitations win.

Discipline.

What if I hadn't stuck to my plan? I might have failed in Boston. The pain from being unprepared could have left me injured, humiliated, and haunted by regret. But I *chose* to get the work done, and crossing that yellow and blue finish line on Boylston Street felt glorious.

Discipline also means knowing when to pivot. If you're sick on race day, scale back to a shorter distance or skip it altogether. That's not quitting; that's wisdom. A true champion knows when to push and when to pause.

Let's also talk about perspective. Had a rough day? Sure. But someone else lost a limb or their child. Perspective won't erase your pain, but it helps you survive it without sinking. Do not let oppositional forces disrupt your mission. If you want results, skip the drama. Skip waiting to "feel like it." **Decide to show up for yourself every time.** That's where the progress lives. That's where transformation begins. Discipline over motivation. Every. Single. Time.

Now that you're committed, here are some tactics to support your journey:

- **Make a plan and stick to it.** Write down your goals. Post them somewhere visible. It's like a contract with yourself, making follow-through more likely.

- **Tell everyone.** Accountability works! Announce your plans. Let your people cheer you on instead of unknowingly sabotaging you. Get your ego involved, it's powerful. Nobody wants to fail publicly.

- **Ask for help.** Most folks want to support you. Ask them for encouragement, advice, or time. You might be surprised how much they lift you up.

- **Set short- and long-term goals and reward yourself.** Checking boxes is wildly cathartic. Don't just chase the big win, stack up the little ones and celebrate each milestone.

- **Sign up (and pay!) for big goals.** Whether it's a race or a hiking trip, money on the line keeps you committed, skin in the game matters.

- **Use tech.** Trackers, apps, fitness watches, and free video content on Fitzness.com can help keep you focused. Data is power!

- **Keep your eyes on the prize.** Visual motivation works. Hang up your goal outfit. Take progress pics. Watching your body change is straight-up fun.

- **Put your money where your mouth is.** Trainers are valuable for three big reasons: knowledge, encouragement, and, yes, accountability. Pay in advance. You'll show up and give it your all because you won't want to waste your money.

- **Workout besties.** A buddy can make your workouts fun, social, and challenging. Whether they know more or less than you, you'll both benefit, and *nobody* wants to be the flaky friend who bails on a workout.

- **Put me in, Coach!** Joining a team turns fitness into playtime for adults. From corporate softball to charity races or bowling leagues, the combination of goals, community, and competition is magic.

- **Online support.** Join a group like my Hottie Body Fitness Challenge on Facebook. It's full of kind, motivated people cheering each other on.

Discipline to the Rescue!

Sometimes you'll slack off on your workouts or veer from The Formula. Of course, we both wish it wouldn't, but let's prepare for the worst. This is precisely when discipline becomes your lifeline because the undisciplined often spiral when motivation disappears. What took a year to build in fitness can unravel in just three months of slacking.

Start by acknowledging the change in your behavior. Be honest about the consequences if you don't get back on track. Instead of making excuses for poor eating habits or skipped workouts, write down the reasons you committed to fitness, nutrition, and The Formula in the first place. Then go further; add all the positive things you've already accomplished. Once you've reminded yourself of what you've gained and what's at stake, recommit. The sooner you return to your routine, the easier it is to reclaim your momentum.

Another powerful step? Ask for encouragement. Reach out to friends, especially those who also have fitness goals. My free online training group is filled with thousands of like-minded, supportive grown-ups who show up for each other. Sometimes, a member who lost a ton of weight and became super fit vanishes, slips backward, and only resurfaces after regaining 75 pounds. If only they had asked for help when they first noticed their good habits waning. If only they had spoken up after five pounds instead of seventy-five. All they had to do was say something.

So that's what I'm begging of you: speak up, reach out, and join The Hottie Body Fitzness Challenge Group on Facebook, a powerful place where good people accomplish great things with my guidance. It's free, and I'd love to have you as part of my crew.

Fail Like the G.O.A.T.S

Failures and struggles prepare you for the next thing. Losing sucks. Failing sucks. Making a mess of things sucks. I've done each a million times, and so did Michael Jordan and Abraham Lincoln on their way to G.O.A.T. status. You always have the opportunity to turn things around until you do something that leaves you dead. It's likely impossible that you are the one person on earth who is officially incapable of doing and being better. That would be weird, right? There are a whole bunch of quitters on this big blue planet, but since you're reading this book, I am pretty sure you are not one of them.

Instead, you're probably a plugger. Someone who cares about their success in multiple areas of life and is willing to put in the time and effort to improve. If that describes you, welcome to our club. The "Abe Lincoln, Michael Jordan, and Fitz Koehler Club!" Yes, I just put myself in a club with two of the most iconic men in history. But that's only because we have legit stuff in common, like supercharging our lives, and so do you! We have each made bad choices, faced rejection and loss aplenty, but continued in the right direction to eventually find success. I would dare say that failure only made The Abester, Mikey, and Fitzy better (we have these cute nicknames for each other).

Some of my lowlights include being cut from a dozen sports teams in high school, rejected for tons of paid and volunteer opportunities, mean-girled a bunch, brutalized by cancer, and being told that I looked like I was a victim of the Holocaust! Still, I've built my dream career, authored five books, announced hundreds of iconic events as a race announcer, served as a keynote speaker for hundreds of corporations and associations, traveled the world, and am fitter post-cancer than before. And those mean girls - they're stuck living with themselves.

When I faced constant rejections as a kid, my mom would tell me that I was "building character." I loathed hearing that because I felt for sure that I was enough of a character as I was. Eventually, chemotherapy started showing up on my calendar every three weeks for 15 months, and I started to find value in my previous hardships. It became crystal clear that every one of my failures and disappointments was steeling me up to handle the big stuff. And they did. I can only imagine Mike and Abe's parents were encouraging them similarly.

Getting knocked down and getting back up is a skill. And it's a requirement of life because staying down is not an option! Remaining unfit and overweight is not an option either. If you have failed to become fit before, fear not. You were probably misguided, uninformed, trying hokey, unmaintainable diets, or worse. Now that you have accurate information and a much-needed kick in the can, your odds of success are infinitely better.

You've rebounded before, and you will do so again. You have been disrespected, rejected, fired, and cut. But there you are, still moving in the right direction. Now that you're a part of this club, I'm telling you, every single disappointment you've ever experienced is an integral part of your armor and an essential piece of your weaponry. You are resilient, experienced, wise, unafraid, and the most badass you've ever been. You are ready to weaponize all that and use your fierceness to conquer most of the battles that lie ahead. Your previous failures will become your future victories! Mikey, Abe, and I can't wait to see you succeed; secret handshake instructions on the way.

Chapter 11 | Motivation vs Discipline

Did you know?

As a sophomore, basketball legend Michael Jordan was cut from his high school basketball team. He missed over half of the shots he took as a pro and had a failed pro baseball career during a 17-month semi-retirement from basketball. When he un-retired, he won three NBA championships with the Chicago Bulls.

President Abraham Lincoln lost seven political campaigns before being elected President of the United States. He was also fired from jobs, failed as a business owner, went bankrupt, and suffered a nervous breakdown. He used those failures to become one of the most impactful presidents in American history.

Talk about refusing to take no for an answer! Jordan and Lincoln chose to supercharge their lives because even when influential people rejected them, they relentlessly stayed on their chosen courses. Ultimately, responsibility for your success is yours, and I hope that thrills you. Imagine if your health depended on someone else. Do you think they'd do the work for you? **No way.** Taking complete control of your outcome is empowering. When you own your failures, you earn the right to own your successes.

I can't wait to see you commit, persevere, and succeed.

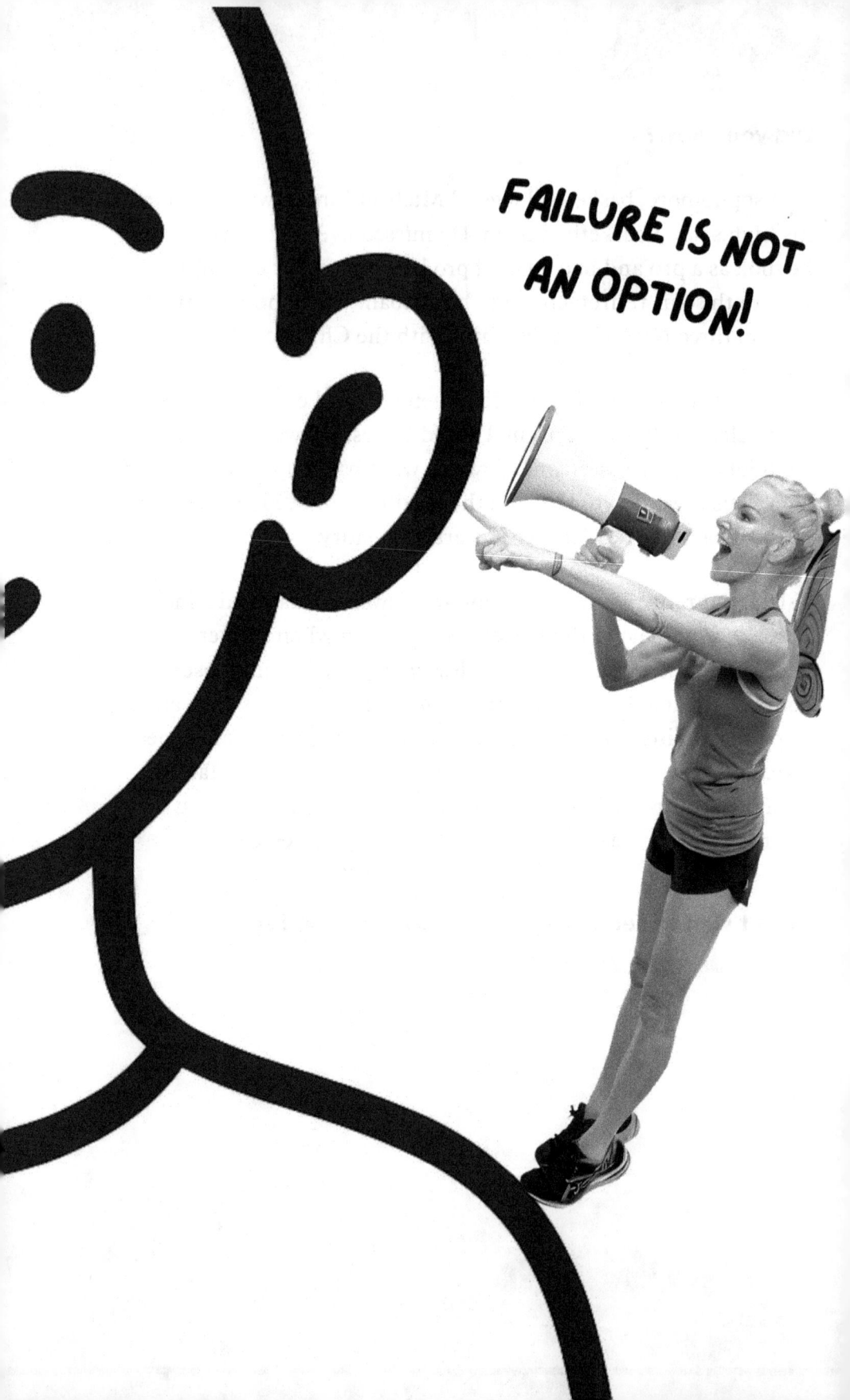

Chapter 12

RIPPED ABS & GORGEOUS GLUTES

You. Supercharged!

Want lean, hard, curvy muscles? I bet you do! They will be an obvious sign of your supercharged body. Sure, they're not on everyone's wish list, but if they're on yours, I've got you covered. Strong shoulders, a plump booty, bulbous biceps, chiseled calves, and, of course, defined abs are absolutely attainable. You simply have to do the work. Everything else I've said in this book still applies, but now's the time to go all in on your goal setting, Formula, nutrition, and workouts.

Let's be honest. Losing seven pounds when you're obese can be pretty easy, but losing the last seven pounds on your way from fit to ripped can be pretty hard. In fact, the closer you get to Adonis status, the more intense you'll have to be. You've got that fire in your eyes, though, so let's make it happen.

They say that shredded abs are made in the kitchen. Why? Because every human already has abdominal muscles. And most folks who work out consistently have reasonably strong ones. But strength doesn't equal visibility. No one can admire your six-pack if it's hidden under a large or small layer of fat. The same goes for the 650+ other muscles in your body. To make them pop, you've got to build those muscles and burn the fat off.

Chapter 12 | Ripped Abs & Gorgeous Glutes

Six-pack abs are connected with elite fitness. **If you want to look like an athlete, you've got to behave like one.** Moderate workouts and eating habits won't be enough. Strength training should be intense. Prioritize resistance over repetition. Challenge your muscles to grow, and they will. Always increase weight gradually to avoid injury, but know that more resistance = more pronounced muscles. Ladies, you don't have to worry about bulk; unless you're fueling like a bodybuilder, your muscles will pop, not bulge.

Strength training increases your muscle mass and throws your metabolism into high gear. The more muscle you have, the faster you incinerate the fat covering it. Why? Because muscle is metabolically active tissue, it burns calories even when you're sleeping, scrolling, or binge-watching your favorite show. A pound of muscle burns significantly more calories at rest than a pound of fat, which means your body becomes a fat-torching furnace 24/7. Plus, strength training triggers the "afterburn effect" ("EPOC," Excess Post-exercise Oxygen Consumption), which elevates your calorie burn for hours after you finish working out. Bottom line? The more you lift, the more you burn. It's a beautiful cycle of strength, sweat, and results.

Boost your athleticism and fat burn with High-Intensity Interval Training and circuit-style workouts (see the *Everything Exercise* chapter for more). These training styles build muscle and torch fat efficiently, leaving you gasping in the best way.

Getting ripped means shedding your body fat. That happens by fiercely sticking to your Formula and eating whole, clean foods that fuel muscle growth and boost energy. If your only goal were weight loss, you'd have more wiggle room. But here in Rippedville, we're laser-focused. Cut excess calories by ditching alcohol, sugary drinks, and processed garbage. Load up on produce, lean proteins, whole grains, beans, nuts, and seeds, and drink a ton of water.

Also: rest. Yes, rest! Muscles don't grow during your workouts; they grow in the 48 hours after. If you're hitting every muscle every day, you're sabotaging your progress. Want to lift daily? Great. Just alternate body parts so each gets that crucial two-day break before being worked again.

Track your progress like a pro. Take monthly photos in the same lighting, outfit, and poses, front, back, and side. Flex like a bodybuilder to show off those gains. Measure key areas (waist, hips, arms, thighs) once a month. Log your workouts, weights lifted, reps completed, cardio durations, and improvements in flexibility and balance, too.

Ultimately, building a visibly-lean and strong body isn't drastically different from reaching moderate fitness goals. You just have to crank up the intensity, consistency, and discipline. Big goals demand big effort. Depending on where you're starting, this journey might be a sprint or a marathon. Either way, it's doable. The lean, hard, curvy body you've been dreaming of? It's within reach. The only thing separating you from the shredded crowd is time and effort; now you know precisely how to invest both. Get to work!

Chapter 13

BREAKING UP WITH BODY SHAME

You. Supercharged!

Our bodies are miraculous, but I didn't fully grasp how much until I started making humans. That's right, I made two phenomenal humans from scratch. Spinal columns, brains, digestive systems, bones, joints, eyes, taste buds, all of it. There was no instruction manual or YouTube tutorial, just pure magic. I must be some kind of superhero, right? I share this not to brag, but to remind you that your body is also an impossibly cool creation. Our bodies and brains are spectacular gifts, and even though I'm a science-loving chick, I'm still flabbergasted by the complicated components and systems that we're made of. Maybe that's part of the reason I'm so passionate about helping you care for yours.

I want you to feel excited and grateful for your body. That starts with respecting every remarkable piece formed in your mother's belly, and everything they do each second of every day. Your body houses your mind and soul. It takes you places, helps you work, love, create, explore, and play. It's more impressive than a Ferrari, a jet ski, or even a private jet, because those things came with instruction manuals and can't function independently like you can. It's time to stop nitpicking and start appreciating your extraordinary self.

Reading this book, getting your workouts in, and consuming nutritious foods are all meaningful ways to show your body the

Chapter 13 | Breaking Up with Body Shame

love it deserves. And that love should never involve punishment, shame, or abuse. We are not cookie-cutter copies of each other, and that's something to celebrate. Too many people waste time obsessing over looking a certain way or trying to look like someone else instead of appreciating their unique features. Isn't it wonderful that humans come in different colors, shapes, sizes, and abilities? Wouldn't life be dull if we all looked the same, like plastic Lego people? We need diversity, not just in appearance, but in talents and perspectives. I mean, would the world really be better without the unique gifts of Michael Jordan, Jerry Seinfeld, or Taylor Swift? I think not.

Throughout this book, I discuss fitness and weight loss extensively, but please remember that my mission is to help you live longer, feel better, and move more comfortably. I'm all for improving your appearance if that excites you, but I hope you'll do it from a place of pride, not punishment. I've walked the dark road of body shame, and I don't want you to go there or stay there, either.

As a teen, I was overweight and struggled with an eating disorder. I was a good kid, a great friend and a strong student, but insecurities overwhelmed me. My 40 extra pounds felt like a curse because thin was the beauty standard, and I didn't understand how to lose weight in a healthy way. I exercised like crazy because I taught fitness classes and played sports, but my eating habits were abysmal. What I regret most isn't the weight, it's how cruel I was to myself. Bulimia, which lasted for years, became a form of punishment I didn't deserve. Eventually, and thankfully, I decided I'd had enough. I started talking to myself with kindness and focusing on the traits I loved. I looked at my friendships and realized I didn't value people more or less based on their bodies. I loved them for who they were, and it clicked that I deserved that same love from myself.

These days, the pressure to look a certain way is louder than ever. It's not just about being thin anymore. Now it's big muscles, bubble butts, thigh gaps, and perky everything, coming at us nonstop through social media. The pressure affects everyone. So, how do we resist it? I believe it starts with a deep appreciation for the body you already have and a strong focus on the beautiful non-physical things that make you, YOU. That's what helped me ditch disordered habits and chase real, lasting health.

If you're working toward weight loss or building muscle to feel better and be healthier, I'm thrilled for you. But if you're name-calling yourself or trying to 'fix' your body through extreme diets or punishing workouts, it's time for a serious reset. That toxic mindset won't lead to long-term success, and it certainly won't lead to joy. If you're stuck in that pattern and can't break free, please consider reaching out to a licensed mental health professional who specializes in body image and eating disorders. There's no shame in getting help; there's power in it.

As a mom, I've made it a point to create a home where skinny isn't idolized and the word "fat" isn't used to describe people. Sure, it's fine to call an elephant or a pumpkin fat, they are. But humans? Nope. In our house, we talk about health. We talk about earning strong, flexible, resilient bodies that last a century. We discuss the dangers of being overweight, like heart disease, diabetes, and joint pain, and we also acknowledge the serious risks that come with being underweight, whether due to illness, malnutrition, or extreme dieting. My kids know that Mommy is smaller than some folks, but not because we worship being skinny, it's just who I am. We don't praise or shame people for their size.

We also never, ever pick on our bodies. I saw adults do that growing up, people I looked up to, constantly putting themselves down: "I'm so fat," "Do I look fat in this?" And I repeated that behavior for a while, until college, when I lived next to a gorgeous

Chapter 13 | Breaking Up with Body Shame

girl who obsessively asked if she looked fat. All day, every day. It was exhausting, annoying, and honestly, a wake-up call. I realized I didn't want to live like that. So I quit insulting myself cold turkey and never looked back. If you do this, I encourage you to stop for your sake and everyone around you.

Loving your body starts with gratitude, a clear head, and a supercharged attitude. Make it a habit to notice and appreciate what's wonderful about you. When you glance in the mirror, show up at the gym, or climb into bed at night, take a moment to thank your body for what it's done for you. It's been with you since the beginning, carrying you through the highs and lows. It's strong. It's unique. It's a miracle. Treat it that way.

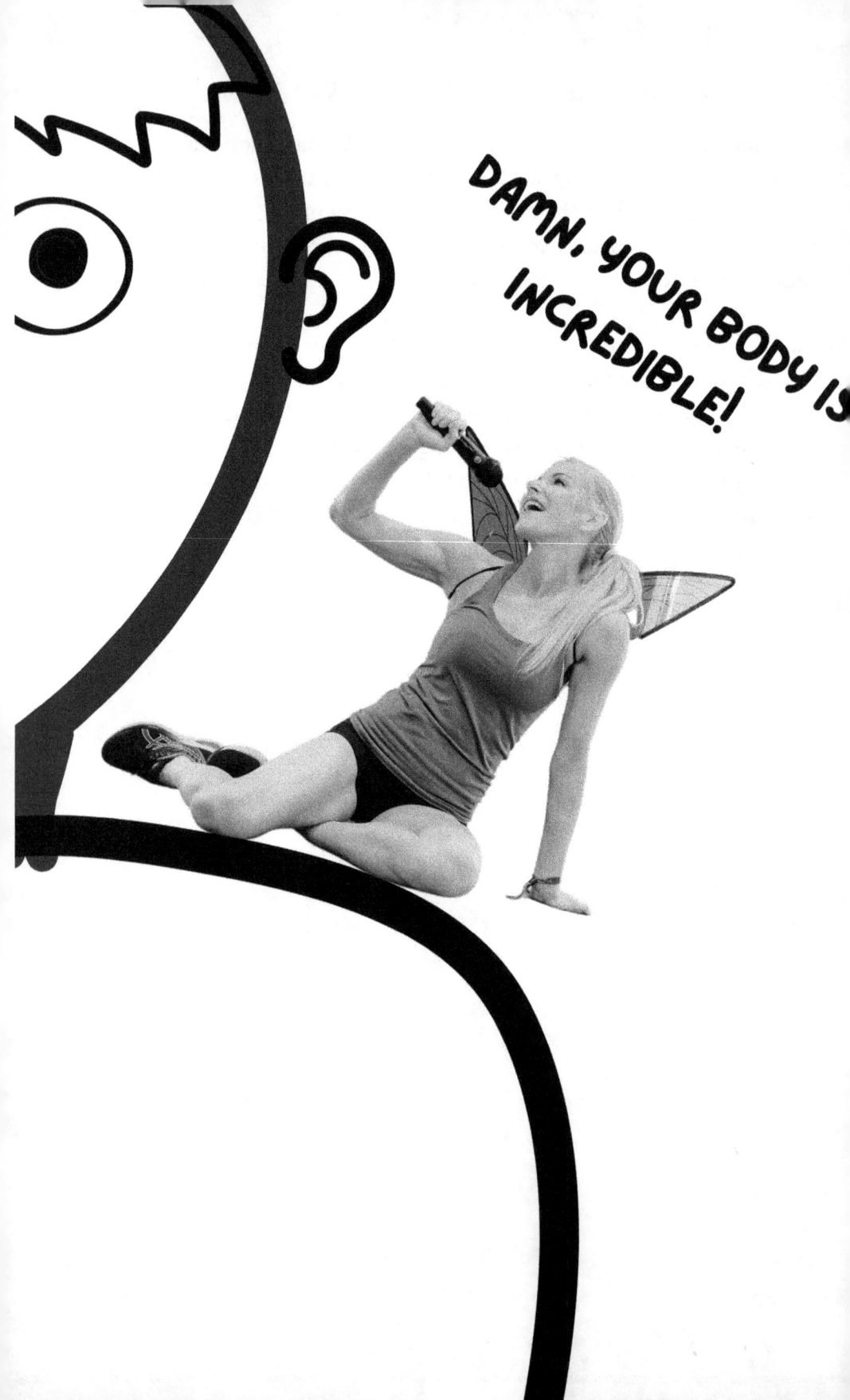

Chapter 14

GET COMFORTABLE BEING UNCOMFORTABLE

You. Supercharged!

You're not reading this book because you're okay with settling for the status quo. You saw the word supercharged and thought, "I could go for that!" You're eager to make progress, and with that comes risk. Being satisfied can feel good for a moment, but inevitably will turn any experience stale. Instead, I encourage you to be proud while always aiming for more, because there is a drastic difference between "happy" and "satisfied." Happy means you can appreciate your successes and special moments. Feeling joy is important. But satisfied means you're done. Finished. Complete. Until you're dead, you shouldn't be. To continue improving and, at minimum, prevent decline, you have to keep pushing the envelope, because stagnation will only lead to a decline.

If you feel stuck in the "I am what I am" mindset, or as Popeye says, "I YAM WHAT I YAM," fear not. You can change. I certainly have. I'm ashamed to say I used to feel proud that I was stuck in my ways. "This is me! I won't budge, and that's awesome!" No. That wasn't awesome at all. Maintaining that attitude would have left me experiencing, learning, and accomplishing so much less. The stubborn me of yesteryear makes me cringe. I seriously cannot fathom why I took so much pride in being an old dog who wouldn't learn new tricks (at 20 years

Chapter 14 | Get Comfortable Being Uncomfortable

old). Perhaps you have some cringeworthy hangups as well? I'm guessing you do.

If you only do the things you're already good at or know, you've imprisoned yourself. You've built walls around your life that prevent you from doing anything else that might make you feel "gasp!" uncomfortable or unfamiliar. But those two feelings are the precursors to wonderful things like surprise, delight, exhilaration, enlightenment, and many other fantastic experiences. Remember your first kiss? How about your first kiss with that hottie you met on vacation? Even though kissing someone for the first time can be incredibly awkward, it can also be magical, right? The same holds true for firsts in other areas. First karate lesson, dance class, or triathlon. The first time trying a healthy dish at a restaurant or cooking one yourself. First-time zip-lining, whitewater rafting, or snow skiing. Sure, you may not be great initially, but risking unfamiliarity is required for a richer life.

In order to supercharge your body and mind, you'll need to start pursuing things you've never tried before and things you are bad at. That might sound intimidating, but the bright side of trying something new is that you have no obligation to be good! While there may be pressure to perform at a certain level, doing things you're known for, you get to enjoy complete amateur status when trying something foreign. Wouldn't it be weird if you were a badass on a surfboard on your first try? It sure would. So take the pressure off, leave your ego behind, declare your newbie status loud and proud and see what happens. When you untether yourself from your obsession with being the best, you'll laugh more, enjoy the learning process, and take pride in every triumph, even the little ones.

Pride is an important emotion, and expanding your horizons is a clever way to pursue it. I recently accepted a challenge to compete in a Dancing with the Stars ballroom dance competition for a charitable cause. I agreed to the opportunity without hesitation, even though I had zero dance background beyond shaking my thang at the occasional wedding reception. I didn't even consider rejecting the invitation because I knew every step I took would be a significant accomplishment. I also knew the expectations of me were very low since I was a non-dancer. From rehearsals to performing in front of a massive live audience, my DWTS experience was among the most delightful I've ever had. I adored struggling to learn the jive, laughed at my missteps, celebrated my progress, and arrived at the gala eager to perform. I took so much pride as I stepped onto that stage with my professional dance partner, knowing how far I had come. The audience of 600 lost their minds as we performed to Tina Turner's "Proud Mary," and I beamed. Not because I was the best jive dancer on earth, but because I lived without fear, expanded my skillset, met personal expectations, and did so through quality exercise. Win! Win! Win!

Many friends have told me they would be too scared to do something like that. Really? Scared of dancing? Scared of dancing in front of people? A reality check may be in order. Folks, cancer is scary. War is scary. Tornadoes are scary. Dancing in front of people doesn't make the Top 1,000 list of scary things. Please remind yourself of that next time you start to cower. Don't live in fear of mundane activities. Don't limit your adventures by the threat of other people's opinions. Truth is, those other people's opinions are none of your business. And even if they were, you couldn't please or impress them all. Stop trying.

I often share that message at the start lines of the many road races I announce across America. Standing before 10,000-20,000 people, I'll ask if anyone is nervous, and a sea of hands rise into the air. When I remind them of real-world fears and ask "What's so scary about going the distance with a bunch of cool people?" I can hear a collective sigh of relief. Many tell me they remind themselves of that message during their run, which helps. So I hope you'll do the

Chapter 14 | Get Comfortable Being Uncomfortable

same. Put a little Fitzy on your shoulder and let me into your head when you start doubting yourself. Together, we can do phenomenal things!

The more variety in your life, the better your physical and mental health will be. Activities that challenge our brains can improve processing speed and memory. When you vary your workouts, your body benefits by adjusting to the burdens you bestow upon it. If you'd like to get fit, stay fit, and prevent decline, you've got to get comfortable being uncomfortable.

Make your transition from the person who is great at everything to a person who's up for anything.

- Adopt the mantra. "Perfect is boring". Say it often and mean it. Perfection is almost completely unattainable and rarely comes with giggles.

- Make a list of 10 things you wouldn't mind giving a go, even just for once. If nobody was watching and no one knew what you were up to, what would you do? Once you've made your list, make plans to give each a shot. Remember, you're not afraid of the opinions of others.

- Boost your ego by declaring, "I'm excited to try something new" when you attempt a new feat. Let people around you know that you're a beginner. Instead of judging you, they'll be excited for you and likely eager to help. Your successes will be their successes.

- Start at the start. Instead of jumping into the pool's deep end to learn how to swim, ask a friend or hire a coach to teach you ... in the shallow end. Start small, learn a few skills, and advance with baby steps. Take pleasure in the learning process and progress gradually.

- Take videos, photos, or notes to record your progress. It'll be cool to have proof of how far you've come.

- Invest in some equipment if necessary. My first month of ballroom dancing was tough because I was dancing in running shoes. The second I put on a proper pair of dance shoes, I spun like a top instead of tripping clumsily. Don't spend a fortune immediately; just get whatever you need to make your chosen activity less complicated and safe.

- Enjoy your new activity until it becomes unenjoyable. If that happens, move to another item on your list.

As you open your world to more opportunities, know that your body and mind won't be the only beneficiaries. Your spirit will soar as you spice up your days. Each new venture will likely bring new friends and acquaintances. Perhaps you'll add a new bestie or romantic interest. You may also make valuable professional connections. Golf is renowned for inspiring business deals on the green, but the same goes for pickleball, mountains, and yoga studios.

My final thoughts on expanding our horizons are connected to our final days. As we grieve people we know who died at any age, we tend to think about their time here on earth. I always find it comforting when a person's life had been filled with wonderful people, passions, love, and adventure. It's rare for us to think our friend's time was "enough." However, I find it comforting when I believe that person made the very most of the time they had. When you die, will you be remembered as someone who had a life well-lived? I hope so.

Chapter 15

FLAWLESS-ISH

Go Above and Beyond

As you strive to supercharge your life, I encourage you to extend your ambitions beyond fitness. Obviously, your health should be your top priority, but gosh, there are so many other ways to support your physical and mental health in meaningful ways to enhance your quality of life. Take small steps and big leaps to update and upgrade everything about how you look and feel, whether experimenting with a new haircut, investing in comfortable clothes that make you feel confident, or simply dedicating time to relax and recharge.

Glow Up

With your epidermis, AKA skin, being your largest organ and thankfully, the only one we can see, it's a pretty cool starting point. A thoughtful skincare routine is a bright idea for health and beauty, something even the macho macho men reading this book should pursue. The basics include cleansing your skin, moisturizing, and using sunscreen. These three steps alone can minimize breakouts, wrinkles, sun spots, and skin cancer. It's recommended that we wear sunscreen daily, even when we're not at the beach, pool, or an outdoor event.

Beyond the basics, you could learn about extra measures you can take at home, including exfoliation and serums that brighten and even out skin discolorations. You could also check out professional options such as chemical peels, laser treatments, and microneedling. Talk to a dermatologist or esthetician to discover what treatment options might be best for you.

Hair

A fresh haircut, color, or extensions can refresh or completely change your look. If your coif has become a bit stale or you're just looking to update your appearance, some time at a salon might work magic. Before committing to a drastic change, use an app to show you what you would look like with a particular new hairdo. Upload a selfie and the app will give you an idea of what you do and don't like by superimposing various hairstyles on your head. Even though losing my hair to chemo wasn't cool at all, I got to experiment with all sorts of different looks as my hair made its delightful return. From my buzz cut to the shark fin (spiked up) to braids of all sorts, I did my best to have fun with it and did appreciate each stage and length. Maybe you should have some fun too!

Nails

Whether you try gel nail extensions or just keep them clean and shaped, cared-for nails look great and show a lovely attention to detail. Men and women alike can benefit from trimming and filing to avoid looking unkempt. Adding color and length can be pretty, glamorous, and fun. Whether you care for your nails at home or get manicures and pedicures at a salon, remember that your hands, at minimum, are almost always on display.

Update Your Wardrobe

No matter where you are in your fitness journey, it's a stellar idea to dress in attire that fits comfortably and gives you confidence. Of course, what's inside is most important, but prioritizing fashion is lovely too. Clear out clothing you've shrunk out of immediately. Donate or sell your too-big clothing immediately if you're on a mission to lose weight and have done so successfully. It's a lot harder to let yourself regain weight when you have nothing that fits in the closet. This alone may be a terrific motivation to return to healthy habits and lose weight.

A new outfit or accessory can be the perfect reward for your efforts towards a fitter body. As you progress, invest in a few items here and there, new pants, shirts, swimsuits, or dresses. Wardrobing a fitter body can be a heck of a lot of fun and is certainly a wiser reward than indulging in unhealthy foods and drinks. Will you try completely different cuts/styles from fancy, to fitted, classic, punk, professional, western, nautical, or sporty? Play around with colors, patterns, or accessories! Whether you purchase one piece at a designer retailer or an entirely new apparel at a thrift store, updating your apparel is a rewarding way to change up your look with little consequence.

Facial Hair

Growing and sculpting facial hair can do as much for a man as makeup can for a woman. Want to look older, younger, tougher, more glamorous, or natural? Even though our faces are mostly set in stone, we can still change things up. A beard, mustache, Fu Manchu, sideburns, or a complete shave can give men ever-changing looks. Perhaps you'll look 20 pounds trimmer with a sweet 'stache or 20 years younger clean-shaven. You'll never know unless you try. Invest in a beard-trimming kit so your face gets the care it needs as you trim and sculpt. Surround that gorgeous

Chapter 15 | Flawless-ish

mouth of yours with some scruff, or don't. Just keep smiling, you handsome devil.

Makeup

Supercharging your face by knowing how to wear makeup can be a game-changer. The ability to brighten, highlight, sculpt, conceal, and shape our faces is a skill worth working towards. Growing up on Fort Lauderdale beach, I had little use for makeup and was never taught how to use it. As an adult who spends my life on stages, I've had to invest a lot of time, energy, and money to figure it out. Mad respect to those of you who choose to go au naturale, but for the rest of us, a little bit of know-how in this area can be helpful as we try to look our best.

Makeup can be purchased at all price points, from drug stores to designer brands, and learning has never been easier. Most makeup specialty shops and department stores offer free consultations or hire a professional makeup artist to teach you. Social media is packed with an endless array of online influencers sharing videos on all sorts of makeup tricks. I watch and try out their suggestions all the time. Whatever you choose, know that a beautiful face starts with a smile.

Teeth

Making our teeth brighter or straighter has never been easier. Braces still work, but orthodontia has become far more sophisticated with ceramic options that match the color of your teeth, known as "clear braces." They are a much nicer option than the silver variety that earned me "metal mouth" status as a kid. Then, there are removable clear aligner trays, which adjust teeth gradually and are relatively unnoticeable. Both braces and aligner trays cost a few thousand dollars and deliver long-lasting results, which makes them a special investment at any age. Tooth brightening is a far easier and less expensive process. Whether you spend a few hundred clams at the dentist for an official whitening procedure or drop $20 at a pharmacy for whitening strips, a brighter smile can be a big boost for confidence.

Set up a Home Gym

Even if you have a gym membership or play sports, it's wise to have exercise options at home. With a small amount of space, fill a bin with portable equipment like a yoga mat, jump rope, a dumbbell stack, resistance bands, and maybe even a medicine ball. With a little more room, I recommend cardio equipment like a treadmill, a stationary bike, an elliptical, or a rowing machine. Face them towards a television to make your sweat session fly by. If you love to cycle, buy a bike trainer to ride your outdoor bike indoors. With lots of space, you can cover your floor with mats, add fans, a Swiss ball or BOSU, a universal strength training machine, and cover your walls with mirrors. All of this depends on your space and budget, though. Get creative! Decide what equipment matters to you and go shopping. Pro tip! If you're on a budget, shop for fitness equipment second-hand. Garage sales are full of dumbbells!

Clean Up This Mess!

Growing up, my mother would always shout at me and my siblings. "Clean up this mess! It looks like your room was hit by a tornado!" or a bomb; she used bomb and tornado interchangeably. Anyway, I didn't understand the value of being tidy and organized as a kid, but I do now. Decluttering your home can positively impact your mindset and stress level. Walking into a neat room that smells fresh feels good. Walking into chaos with clothes flung everywhere, cups on the counters, and sticky stuff on the door handles feels bad. As with your exercise habits, start making small changes. Put all dirty dishes and cups in the dishwasher nightly.

Put away laundry in the morning. Wipe things down and vacuum every few days. Purge nonessential items like clothes you don't wear, books, games, and bags you don't use regularly. I've been trying to get rid of at least one full garbage bag of things to donate weekly, and each one gone feels so refreshing. If you can afford it, hire a professional organizer, junk removal, or cleaning service.

Yo Homies

Once your casa has been cleaned and decluttered, revitalize the decor to suit your healthy new vibe. Want colors and textures that inspire you to move? Maybe you'd prefer some whites and beiges to help you relax? Whether you make large or small updates, a splash of color, a new couch, or even some new placemats may make your abode feel more fabulous. Also, give your condo, apartment, flat, cabin, or palace a nickname. I call my house "The Koehler Mansion!" It is definitely not a mansion, but all of our friends know its name, and it just makes life a little more fun.

Gym Bag

Grab and go fitness! Keep your bag stocked with your favorite fitness apparel, socks, shoes, an empty water bottle, earbuds for music, a small towel, and anything else you traditionally use. How about weight lifting gloves or belts, a swimsuit, swim cap, goggles, helmet, elbow pads, anti-chafe balm, bandages, or pilates socks? Whether you get an elaborate duffel with lots of pockets or a simple drawstring, having your gym bag packed, at your door, or in your car can be the difference between working out and not.

More Pressure, Please.

Massages aren't just for fancy folks; they are also for anyone who needs a little TLC. They can alleviate pain, increase range of motion, induce relaxation, and feel downright luxurious! Having a licensed massage therapist rub and manipulate your body's soft tissues (muscle, connective tissue, tendons, ligaments, and skin) is an investment in healing and recovery. Using various techniques under or over your clothes, regular or even sporadic massages can help keep your body at its best. Perhaps this will be the reward you provide yourself for accomplishing certain fitness-related goals? As I steer clear of pain medicines, I can vouch for massage therapy as a powerful tool of both healing and maintenance. If you have insurance, check to see if this service is covered.

Needles in your Forehead and Feet?

Acupuncture is an ancient form of Chinese medicine designed to trigger the body's natural healing processes by stimulating the central nervous system, affecting your muscles, spinal cord, and brain. While needles are usually involved, they're incredibly thin and are often hard to feel being inserted. Even needle-phobes (like me) can get comfortable with the practice. Honestly, I used to think this practice was quackery. And then I tried it with outstanding results. Acupuncture has helped decrease nausea during my last pregnancy, diminish neuropathy during chemotherapy, and relieve various aches and pains. Find a licensed acupuncturist, and if you have insurance, check to see if this is covered.

Mental Health Counseling

Just like our bodies, our brains need support too! Exercise is certainly a powerful weapon against stress and sadness, but it's not the only one! Speaking to a licensed mental health care professional proves you are mature and responsible, so never think it's a sign of weakness. Sure, they can dish out advice, but often they serve as a safe place to discuss your feelings without fear of consequence. They can also help you manage anxiety, depression, doubts, and dark feelings. Of course you could book in-person appointments with a local provider in your town. But if you're more comfortable, you can also book counselors online, and video chat from your home or a park bench. If you have insurance, check to see if this is covered.

Schedule Annual Exams

This advice competes as the most important in this book. We all bring our cars in for regular check-ups. You need to be even more serious about bringing your body in. Doctors will not creep into your home in the middle of the night and look under your covers with a flashlight to see if you're okay. Instead, you have to physically bring your body in for the looksies that might save your life! A primary physician is a great place to start for lab work, blood pressure, and reflexes. They'll listen to your heart and lungs and discuss your overall health. This is the right place to express any concerns and ask lots of questions. They've seen it all and have lots of answers. If they see any red flags, they may refer you to a specialist or order more tests.

Dermatologist: For skin cancer screenings and to discuss other issues.

Optometrist: Eye exam, vision test, updating of eyeglasses or contact prescriptions.

Dentist: X-rays, teeth cleanings, oral health examinations.

Gynecologist: Annual pap smear, internal exams, and discussions about sexual health, pregnancy, menopause, and more.

Mammograms: Recommended annually for women 35 and older, but if you find a lump in your breast or armpit, see bumps, rashes, or discoloration of your skin, or experience pain, seek medical support and scans immediately. Self-exams should be done weekly.

Colonoscopy: It is recommended that you start at age 40 and repeat it every five years or more as recommended by your digestive disease specialist.

As of 2025, below are the American Cancer Society's recommended ages for cancer screenings.

Age 25-39 Screening recommendations

- **Cervical cancer screening** for women beginning at age 25.

Age 40-49 Screening recommendations

- **Breast cancer screenings** beginning at age 45, with the option to begin at age 40.
- **Cervical cancer screening.**
- **Colorectal cancer screening** for everyone beginning at age 45.

At age 45, African Americans should discuss **prostate cancer screening** with a doctor.

Age 50+ Screening recommendations.

- **Breast cancer screening**.
- **Cervical cancer screening**.
- **Colorectal cancer screening**.
- People who currently smoke or formerly smoked should discuss **lung cancer screening** with a doctor.
- Discussing **prostate cancer screening** with a doctor.

Chapter 15 | Flawless-ish

See Something, Say Something!

Annual checkups and exams are essential, but they aren't enough. You must also take full responsibility for your health by exploring your body regularly. Pause each week to look your body over, using a handheld mirror for your backside if necessary. Touch your body too! They're your hands, and it's your body, so squeeze your stuff while looking for lumps, bumps, and texture changes. If you see or feel something strange or different on any part of your body, make an appointment to get checked out immediately. Early detection saves lives. In fact, if I hadn't found and reported the cancerous lump I discovered in my breast six weeks after a clean mammogram immediately, I'd likely be dead. Time is of the essence.

Stop Smoking

Smoking cigarettes, cigars, pipes, weed, and vaping all put you at risk for 12 types of cancer, cardiovascular diseases, chronic obstructive pulmonary disease (COPD), depression, and fertility issues, among other nightmarish side effects.

Versatility and Such

One trick pony? Not you! Old Dog? Heck no! Now's the time to try new things to challenge your body and brain. Isn't it weird that most folks stop joining clubs and taking classes in their early twenties? Instead of stagnating, commit to a state of constant learning. Whether it be a new language, art form, sport, instrument, or other skillset, the process of going from complete know-nothing to know-something can be pretty rewarding. In the past few years, I've started taking both guitar and ballroom dance lessons. I'm mediocre at both thus far, but I've had hours and hours of entertainment taking my skills from the struggle-bus to a girl who can ChaCha like a boss. Perhaps you could become a stock market wizard who plays the bagpipes and throws axes on the weekend? The options are endless.

Create a Bucket List

Life can be much more fun, enlightening, and meaningful if you seek to do more and be more than you are. So make plans—big ones and small. Travel, read 100 books, meet your favorite celebrity, take on athletic challenges, sing karaoke, learn to speak a new language, or fit back into your favorite swimsuit. If something sounds wonderful to you, write it down and make a plan to place a big fat checkmark next to it someday. I fulfilled a lifelong dream to swim with whale sharks last year, and I'm still on cloud nine. Your bucket list will be a source of joy, excitement, and certainly enhance who you are. Make it juicy and keep it fresh. When you cross something off the list, add something new.

Supercharged Pets

The same methods for improving your physical and mental health will work for your favorite animals. Ensure your furry, scaly, and feathered friends get plenty of exercise, fresh air, nutritious foods, and mental stimulation. If you want them to live long and well, put in the effort. Keep them moving with daily walks, playtime, and toys. Prioritize fresh foods too! Instead of forcing them to eat processed foods out of a box or can every day for their entire life, offer fresh items approved for your particular animal. Do a little research or ask your veterinarian for recommendations.

Animals experience the same consequences humans face when they're overweight and out of shape. Your fat cat and rotund Rottweiler are not cute, they're suffering. It's hard to play, breathe and sleep when they're too heavy. They're also at risk for heart disease, strokes, certain cancers, type 2 diabetes, and pain. Folks, your pets cannot shop, cook, or even open the packaging on their food. If they're overweight, it's likely your fault. If you've overfed them and played too little, it's time to do better. I know you love them! Your pet is probably an incredible source of joy and comfort. Providing healthier foods, fewer treats, and lots of activity is the most sincere way you can prove your love. They'll also need some baby talk and cuddles, unless of course, your pet is a shark.

My Labrador mix, Piper, has enjoyed two to three miles of daily walks and playtime her entire life. Without naming brands, we feed her dog food from the refrigerated section of the grocery store, consisting of fresh lean meats and veggies. We just celebrated her Sweet 16th birthday, and she's still chasing squirrels and wrestling with her little doggo brother, Joey. This isn't luck. We've supercharged our sweet bestie with a lifetime of exercise, nutrition and love. Healthy habits can certainly extend the length and quality of your pet's life too.

If you're looking to bring a new pet into your family, I hope you'll consider a rescue. Instead of paying top dollar for a designer breed, you can spend a small amount for a bestie that needs you in a big way. Too many cuties are euthanized (doggo and kitty death row) because a loving human hasn't come for them. I promise that if you choose to rescue, you'll soon find that your new bestie rescues you right back.

If you're constantly pushing the needle forward in all aspects of your life, you're bound to become healthier, happier, and more successful. Do better in the places you feel strong, and do better where you're weak. Each upgrade you make will make life less hard, more awesome and bring you closer to supercharged status.

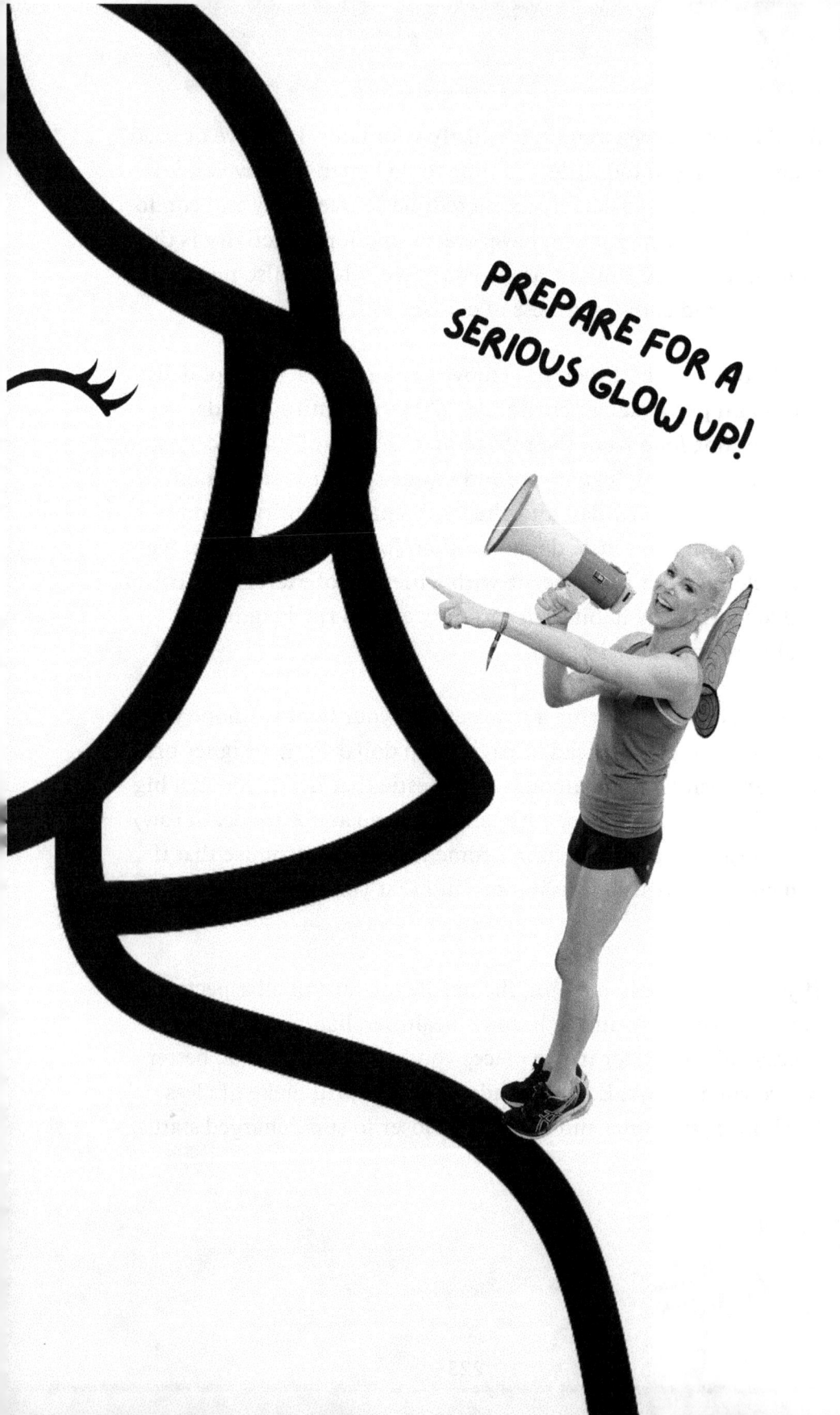

Chapter 16

OBESITY IS SCARY STUFF

Being a little overweight can be frustrating. Being obese can be downright frightening. At least, it should be. I don't start this chapter this way to be discouraging. Instead, I'm hoping to light a fire under you to pursue the type of supercharged transformation that will make every moment of your life better, inspiring others to follow suit. Carrying around an extra 50 pounds or more puts your life in imminent danger, and you should act accordingly. Healthcare providers classify someone as morbidly obese if they have a Body Mass Index (BMI) of 40 or more. Too many people dismiss obesity as an issue of vanity, and if you "love yourself" enough, you should accept your body as is. This is a dangerous mindset! Obesity puts the young and old at risk for an endless slew of medical conditions, including heart disease, stroke, diabetes, and death, among others. If you've been stuck in cycles of frustration, it's time to break free. No more waiting, take immediate action.

Now for the great news. You can make quick and long-term progress using the Exact Formula for Weight Loss. When you have a lot to lose and trade excessive eating habits for moderation and discipline, pounds will disappear quickly, which can be really exciting. The secret here is for you to stay the course. Remember that you are not on a diet. You are not doing anything weird or drastic. You are just trading reckless consumption for measured

Chapter 16 | Obesity is Scary Stuff

consumption. With The Formula, you should finish your day feeling satisfied, not starving or cranky.

I explained this in Chapter 3, but you may choose to start with a modified Formula if you have 100 pounds or more to lose. For example, if Marcia weighs 508 pounds and her goal is 175 pounds, she could start her path by focusing on getting to 400 pounds and setting her caloric budget to 4,000 calories daily. Since Marcia likely consumes at least 5,000 calories daily, a severe drop to 1,750 calories could cause her to feel depleted, hungry, and experience headaches. Committing to maxing out at 4,000 calories daily instead would still give her an enormous amount of food if she chooses primarily healthy options, and her weight would still start falling off quickly.

Your goal is to do better. You don't have to aim for perfection now or ever. A simple switch of habits from reckless to reasonable will be highly effective. Once your reasonable habits become second nature, you can start lowering your budget and increasing the quality of your food choices. Dieters fail because they jump into plans filled with stringent and unreasonable rules. If nothing else, The Formula is precisely reasonable; therefore, you can maintain it for life.

Exercise may be challenging, but it will be necessary. Being obese is uncomfortable, so you're already there. If exercise feels uncomfortable, at least it's the beneficial kind. Instead of focusing on the things you cannot yet do, focus on the things you can. Know that every move you make will better yourself. If you can not exercise on your feet, do so seated or lying down. Dance with your arms and legs while seated. Perform strength training exercises in a chair, in bed, or on the floor. Each of your legs likely weighs 50 pounds or more, so consider your limbs your personal dumbbells and lift them! Forward, backward, up, and to the side. Start with one minute of movement at a time. Do as many one-minute workouts as you can each day until you're ready to increase them to two-minute, five-minute, 10-minute, 30-minute workouts, and beyond. Never focus on what you cannot do. Put all your energy into doing what you can, controlling what you can, and celebrating every effort you make.

Losing massive amounts of weight and getting fit isn't complicated, but it does take some know-how, effort, discipline, and consistency. These are all things you are fully capable of. And do you know what? Your life actually does depend on it. My life's mission as a fitness professional is to tack 10 years of quality life onto everyone I come across. You are the easiest target for my efforts. Obesity kills. If you do not take action, you will lose days, months, or years. And worse, you could stick around for a long time, living a life of pain, suffering, and limitations. Ten extra years isn't a gift unless they are filled with quality. Even if your doctor says your blood work looks good, looking at the bigger picture of your overall health is still important. I implore you to take action immediately.

Get Excited!

You have so many fun days and exciting moments to look forward to, and losing lots and lots of weight is endless fun! Imagine waking up with more energy, moving easily, and feeling confident in your skin. Every pound lost means less strain on your joints, heart, spine, and lungs and more freedom to enjoy life. That's something worth working for. You can also expect to experience some relief from the mental tolls that stem from obesity, which can be all-consuming. These struggles, like finding clothing that fits, not fitting into certain chairs, and fearing judgment, can be intense. But they will diminish as your body becomes fitter and lighter. Instead of focusing on chronic concerns, you'll be able to focus on your progress and all the opportunities that incrementally

Chapter 16 | Obesity is Scary Stuff

become open to you. I hope you'll share your success with me via social media so I can celebrate along with you.

There is no difference between you and the super-fit people you know. They haven't become fit because they were bitten by a radioactive spider like Spider-Man. They are regular people with regular capabilities who have put in the time and effort towards a healthy body. If you put in the same effort, you will likely achieve the same results. Please don't wait for a wake-up call, which would be much harsher than my advice. Take control of your health today. Make small changes, commit to consistency, and trust the process. Your future supercharged self will thank you.

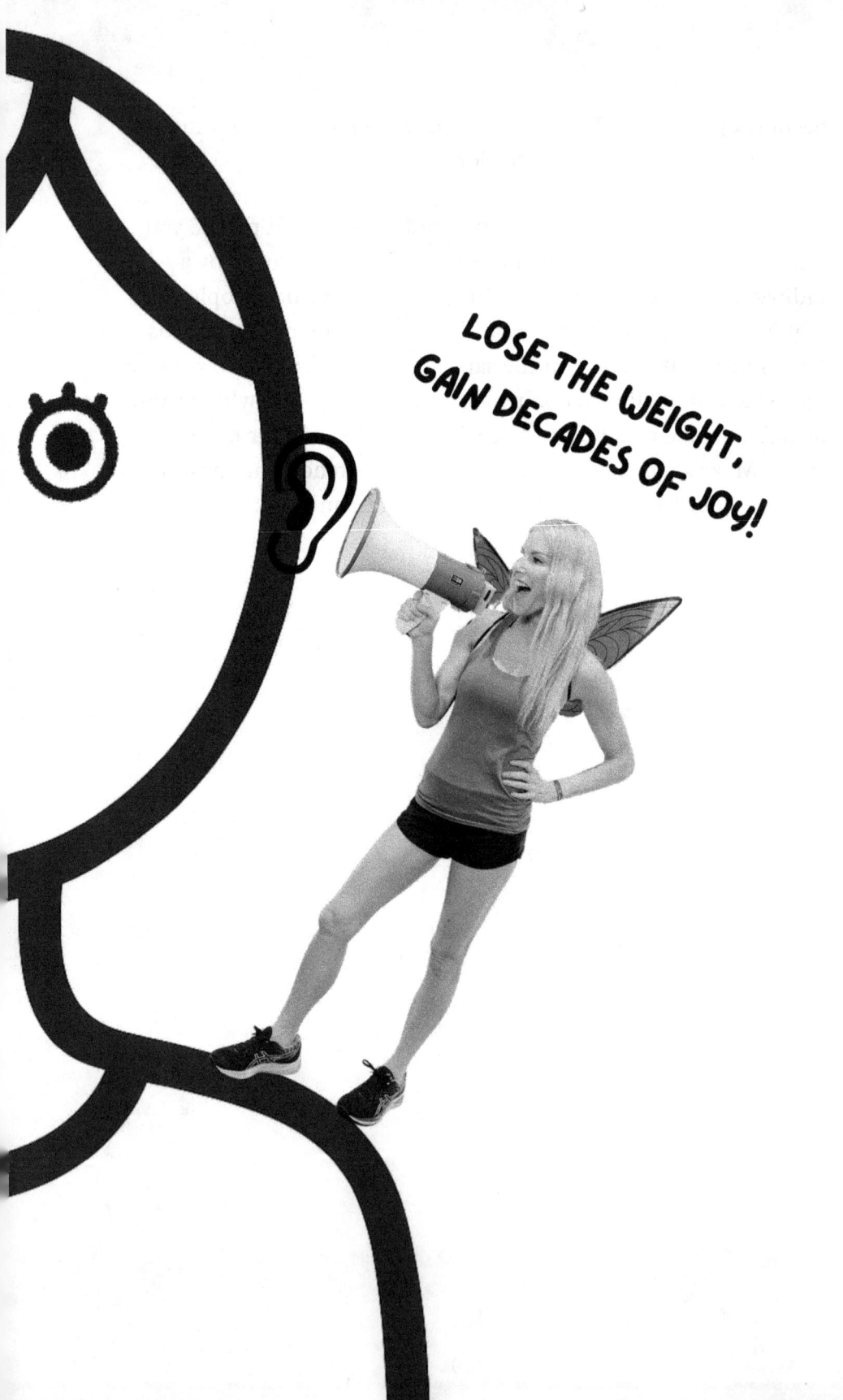

Chapter 17

HEALTH DURING HARDSHIP & MENTAL HEALTH

You. Supercharged!

Your health isn't just important when life is smooth sailing; it's your greatest asset when everything goes wrong. Whether you're facing stress, illness, or crisis, your fitness and nutrition habits can be the difference between swimming and sinking. When a crisis strikes, your health becomes one of the most valuable tools in your belt. Whether you're dealing with divorce, disease, injury, illness, fire, death of a loved one, financial issues, cranky people, and more, exercise and quality nutrition should be considered your protective shields. They will keep your body and brain functioning at a high level, your mind clear, and your stress levels in check. I see far too many people use crisis as an excuse to forgo their healthy habits, but really, it should be your incentive to stick with them more passionately than ever. Your body is strong, resilient, and capable of adapting. Having a fit body is not about perfection; it's about persistence. It's time to stop using life's big and small hurdles as excuses and start seeing them as opportunities to get creative with how you stay active and healthy.

Know that a fit person is far more likely to rebound and recover from illness or injury than an unfit person. Going into any sort of crisis, your previous efforts in health will make an instant impact. I discuss this a lot in my book *Your Healthy Cancer Comeback: Sick to Strong*. If you're going to be hurt or diagnosed with a disease, would you rather your starting point be that of a supercharged

Chapter 17 | Health During Hardship & Mental Health

healthy person or a frail weakling? We don't often think this way, but we should. If we are going to face a decline, let our starting point be from the highest peak possible.

My cancer treatment was brutal, but because I entered it in peak shape, I avoided many complications, hospital stays, feeding tubes, and infections. My oncologist told me outright that my fitness likely saved me from worse outcomes. That's the power of a healthy body.

If you absorb the guidance in this book and follow my advice, you will become fitter. This will happen whether your parents are in the hospital, you lost your job, or if your house burns down. If you take lengthy breaks each time something goes wrong, your situation will only worsen. Instead of sacrificing healthy habits, view them as your sword and shield - your weapons against utter destruction. Don't drop your shield when you're under attack; that's when you need it most! You need quality fuel nourishing your body to handle the stress of your challenge. Your body needs strength to fend off illness, rehabilitate itself, or serve those people and things that need serving. Your mind will REQUIRE downtime to manage stress and conjure up smarter solutions. Exercise is proven to help expel toxic emotions as well as increase creativity, both being so valuable during tough times.

Prepare your body to do battle today because you never know when illness or injury will strike! Nobody gets out of this world unscathed, so start doing the work to protect your future self from the inside out. Every effort you make will eventually pay off in unexpected ways.

Injuries Aren't a Free Pass

Most injuries aren't a mandate to cease exercising. Usually, they're more of a catalyst for creativity. When you've had a sprain, strain, tear, fracture, break, etc, instead of focusing on what's off-limits, focus on what's still within reach. I encourage you to focus on what *is* functioning. If your arm or shoulder is out of commission, don't worry, your lower body can still put in the work. Walking, cycling, squats, lunges, and leg presses are all fair game. If you have a lower-body injury, dumbbell presses, bicep curls, and chest presses can all keep you strong, and you can do them from the seated position. You can also train your core through most limb injuries.

Cardio also doesn't have to stop just because you're injured. Try swimming with a buoy between your legs to take pressure off your lower body, or get creative with seated shadow boxing to keep your heart pumping. It's about working around the injury, not letting it take over your life. The same goes for stretching and balance training. Do what you can when you can, as long as it doesn't negatively affect your healing body part.

If your injury led you to medical care, ask if physical therapy would help. While narcotics mask pain, physical therapists help us overcome it through exercise and other remedies like massage.

No matter what type of injury you face, modify and adapt, but keep moving. Feeling frustrated when you're sidelined is normal, but staying active in any way possible can keep your spirits up and help you bounce back stronger. An injury is a setback, not a stop sign.

Illness Isn't an Excuse to Stop

Feeling under the weather? That doesn't always mean you have to press pause on movement. For mild illnesses like a cold, light activity like walking or stretching might help you feel better. Of course, if your body is screaming for rest, listen to it. But don't let

Chapter 17 | Health During Hardship & Mental Health

a few days on the couch turn into weeks of inactivity. Once you start feeling better, ease back in with gentle movement.

Of course, a cold will pass in a few days, but what if your health battle is bigger? For those facing long-term illnesses like cancer, muscular dystrophy, or Parkinson's, movement isn't just helpful; it's essential. Exercise may stave off physical decline, depression, pain, and debilitation. It isn't about doing everything you used to do; it's about doing the things that you can when you can. During chemo, I spent plenty of time in bed, but I still found moments to move, do leg lifts, resistance band exercises, and stretches. It wasn't about intense workouts but about keeping my body engaged. No matter what you're facing, movement is medicine.

Many people living with chronic illness use exercise and nutrition effectively to stave off negative effects, delaying the full-blown onslaught of symptoms. There are even group classes and online programs targeting folks with various diagnoses. If you're in this category, be proactive! If you're facing a chronic illness, make a commitment today: XYZ will have to fight hard to take you down because you're going to give it everything you've got. Work with your medical team, find a movement routine that works for you, and keep showing up for yourself.

Staying Active Through Life's Obstacles

Life will throw challenges your way, injuries, illness, and unexpected life events, but those obstacles don't have to derail your progress. Let's be honest: a broken arm or a cold isn't a reason to abandon your health goals. Neither is death in the family nor being fired from your job. Setbacks happen, but your response is what matters. Adapt, adjust, and keep moving forward, because your health isn't just a goal; it's a lifelong commitment!

One of the coolest things I get to witness as a professional race announcer and host of massive running events around America is the perseverance of those who seemingly have legitimate reasons to sit things out. I've seen people with zero legs run full marathons, that's 26.2 miles on prosthetics! So inspiring. I've also watched athletes with ALS pushing through start and finish lines using walkers because they refused to allow the disease that will eventually steal their ability to move to take today's opportunities away. I've also celebrated an endless number of athletes battling stage 4 cancers, heart transplant recipients, those with Down syndrome, diabetes, and more. Thoughts of these inspirational people convinced me to accept an unexpected invitation to run the Boston Marathon soon after I finished my cancer treatment. How could I pass up the opportunity to challenge myself after watching these athletes overcome such hardships?

There are opportunities for you, too. Whatever injuries, issues, ailments, diseases, or genetic disorders you may face, the world of sports and fitness is highly inclusive, with so many ways to stay active, regardless of ability level. Did you know we have chair divisions in road races? Athletes with all sorts of limitations that prevent them from running or walking comfortably can race in a traditional wheelchair or racing chairs known as either hand-cycles or push-rims. These chairs move fast! We also have many determined athletes who get pushed the entire way by an athlete on foot in what we call a racing chariot. It's an exciting ride for the seated athlete who is responsible for inspiring the running partner to keep going. Teamwork makes the dream work! I love welcoming all of these athletes through their start and finish lines. When too many people just flat-out quit on themselves, these athletes demonstrate true resilience and tenacity.

There are popular leagues for chair basketball, rugby, and ballroom dance, seated volleyball, adaptive swim teams, sled hockey, and

Chapter 17 | Health During Hardship & Mental Health

more. If you would like to get back to experiencing the thrill, companionship, and camaraderie that comes with sports, you should! Playing will improve your physical and mental health, provide serious stress relief, expand your network of friends, and give you something to look forward to. No matter what you're facing, I encourage you to rise above it and get back in the game.

Health and Healing Through Nutrition

Compounding your existing issues with those that come with poor nutrition won't be helpful. You control what you put into your body, and that's the key to maintaining a healthy weight and lifestyle. Just like with exercise, moments of crisis should inspire you to look to food as part of your First Aid kit. Could you lean on foods high in Vitamin C to boost your immune system, or those high in fiber to get your digestive system moving? Perhaps you'll seek out calcium and phosphorus-rich items to help a broken bone heal more quickly. I can't find any research indicating margaritas and fried cheese as a fix for anything. The cases for fresh produce, legumes, and whole grains are endless.

Beyond aiding recovery, good nutrition also plays a crucial role in maintaining overall health, especially during stressful times. When stressed, it's easy to turn to food for comfort, but that can quickly backfire. I can't tell you how many people have asked me for help after they've gained excessive weight because of a completely-unrelated crisis. Folks, don't do that to yourself. You're just going to make life more difficult. Find a healthy outlet for your frustrations instead. And don't use the unsavory issue you're dealing with as an excuse to eat recklessly. When tough times hit, make a conscious effort to fuel your body with foods that support healing and health. I'm always happy to give you a little push. Find me @Fitzness on Instagram and Fitzness.com

Managing Stress and Grief

Life gets tough, but neglecting yourself in those moments won't make things better. Exercise is one of the most effective ways to release stress, vent frustration, and clear your head. Overwhelmed? Go for a walk. Angry? Hit a punching bag. Feeling down? Take a yoga class or dance around your living room. One of my ambassadors, Pam, asked me what to do after losing a loved one. My advice? Keep going. Exercise doesn't just build physical strength; it heals your mind and soul. Pam and her daughter took long walks together. They grieved, they talked, and they healed through movement. Whether you're suffering or supporting someone who is, movement can be a powerful tool. And if you're a caregiver, remember that staying strong, physically and mentally, helps you show up for those who need you. Professional mental health counselors should also be an option when you're struggling. It's not much different than going to a physical therapist for an injured body part. If your soul is sad, do what you can to help it. Mental health struggles can take a real toll on your body, from weight gain to heart disease. Don't wait until stress overwhelms you; find healthy outlets, talk to a professional if needed, and take action before it affects your well-being.

Becoming a Bright-Sider

Being a bright-sider means seeking out the good in every situation, even the tough ones. It's about finding a silver lining, shifting perspective, and embracing optimism, no matter what life throws at you. I'm a joy addict. Lucky me. My body and mind crave happiness, so I will instinctively do whatever it takes to see the bright side in every situation. Seriously, even when I was diagnosed with breast cancer in 2019 and was told cancer was running through me like wildfire, my brain did a bunch of funky twists and spins until it made me feel fortunate I wasn't a child with cancer or the parent of a child with cancer. Boom! Bright side. Extra points for me. My mom blames my joy addiction on the way-too-personal fact that I was conceived at Disney World (revealed only once I became an adult). If you are a bright-sider, too, congrats. It is so much easier to be us. But if you're not, that's okay, because you can be. It's never too late to start. No matter where you were conceived or what your natural instincts are, you can become a joy-seeking missile. Becoming a bright-sider is a skill that can be learned and practiced until it is who you are. You can train your brain to see the bright side by starting small. When challenges arise, pause and ask yourself, 'What's the good in this?' With practice, this can become second nature.

Perspective

Many years ago, I was standing in the "10 items or less" checkout lane at my local grocery store and in a hurry. Unfortunately for me, the 353-year-old woman ahead of me was removing about 4,052 items from her cart and paying for them with a check. So frustrating! Of course, I would never say anything disrespectful or give cranky vibes to a senior, but on the inside, I was stewing. That is until I looked over to aisle #2. In that line was a teeny little 5-year-old-ish girl wearing a shiny red, blue, and yellow Snow White dress with a very bald head. It pained me to imagine what that poor child must be going through. And then I thought about how much her parents must be suffering.

Instantly, I was so grateful that my greatest burden was waiting patiently in line at the grocery store. I was also embarrassed for feeling so irritated by it. That perspective has stuck with me ever since. In fact, "It's not cancer" became my mantra. If I lost an expensive piece of technology, I'd think, "It's not cancer!" and I'd be over it in an instant. If someone canceled on me or I lost a work opportunity, "It's not cancer", and I'd move on. When most people stuck in a massive traffic jam are grousing angrily, I'm the weirdo who can only focus on how grateful I am not to be the person in the accident that caused the jam. This perspective and mantra have saved me endless amounts of self-induced misery over the years, and I'm grateful for it. Perspective isn't just about finding the bright side when things feel small or inconvenient, like waiting in line at the store. It's about training your mind to find gratitude and strength, even in the face of bigger struggles, like illness, loss, or setbacks. It's about knowing that what feels like a crisis today may not be as heavy as something else you could be facing.

The stress that came along with my cancer diagnosis was inordinate, and I certainly spent time crying and coping with fear. Honestly, I could have basked in the grief. But that would have been miserable, unproductive, and a solid waste of whatever time I had left on earth. Instead, I allowed about 15 minutes of tears each day, remembered how lucky I was not to be a baby with cancer, and forced myself to get on with it: life, work, momming, and fitness. All of it. So when hardship hits, give yourself permission to feel all the feels, but with a limit. Allow yourself a set time each day (like 15 minutes) to cry, vent, or process your emotions. Once that time is up, remind yourself that it's time to move forward, focus on what you can control and find gratitude in the present.

You can do this too. Know that life is going to suck sometimes. Hardship will come your way, small bumps in the road, and big fat doozies. When they do, you must focus on the good things you have and continue to conquer each day. Perspective will prevent stress from eating you alive. Your brain is a powerful weapon in this fight, and you must steer it toward strength and hope. Allow your grief to come out, but don't allow yourself to bask in it. There will always be something to be grateful for, and there will always be something to smile about. Sometimes, you have to look for it.

Chapter 17 | Health During Hardship & Mental Health

Stuart Smalley

Looking for and finding the bright side is step one. Start each day focused on the wonderful things in your life, including yourself. Habitualize these thoughts as you brush your teeth each morning (ideally while standing on one foot for balance training). You can converse with yourself, make a visual list, or make notes on paper or your phone. This is an excuse-free activity. You ALWAYS have 60 seconds of headspace to focus on stuff you're happy about. Set an alarm on your phone to remind yourself to do it while brushing. Eventually, this habit will become so deeply connected that you begin to think grateful thoughts the second you pick up your toothbrush. Once gratitude becomes second nature in the morning, you'll notice it more throughout your day. You might find yourself grateful for the little things, like the sun shining or a kind interaction with a colleague. By starting the habit in the morning, you set a positive tone for the entire day.

Example of your inner dialogue: "I'm grateful to have a safe place to wake up each morning, thoughtful neighbors, funny pets, the ability to work and earn, and a free country to live in."

Sample happy thoughts:

I love my new neighbor.

No car payment.

Excited about dance class.

My dog has the softest ears.

I paid off that annoying credit card.

My eyes are extra sparkly today.

You can also go crazy and just repeat the "daily affirmations" phrase the goofy "Saturday Night Live" character Stuart Smalley said as he sat in front of a mirror, "I'm good enough. I'm smart enough, and doggone it, people like me!"

Passions

Part of being a bright-sider is knowing what makes you happy. Things you enjoy doing, seeing, smelling, hearing, and tasting. People you feel great around or places you like to be. Of course, you have daily task-oriented obligations, but you can and should force things you like or love into each day. Know this: you are NOT a robot! Robots are cool with being programmed, getting stuff done, and shutting down. Good for them. You are a thinking, feeling, and emotional being who will do better and be better with joy. Engaging in your passions isn't just about having fun; it's about taking care of your mental and emotional health. Studies show that doing things you enjoy can reduce stress, boost mood, and even improve cognitive function. It's like giving your soul a daily workout.

Your passions are personal to you and can appear in massive or minuscule ways. If you force, shove, and cram as many of them as possible into your days, you'll experience more joy. And I'm not talking about weekends and holidays. I want you to pursue your passions every single day, through good days and bad. You should ALWAYS be hunting for and engaged in things that bring you joy. My list includes animals, family and friends, fresh air, the outdoors, music, podcasts, playing guitar, working (I adore my career), exercise, cozy blankets, patriotic things, Gator sports, and learning. Take a pause from reading and make your list right now. Store it as a list in your phone or write it on paper and hang it on your fridge.

Chapter 17 | Health During Hardship & Mental Health

Sure, I can enjoy almost all of these passions on my days off. But I can also enjoy many of them on my worst days. When tragedy or hardship strikes, I lean harder into my passions because I know they'll provide relief. When I'm sad, I find solace in exercise, the outdoors, cuddling my dogs (and everyone else's), listening to music, etc. You have to prioritize and practice being your own rescue squad. Your instinctive response to frustration or sadness should be doing things you know make you feel good. Trust that this move is more productive than wallowing in misery. If your leg were swollen and aching, you would likely seek help from anti-inflammatories, ice, and rest. Those things are known solutions that provide relief.

You can alleviate emotional strain similarly by doing things that make you feel good. I get it, life can be busy, and pursuing passions can sometimes feel impossible. But even if you can only find 10 minutes to immerse yourself in something you love, make that time count. Maybe it's listening to a podcast while you cook dinner or taking a walk outside on your lunch break. You don't need hours or money to reap the benefits of joy; small moments add up. Imagine if everyone were taught the skill of prioritizing joy and helping themselves out of emotionally difficult situations. We'd likely see fewer suicides, acts of violence, and disputes.

Boo-hoo Bullshit

Rejecting self-pity will prevent you from landing in the emotional gutter. To a natural bright-sider like me, this seems obvious. Still, I know and love so many wonderful people who seem to be magnetically attracted to drama and revel in the aftermath of arguments, injuries, and tragedy by propagating them exponentially. Those who twist their ankles rushing to social media, notifying the world of their every injury or that they've been wronged. Those who show up at their office, meeting, or family gathering reiterating every detail of being stuck in a traffic jam or overcharged at the mall. These folks could benefit by dealing with their negative experiences and moving on without broadcasting the bad news to everyone who will receive it. "Celebrating" negative experiences this way actually does increase the likelihood that one will seek out more negative experiences because they lead to attention. Attention over negative things can feel equally rewarding as the kind we get for doing or sharing greatness. The popular saying "All press is good press" does not apply to your personal life.

Social media is another place to avoid spewing misery because publicly posting about a negative experience is never an actual remedy. In fact, it upsets other people, causing concern, irritation, or anger. Comments of pity won't heal your wounds or repair your relationships. Posting about that jerk who sped past you won't slow anyone down. Trashing the waiter that screwed up your order will likely only do harm to a struggling business owner. However, posting something positive can lift spirits, broaden smiles, and enrich relationships. I'd like for you to focus your public shares on good things and appreciate how the responses you receive make you feel. Know that your social circle creates an opinion of who you are based on your posts. Would your followers describe you as a grump or a delight? Fight the urge to gripe and spread sunshine whenever possible. It's better for everyone involved!

When something significant happens, it's okay to vent to close friends or family. The key is ensuring that venting doesn't turn into a constant loop of negativity. Share your frustrations with people who offer support, but don't allow it to become a habit that keeps you stuck in the problem. We all face moments when we feel down, frustrated, or upset. Acknowledging those feelings is healthy. But wallowing in them or endlessly rehashing them isn't productive. It's important to give yourself permission to feel and then move forward, focusing on solutions or better experiences.

Chapter 17 | Health During Hardship & Mental Health

Practice letting it go instead of harping on your negative experiences and dragging down everyone around you. Sure, you can address egregious acts of poor service with a manager, but once your appropriate action has been taken, move on! Focus on more positive and productive things and leave irritation behind. If you don't, your psyche will pay the price, and you'll drag everyone else down with you. Learn to LET IT GO! That's right. Anything you likely won't remember in 10 years is not worth ruining even one day over. LET IT GO! **If you'd like to use my mantra, "It's not cancer!", it's yours.** Have it.

Choose Joy

If you want to be a happier, healthier person, you will have to force it. Day by day, hour by hour, happiness is a choice. You must CHOOSE to find the bright side in every situation. Sometimes, choosing joy feels like a challenge. And that's okay. Embrace those moments as part of your growth process. The goal is progress, not perfection. Choosing joy doesn't mean ignoring or suppressing your emotions. It means that after acknowledging your frustration or sadness, you consciously decide to shift toward a more positive perspective. It's not about forcing a fake smile but choosing to rise above negative situations for your well-being.

Stuck in traffic? That's cool. You'll have more time to listen to your favorite podcast, probably The Fitzness Show.

The cat jumped on your glass of red wine, spilling it on the carpet? The perfect motivation to finally get those carpets cleaned, because it's been too long.

Sitting on the tarmac in a plane that's delayed? Thank goodness the airline is making sure your plane is safe. A delay is always worth it if you land at your final destination in one piece.

Did you lose your job? A fantastic opportunity to make a fresh start and negotiate better terms!

Broke your arm? You will use this time to strengthen your lower body and abs!

Pretend you are your life's publicist with the mission of spinning everything negative into a positive. Throw some ego into it and refuse to let any person or thing get the best of you. You're far too good for that! Amaze yourself with the grit and grace you show under pressure. The ability to laugh off aggravation and rise above it will make your life sweeter, and you may inspire others to do the same. Choosing joy is contagious. What a lovely gift to spread to your sphere of influence.

Exercise doesn't just improve your body; it profoundly impacts your mind. When you move your body, your brain releases neurotransmitters like serotonin and dopamine, which are directly tied to feelings of happiness and well-being. This biochemical response doesn't just make you feel good at the moment but also helps you better manage stress, improve your mood over time, and build emotional resilience. Happiness increases your propensity to eat healthy food and exercise. It's an undeniable cycle of excellence. So, when you consider whether or not to let that fool in the cubicle next to yours ruin your day, choose to let it go. He's not worth your mental or physical health, and if you let him get to you, you'll pay the consequences, not him. On the best and worst days, supercharge your life with perspective, passions, and joy!

Combining a healthy body with a healthy mind will make you unstoppable!

Chapter 18

PERSEVERING THROUGH PAIN

Setbacks suck. Whether you're dealing with sprains, strains, tears, fractures, breaks, brain injuries, degenerative diseases, cancer, or other conditions, nobody likes pain and suffering, whether temporary or permanent. Physical setbacks can be tough on your mind, body, and soul, and certainly make you second-guess your efforts to get supercharged. However, they are never, and I do mean never, a justification to slack on fitness. Instead, they should increase your motivation tenfold. Nothing brings into focus the importance of health like injuries, illness, and pain. I, and millions of other cancer patients, can tell you that when we heard those words, "You have cancer," we no longer cared about fancy cars, clothes, or trips. All we wanted was our health. I imagine folks who've been hit by vehicles feel the same. Health is often taken for granted, until it's not.

If you are fit and strong going into any sort of physical crisis, know that you will be far more likely to rebound and recover more effectively and efficiently than an unfit person. I recommend that you prepare your body to do battle today, because one never knows when illness or injury will strike. A fall, crash, or illness could be on the horizon. Will you be at your best when it does? If the answer is "no," get serious about your training, nutrition, and sleep immediately.

Chapter 18 | Persevering Through Pain

If you are already living with pain, it's time to lean in. Of course, pain can be a real deterrent! Who wants to move when you feel bad? I know, I know. But the solution to illness and injury is strength, stamina, mobility, balance, quality rest, and nutrition. Everything I've been preaching throughout the pages of this book pertains to people with and without pain. Health is the solution! This is why doctors write physical therapy (PT) prescriptions and send patients to registered dietitians to discuss nutrition. Physical therapists are kind of like medically-savvy personal trainers. They assess where their patients are tight, weak, and off balance, and devise a plan to get them past it. Those plans often include a ton of strength training, stretching, balance training, and cardio. Sometimes people do PT just a few times before being released. Some folks do PT for life. That's because exercise is essential to recovery. If you are released from PT with a list of exercises to continue doing, do them. If you stop, you may backtrack.

If pain prevents you from exercising, know that in most circumstances, this pattern will only make you worse. Without challenging movement, your entire body will become tighter and weaker. You will lose stamina and balance. Every move you make will become more difficult, and your chances of injury via falls and strains increase dramatically. Arthritis is a terrific example of this. Arthritis causes inflammation and stiffness in joints, which can be excruciating. That pain obviously deters people from wanting to move, which makes sense! However, the phrase "motion is lotion" was likely invented for these folks because movement increases circulation and keeps the muscles surrounding the joints strong and flexible, thus diminishing inflammation and pain. Exercise is relief, but it takes a lot of discipline to get started despite pain, in the hopes it will make things better.

Whether you have arthritis, multiple sclerosis, scoliosis, or any other issue making movement more difficult, I encourage you to fight nonstop to stay mobile. Every effort you make will serve to prolong the progression of your ailment. In fact, if you look at any guidebook for dealing with any physical disease or disorder, you'll likely find that exercise and nutrition are part of the recipe for success. Shoot, you can find fitness classes just for people with Parkinson's worldwide.

Exercise can come in so many forms. Sometimes it's the act of wiggling fingers after experiencing a spinal cord injury: the tiniest movements can lead to so much hope and progress. Sometimes it's the use of spirometers by patients suffering from respiratory issues to help their lungs grow stronger. And sometimes it's doing plyometric box jumps for an athlete making her way back onto the field.

In the Everything Exercise chapter, I referenced strength being superior to weakness. Physically, weakness has no benefit. I've been weak due to illness and injury, and I loathed it. This is no slam on you if you're weak due to either. However, I want to compel you to be proactive and combat weakness with all your might. Do so with tiny and massive efforts. Discipline and consistency. Be creative too! Whether you are gritting your way back from injury or working to slow the progression of something bigger, fight like hell to become one percent better every day. What if your comeback actually is better than your setback? What if you live so much better than people in the same predicament? What if you defy all odds and make your medical team regret telling you that you never could? What if you write your story of success by controlling what you can and doing everything you can to be healthy despite pain and limitations?

Food is medicine. Think about how many people consume extra vitamin C when they get the sniffles. That's because they know it can help boost their immune system, possibly fending off their impending cold. Smart, right? Well, most whole foods are packed with beneficial nutrients to help you out of predicaments. If you get most of your calories from produce, whole grains, beans, nuts, seeds, lean protein, and lean dairy, your body will likely be a healing machine! Processed, sugary foods and those packed with unhealthy fats will make you worse. Want to get weaker and sicker in a hurry? Drink lots of alcohol and smoke. Easy peasy.

Use food to decrease inflammation, heal bone breaks, repair muscles, regenerate neurons, and increase energy. It's all there in the Supercharged Nutrition chapter, you just have to use it. And not just when you're suffering. Use it all the time to fend off aches, pains, and injuries. Combined with exercise, nourishment can have magical effects.

Rest can be rewarding too. If you are injured, recently out of surgery, or ill, extra downtime can be exactly what your body needs. Sometimes you should let all of the energy your body has be used for natural repairs. Sometimes, stillness is the right choice. Sometimes resting on an ice pack or heating pad works wonders. Sometimes, a few days of sleep can be rejuvenating. For the folks shaking their heads because you normally reject downtime, don't be ridiculous. You're human too. Skipping a run, workout, or day of work isn't going to kill you. It might just make you better!

Detours. There's a difference between needing to rest and needing to rest a particular body part. Know the difference, because excessive rest can often contribute to the problem. When your doctor says to stay down for a certain number of days, do it. But ask if you have to rest your entire body, or if you can move the parts that aren't recovering. For example, if your ankle is broken, there's probably no reason you can't do seated bicep curls, crunches, or stretching. Your doc may be delighted that you're so committed to health and looking to avoid becoming weaker all the way around. Knee trouble? Swim laps in a pool with a pool noodle between your knees to help your lower body float. Cranky shoulder? Walk, do lunges, or use an elliptical trainer! Sometimes injuries sideline us completely; sometimes they only force us to be creative.

Active Rest. Sounds contradictory. I know. But when I was going through chemo, 15 long months of chemo, I lived through many stuck-in-bed-sick days. Not because I was ordered to, but because my poor little body needed to stay down. Even still, I knew that lying still for days would have its share of consequences. Since I was still mentally supercharged, I got creative. Instead of doing nothing, I would force little movements like leg lifts, bridges, and Supermans into my rest routine. Yes, I was horizontal in bed, but I was still making efforts to slow the decline. I wasn't preparing for a bodybuilding competition. I was fighting to maintain every last bit of strength, mobility, and stamina I could. If you're freaked out by the not-so-good changes you see in your body, follow my lead. I also stretched in the shower. Bending and twisting while hot water poured over my body felt incredible.

Handle with Care. Exercise appropriately! Aggressively pursuing strength and stamina can still come with caution. If you are fragile in any way, respect your limits and choose exercises that are safe and beneficial. For example, if you've been diagnosed with osteoporosis, it might be time to switch from a road bike to a stationary bike to limit your fall risks. If your cardiologist has put you on heart rate restrictions, switch your uphill runs to downhill runs. You exercise to get better, not worse, so yield to your doctor's safety recommendations.

Know When to Say When. Ignoring a doctor's orders designed to help you heal doesn't make you heroic; it makes you foolish. I can't tell you how many runners show up at my races and tell me that despite their horrible XYZ injury, they will run their marathon. I do not respect that at all. Why put your health at risk for sport? I love sports. But I'd rather heal fully and get back to it than risk further or permanent injury for one event. There may be

Chapter 18 | Persevering Through Pain

little to gain, and potentially a ton to lose. Unless you're the key ingredient to winning the FIFA World Cup soccer championship and your team and an entire country are relying on you to score some goals, dial it back. Health trumps sports. Sitting things out while you're resting up and plotting your return to greatness is okay.

Shifting Focus. Pain can be all-consuming. If it is, I encourage you to seek help managing it. Talk to a counselor or join a support group to help you learn some coping and distraction tactics. The human spirit is extraordinary, and our ability to thrive under challenging circumstances is unique. As I advised in the Health During Hardship and Mental Health chapter, maintain perspective and pursue your passions as much as possible. If you love bowling but can't do so, read about bowling and listen to bowler podcasts. Forcing joy and healthy hobbies into each of your days might be the perfect distraction, shifting your attention from the "ouches" to the "oh yeahs!"

Get Diagnosed! I hope that if you're dealing with acute or chronic pain, you've seen a medical professional. With an accurate diagnosis, there may be a solution for what ails you. If there's any question mark over your head regarding why something hurts so bad or why your body isn't working properly, you may be screwing yourself out of instant or long-term relief. Perhaps you might need physical therapy, acupuncture, a brace, surgery, or any number of measures to set you straight. But there's probably no benefit to you roaming around suffering. It doesn't make you brave, it makes you foolish. Ouch, right? #SorryNotSorry I want you to be well and to feel good. I'm not going to sugarcoat something so important.

Mayday! Mayday! Pain can be a red flag warning you're about to have a heart attack, the discs in your spine are herniated, or that cancer is lurking. When those red flags appear, your job is to acknowledge them and seek help. If you don't, you could be facing catastrophe. Too many people ignore red flags, sirens, and foghorns because they're embarrassed to go to urgent care or the hospital, or worried about the expense. But what good is money and pride if you're dead? So be respectful of your body and take action when necessary. Please.

Just Say No (Probably). I'm also going to pipe up here about the overuse of opioids, also known as painkillers. My dad was addicted to Percocet and OxyContin, and they wreaked havoc on him and our family. These drugs are highly addictive and, in my completely non-medical opinion, are prescribed too often. So be wary.
These drugs that numb pain will also numb your mind. If you've received a prescription for painkillers, know that you don't have to fill it or take the pills. Sometimes doctors prescribe them "just in case" your suffering escalates. Perhaps instead, you'll be able to manage your pain with simpler tools like ibuprofen or aspirin. I don't know. Maybe you can just endure some discomfort? The suggestion that any level of pain must always be masked seems a bit reckless to me. Maybe the throbbing in your hip will prevent you from doing too much on it or encourage you to get the rest you need. Who knows? What I do know is that opioids terrify me. Too many wonderful people have had their lives destroyed or have died because of them. However, I've never heard of anyone's life being ruined because they were addicted to ibuprofen or ice packs. Have you?

While many medications can have some tremendous benefits, an equal number have heinous side effects, the worst being that they diminish your decision-making skills. They'll make you dumber, slower, more likely to say things you shouldn't, irritable, a safety hazard if you're driving, and more likely to fall. The "depressing" effects may also slow down your heart, your lungs, and your digestive system, making you constipated, or, if you're like me, make you throw up. Again, I'm not a doctor, but I am a health expert, and my advice is to tread cautiously when it comes to drugs

Chapter 18 | Persevering Through Pain

of any sort. Do a cost-benefit analysis every time you're offered a prescription, and if you can find an effective natural or less-risky alternative, please do.

A constant commitment to health under any circumstances is the no-holds-barred recipe for the success your body is craving. I've seen men with zero legs run marathons, cancer patients outlive their diagnosis, and women take on triathlons after devastating injuries. Equally impressive is seeing people grocery shopping independently 25 years after a Multiple Sclerosis diagnosis (which comes in many forms). As always, control what you can when you can with thoughtful exercise, nutrition, rest, and stress management. No matter what form your physical pain arrives in, you have a success story inside of you, too.

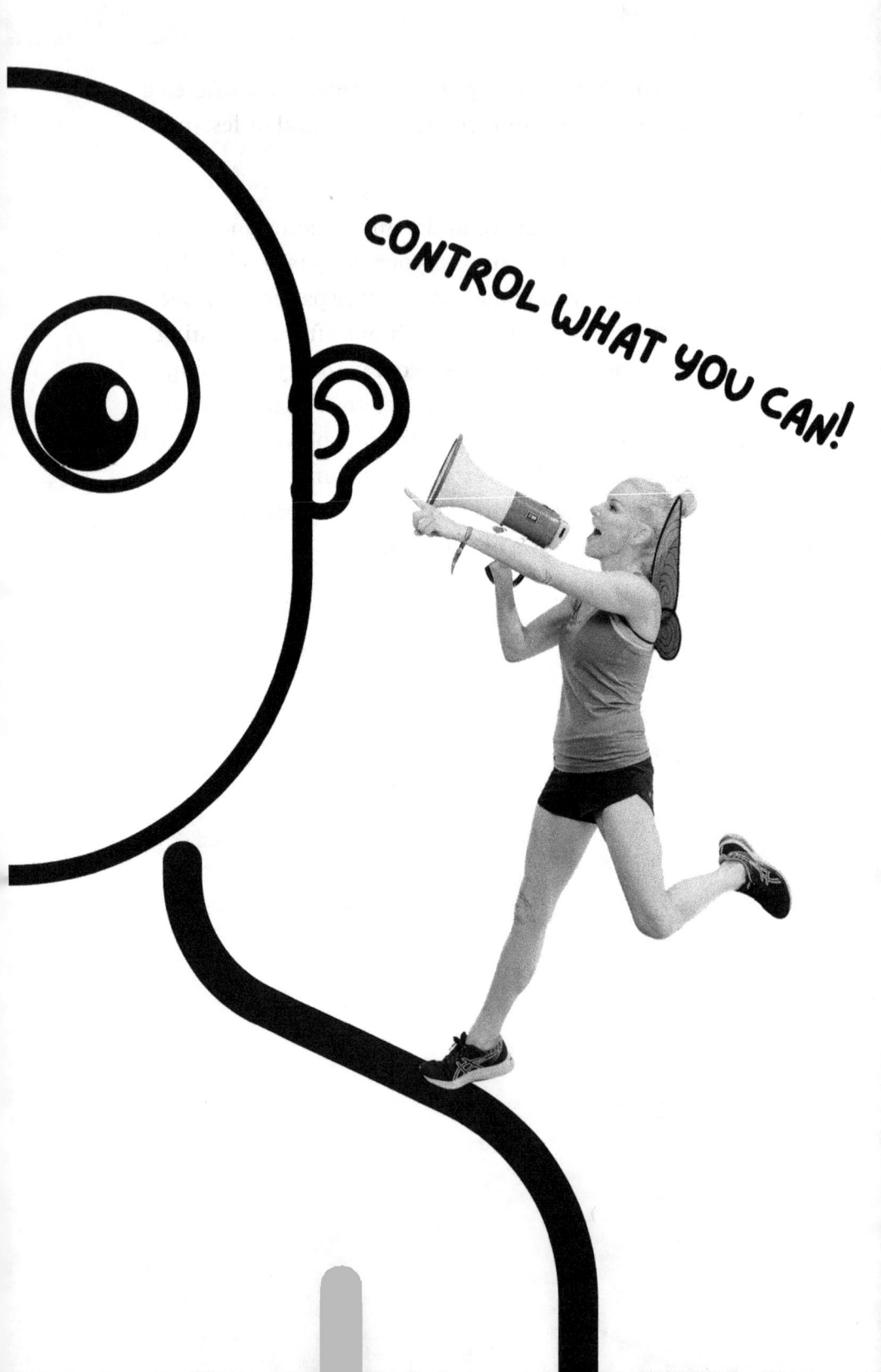

Chapter 19

BRAIN GAINS

Exercise, healthy foods, and spectacular sleep make us smarter. Well, at least they can. And if you've spent your life shunning sports and workouts because you're just too "cerebral" to engage in that nonsense, you've sold your uptown IQ short. Why? Because endless studies have proven that physical activity is fantastic for your noggin. If you'd like to supercharge that big, round, squishy blob between your ears, combine huffing and puffing, grunting, wincing, and wobbling with nourishment, intellectual stimulation, and revitalizing sleep.

Memory Boost

Becoming forgetful as we age or suffering from dementia is pretty scary. But when you do aerobic exercise, even at a moderate level, your heart pumps harder and faster, sending oxygen and nutrient-rich blood soaring through your body. That blood eventually hits the seahorse-shaped superstar in your brain, the hippocampus, which is responsible for learning and memory. Studies show that people with the highest fitness levels tend to have a firmer, larger, and more elastic hippocampus and consistently score highest on memory tests. Translation? The more you exercise, the lower your risk for cognitive impairment. Conversely, if your brain doesn't get enough blood flow, your hippocampus and your ability to learn and retain information can shrink. With dementia and Alzheimer's having such a frightening grip on our older population, isn't it empowering to know you have some control?

Sweat-Fueled Smarts

Exercise isn't just for muscles: it's brain fuel for learning. You know how little kids seem to learn at warp speed: languages, math, and new concepts? That's because their hippocampus is buzzing with activity, firing on all cylinders; no wonder they absorb knowledge like sponges. But just like the rest of our bodies, our brains age too, so we often notice a slowdown in learning as we age. The good news? Just as exercise can keep your legs and back youthful and firm, it can also strengthen your brain. When your hippocampus is well-fed with oxygen and nutrients, it stays sharp, helping you absorb information faster, remember it longer, and stay confidently in the know. It turns out that an old dog who moves can master every trick in the book and maybe even concoct a few new ones.

The Comeback Cortex

Scientists used to believe that once brain cells died off, they were gone forever. Fortunately, that theory has been debunked! Our brains benefit from a special gift called *neuroplasticity*, the incredible ability to adapt and rewire by forming new neural pathways. Even more exciting? In certain areas like the hippocampus, the brain can generate new cells through a process called *neurogenesis*. That means we're not doomed to get dumber or more forgetful as we age. We can maintain, or even improve, brain function if our lifestyle supports it. Healthy foods, regular exercise, and quality sleep all fuel vibrant brain activity. This is especially encouraging for those who've experienced brain trauma. Depending on the severity, many people can recover well through the smart habits I've been pushing you to adopt, along with occupational therapy.

Down with Cortisol!

Cortisol, the hormone generated by stress, is your brain's mortal enemy. It prohibits the growth of new neurons, those crucial nerve cells that communicate with every part of your body, telling it what to do. Neurons are our brain's besties, and we want as many healthy ones as possible. Cortisol can kill those besties, causing us, over time, to lose precious abilities. So instead of allowing stress to escalate and marinate, use proven stress management tactics like exercise, which helps lower cortisol levels and improves emotional regulation. Meditation, journaling, and counseling are also wise weapons in the fight against cortisol.

Happy Hormones

Moderate to vigorous aerobic exercise releases the happy hormones: endorphins, dopamine, and serotonin. This crew boosts focus, creativity, motivation, and happiness. It's often called the "runner's high," but the same benefits can come from any cardiovascular exercise you choose: cycling, swimming, dancing, you name it. Besides getting your "huff and puff" on to increase your heart and lung capacity and burn lots of calories, do it to fend off depression and boost your energy.

Clear Mind, Strong Body

By keeping happy hormones high while decreasing cortisol and inflammation, exercise can prevent mental fog and boost creativity, focus, and problem-solving abilities. When people say they're going to work out to "clear their mind," they actually *are* clearing out the bad stuff while making room for the good. What a powerful way to enhance your intelligence, your ability to multitask, and your capacity to crush daily tasks.

Chapter 19 | Brain Gains

Power Down to Power Up

Sleep is essential for brain power. Just like your prized tech devices, quality rest allows your mind to recharge. Sleep is when your brain handles important tasks like memory filing, emotional housekeeping, and creative idea-building, especially during REM sleep, when your brain activity ramps up and creativity soars. Regular vigorous exercise increases your chances of nodding off quickly and staying asleep until your alarm goes off.

Nourish Your Noggin

Your brain is more sophisticated than the fanciest computer, and it requires premium fuel by way of nutrient-rich foods, for proper function and maintenance. When it comes to the body parts I want operating at their absolute best, I put my brain at the top of the list. So feed it in a way that keeps it humming along, generating new neurons while collecting memories, ideas, and information. Natural sugars from fruits, veggies, and whole grains keep your energy levels stable, while omega-3 fatty acids from foods like salmon and walnuts help build strong, flexible brain cells. Antioxidant-packed produce fights inflammation and oxidative stress, protecting your brain from damage. Nutrients like B6, B12, and folate boost mood by helping produce feel-good chemicals like serotonin and dopamine, and minerals such as zinc, magnesium, and iron are essential for sharp memory, focus, and learning. Even your gut health matters; fiber and probiotics help regulate brain function because a large portion of your body's neurotransmitters are produced in the gut. Simply put: when you eat well, you think better. Feed your brain junk, and it'll start running like an outdated desktop computer from 1997.

Brain Games

These activities support the growth of new neurons, which are critical to learning and memory. Besides doing puzzles, reading, and playing musical instruments, you could learn a dance routine, play pickleball, or pursue obstacle course racing. Getting enough sleep and eating nutritious foods also support neurogenesis, the process by which your brain creates new neurons or cells. It's like your brain growing tiny new helpers to think, learn, and remember. Isn't it remarkable that your brain can keep improving, even as you get older?

If you put in the effort for a body that will last the test of time, you can be the stud at the senior center, standing tall, shaking your thang, and living independently. The same measures will enable you to find your keys, have clever conversations with your grandchildren, manage your house without help, and remember loved ones. If a pain-free, mobile body isn't enough incentive to eat wisely and exercise, I hope a priority on cognitive function will do the trick. Kinda like constantly rebooting and upgrading your hard drive!

I've said it before, and I'll say it again: when you pair a strong body with a strong mind, you will be unstoppable!

Chapter 20

FULL-THROTTLE FEMININITY

Ladies, I hate to gloat, but we are magical creatures. Our bodies can do all sorts of mind-blowing things, while we multitask our butts off, care for those we adore and still find time to shine. I do love being female, and I hope you treasure it too. However, some of the nonsense that comes with our audacious capabilities is over-the-top bullshit. Right? Menstruation, making humans, and menopause: not so easy. But easy is not the path we were born to take, and you know darn well that we can do hard things. So let's discuss ways to take control of our outcomes and support our beautiful bodies and brains in every way possible.

Blood, Sweat and Tears

Some say menstruation is a beautiful part of being a woman; I'm guessing the people who say that are men. Even though periods eventually yield some epic sorcery, the process leaves much to be desired. Cramps, headaches, fatigue, mood swings, nausea, a dip in iron levels, and bloating are just a few of the "beautiful" things we deal with monthly.

You can fight against these side effects with exercise, nutrition, and quality sleep. Has your energy tanked from heavy bleeding? Double down on iron-rich foods like spinach and soybeans. Can't zip up your jeans? Cardio can help you sweat off some of the water weight you're retaining. Sobbing, screaming, and laughing uncontrollably every hour on the hour? The endorphins you'll generate from punching a heavy bag or twerking through a hip-hop fitness class will help level you out. Instead of vegging out on the couch or downing ice cream sandwiches, throw on your period panties and get to work. Maybe your "friend" doesn't have to be such a nasty bitch after all.

Menopause

Menopause kicks in as estrogen and progesterone levels decline, natural hormonal shifts that send your body and mood on a bit of a rollercoaster ride. And not the fun kind. We're talking hot flashes, joint pain, vaginal dryness, mood swings, and more. Are you F'ing kidding me? The whole experience feels like a rude joke. Ha ha! No one's laughing.

But here's the good news: like most challenges, you can make this phase way more manageable, and even empowering, by focusing on your fitness. That's right. Your bestie, Fitzy, has some solid solutions, and if you use them, this wild ride might still be weird, but it won't be the boss of you. With the proper habits, you won't just survive menopause, you'll thrive through it, flipping it the finger in fabulous fashion.

You've seen these strategies throughout the book, but now it's time to revisit them through the lens of menopause. When you understand how to care for your body during this stage of life, you can stop merely coping and start reclaiming your power.

Make Muscles

Strength training doesn't just sculpt your body, it helps preserve bone density, boost metabolism, reduce injury risk, and fight age-related muscle loss. That's some serious long-term return on investment. Consider "making muscles" your most essential pillar of fitness. Do various exercises, from pumping iron to bodyweight exercises, resistance band work, pilates, and plyometrics. Aim to train every other day, but if that doesn't happen, no sweat, just try to fit in a session at least every third day to keep your progress on track.

Huff and Puff

Cardio is excellent for burning calories, gets your blood flowing, boosts oxygen delivery, and releases feel-good chemicals like endorphins, that's why it helps you sleep better, feel more energized, and stay in a good mood. Menopause can increase a woman's risk for heart disease and high blood pressure, and the loss of estrogen can increase inflammation in her joints. Keep your heart, lungs, and joints healthy with multiple 30-minute sessions of swimming, dancing, hiking, or anything else that gets your heart racing weekly. If you're huffing and puffing, you're doing it right!

Be Bendy

Menopause-related hormone shifts can affect coordination, stability, and joint comfort, so regular stretching and balance work can help prevent falls, reduce stiffness, and improve overall mobility. Commit to yoga, pilates, or some standard stretches throughout the day, and stand on one foot as often as possible while doing mundane things like waiting in lines to improve balance.

Cooler Workouts

Guuuuurl: Hot flashes are rude! Are you sweating for no reason in the middle of a snowstorm? I wish I were there to pamper you with ice packs. Don't let heat surges derail your fitness goals.

Instead, be strategic: exercise in air-conditioned or cooler outdoor spaces, wear breathable fabrics, and keep ice water nearby. If you like to train outdoors, beat the heat early in the morning or as the sun sets. And if you want to level up to genius status, exercise in a pool, the perfect refuge! Lastly, keep a hoodie handy in case chills follow your hot flashes. One must be prepared for anything!

Sleeping Beauty

Insomnia and night sweats can make falling and staying asleep difficult, so that handsome prince had better not even think about waking you up! The best way to improve sleep is to exhaust yourself with quality exercise, activity, and mental stimulation. Avoid caffeine later in the day, and set up your sleeping situation to be as peaceful, cozy, and cool as possible. Wind down with calming activities like light stretching, journaling, or a warm bath to signal your body that it's time for rest. Bonus tip: Opt for bedding that helps regulate temperature, like breathable "cool" fabrics and lightweight blankets, especially if hot flashes are part of your nighttime routine.

MEANopause

If hormone changes have turned you into a basket case, you're not alone. Women around the world are struggling with anxiety, mood swings, and depression. Regular exercise is a proven mood-booster, flooding your body with endorphins that can help lift your spirits. It also provides a healthy distraction and a powerful release of built-up tension. Find peace pursuing hobbies, meeting with an understanding friend, or spending time at your local axe-throwing entertainment center. Yes, it's a real thing, and yes, it's the perfect outlet for all these yucky emotions. Remember, if your feelings are ever too heavy to manage alone, there's no shame in seeking help from a mental health professional; it's one of the bravest moves you can make. Whatever your outlet, give yourself grace and know you deserve support, movement, and moments of joy, even in the middle of MEANopause.

You Control Your Weight

Menopause can lead to muscle loss, which slows metabolism, and with stress eating, can lead to weight gain. Despite what many may lead you to believe, you still have a ton of control over your body. If you do the things I've instructed you to do, you can and will achieve your desired weight and fitness goals. If you consistently apply the pillars of fitness with purpose and enthusiasm, The Formula, and utilize nutritious foods to serve your health, you should be able to maintain a weight that makes you happy.

Dem Bones

As estrogen levels decline, so does bone density, making us more prone to fractures and breaks. I implore you to take this call to action seriously to avoid conditions like osteopenia (bone thinning) and osteoporosis (brittle bones). Prioritize strength training and weight-bearing exercises like walking, running, or hiking, as they help build and maintain bone density. Consuming foods with calcium and phosphorus, like dairy, fish, whole grains, nuts, and leafy greens, can also benefit your bones, so work them into your meals regularly and discuss supplements with your doctor.

Vajayay of Steel

Often instigated by childbirth, many women have to deal with leakage, little annoying and embarrassing releases of urine, caused by running, jumping, strength training, coughing, sneezing, laughing, and more. Hormonal changes and muscle loss can weaken the pelvic floor, leading to leaks, discomfort, and decreased sexual sensation. If you find yourself peeing when you don't want

Chapter 20 | Full-Throttle Femininity

to or not enjoying sex the way you used to, it's probably time to throw on a leotard and give that hoo-ha a workout! Kegels are pelvic floor exercises that require zero equipment and can be done anywhere at any time.

Sitting at a red light on your way to work? Supercharge that coochie with Kegels, baby! Flying cross-country? Kegel to join the Mile High Club solo. Video chatting with your pals or colleagues? Squeeze, squeeze, squeeze! Aim for multiple sets of 10-15 reps daily. As you strengthen your mighty kitty, I encourage you to connect with a urologist who may offer treatments including physical therapy, pharmaceuticals and surgical options. I recently had a urologist as a guest on my podcast, The Fitzness Show, and he shared the motivational message that women do not have to tolerate leakage. Solutions exist!

Bringing Sexy Back

You are too damn gorgeous to let a drop in estrogen kill your libido or let vaginal dryness deter you from sex. Sex can be a game-changer for mood, self-esteem, and energy, so if you can do it, with someone else or by yourself, know that it could be beneficial. And fun, right? Instead of just accepting a life without sex, talk to your doctor, who may recommend things like hormone therapy, vaginal moisturizers, or non-hormonal treatments; there's more help out there than you might expect. And don't be shy because your doctor has heard it all and can likely help with medical support. Once you've done that, talk openly and honestly with your partner and ask for help. Perhaps extra foreplay and fun might help get you in the mood. Or maybe you just need some relaxation and alone time to de-stress and ready yourself for a romp? Candles, music, lingerie, and massages are classics, but do what works for you.

Last but not least, invest in lube! If your cute little vaginal walls have thinned and sex has become painful, lubrication has got to be part of the solution. Whether you use a fancy lube brand or a natural fan favorite like coconut oil, this simple step can turn "ouches" back into "oohs and ahs." Grab a few bottles and stash them wherever you're likely to get freaky.

Brain Fog

No. You are not a dummy. You can't remember why you walked into the room because your hormones walked out first! Combat brain fog with exercise and brain games like crossword puzzles. Omega-3s help reduce inflammation, support memory, concentration, and overall mental clarity. Consume foods like salmon and mackerel, flaxseed and chia seeds, leafy greens, and berries to help with cognitive function. Write important things down in your phone or favorite notebook to keep you on task, keep your life on track, and let fewer balls drop. Good sleep and stress-reduction habits, like meditation or unplugging before bed, can also help keep the brain fog at bay.

Focus on Fun

It's time to make all the places you go and the things you do inspire joy. You're a grown-ass woman, and I insist that you make time for all the things, people, and opportunities that fill your heart with glee. From goat yoga to coffee with friends, cloud watching, swimming with dolphins, playing an instrument, iconic concerts, and beach weekends, it's time to prioritize your health and soul. Girl, make both big and small plans; you deserve this!

Pregnancy

Honestly, this section deserves its very own book because a pregnant woman and her child are so damn precious. I'll simply share that a healthy mother is likelier to carry a baby to term and less likely to suffer complications. Fitness is in the best interest of both of you. Just make sure that safety is always the priority. You can still have fun and challenge your body while minimizing the risk of falls and contact injuries. Dancing, running, walking, stationary cycling, swimming, strength training, and stretching are all great choices. Skateboarding and boxing are not. Nutritious foods will help the baby grow and the mommy thrive, but I will stop there, because you need to talk with your medical provider. Congrats! Babies are the best.

Slay

Menstruation, menopause, and pregnancy affect each woman uniquely. Our role in each phase is to listen to our bodies and use our smarts to support our needs, promote health, and improve our outcomes. You absolutely can be healthy, fit, strong, and fabulous throughout each stage of your life. So go dance, laugh, rest, or finally book that trip. Whatever fills your cup, make it happen. You've got this, besties.

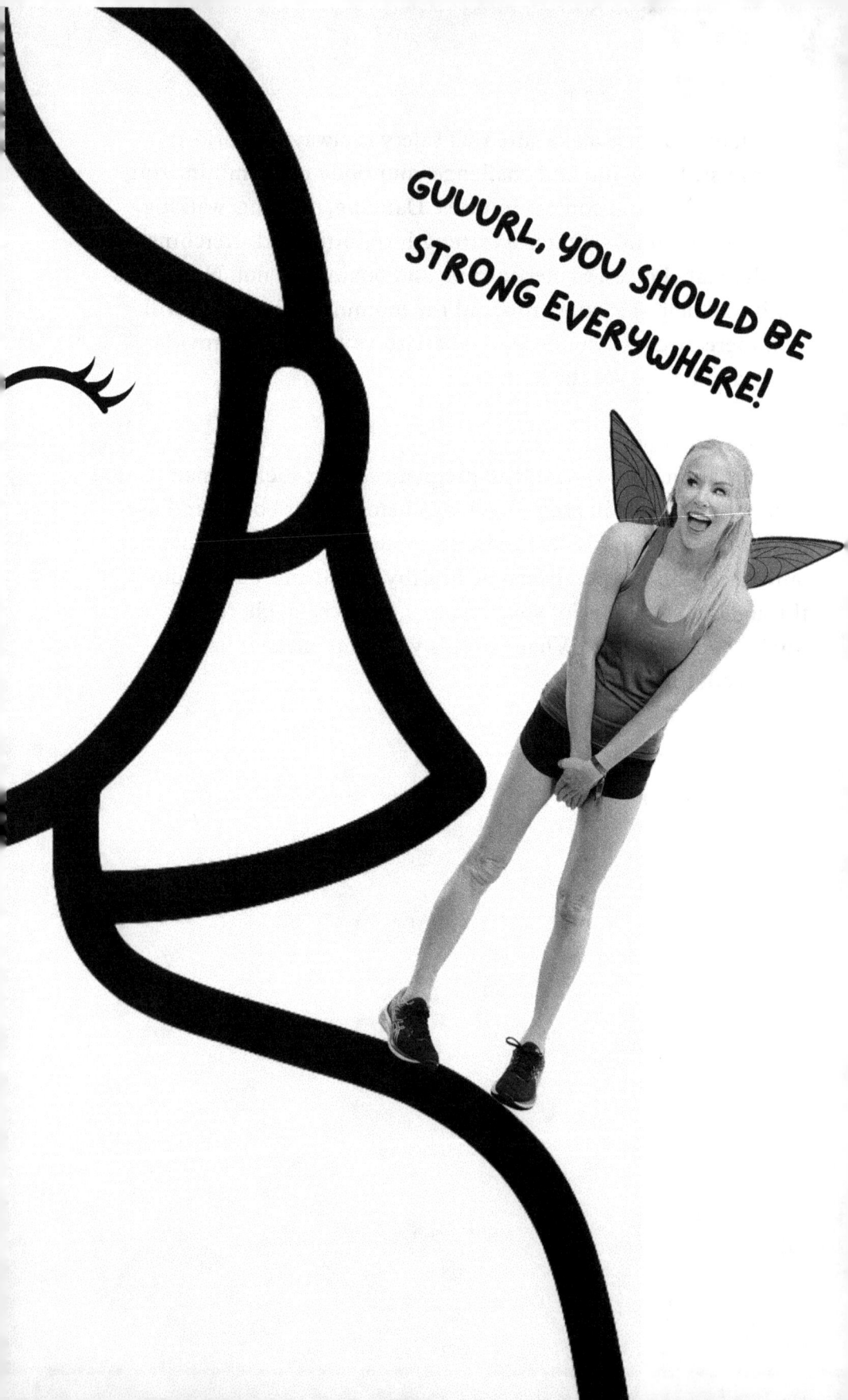

Chapter 21

MAN MODE

Gentlemen, I adore you and am excited to share a little bro time together. From muscle mass and testosterone to andropause and the infamous dad bod, y'all are worthy of your own chapter too. This isn't about six-packs or ego lifting, it's about keeping your body powerful, your mind sharp, and your life on track. Sure, you might've picked up this book thinking you just needed to drop a few pounds or get back in shape, but here's the truth: men's health is a complex machine. As you age, your testosterone levels decline, your recovery slows down, and belly fat moves in like an uninvited houseguest. But none of that means you're doomed. With the right approach to fitness, nutrition, sleep, and stress, you can stay strong, energized, and sharp for decades to come. So buckle up, because we're about to tackle your body from the inside out.

Truth About Testosterone

The big T is a hormone that positively impacts your muscle mass, fat storage (especially around the belly), libido, mood, energy, and mental sharpness. It's the secret sauce that makes you feel so good, which is why you should do everything you can to keep levels high. Strength training, clean eating, and quality sleep can naturally boost testosterone, helping older men feel like younger versions of themselves, even when their birth certificate says otherwise.

Andropause = MANopause

In your mid-30s, testosterone starts to decline by about one percent per year. Over time, this gradual dip can lead to andropause, the male version of menopause, which may cause fatigue, mood shifts, reduced strength, erectile dysfunction, and trouble focusing. Sound familiar? You're not broken, you're just overdue for a reboot. The great news is that with a strong commitment to testosterone-boosting habits, you can reduce or erase the negative side effects entirely.

Unsurprisingly, many symptoms of low testosterone overlap with obesity and type 2 diabetes. If you're nodding your head, connect with your physician and make a plan to reach your ideal weight by upgrading your workouts and nutrition. This is the perfect opportunity to control what you can, when you can. A fitter body might just be the answer to most of what's ailing you.

Important Note: Testosterone Replacement Therapy (TRT) isn't a magic bullet and does come with potential side effects. So do your part with exercise, nutrition, and sleep, do your research, and have a long talk with your doctor before jumping in.

Save the Man Muscles

Sure, men and women technically have the same muscles, but let's be honest, men's muscles are often so much *extra*. And that's exactly why you should protect them. Strength training will help you fend off age-related muscle loss, which tends to kick in around 40. But not you! You're lifting regularly to keep your muscles strong, metabolism fired up, posture confident, and joints feeling good. If you want to look and feel young, put your muscles to work, even if you've never strength trained before. Today is the perfect day to start. Just check your ego at the door. If you're chasing the title of deadlifting champion of your gym or house, you might blow out your back and spend the next 50 years on the bench. Instead, start where you are and make steady progress. The weight room isn't a place to show off. It's a place to show up, stay consistent, and earn injury-free, powerful awesomeness. Note: *Deadlifts make me nervous because I've heard too many horror stories. My physical therapist friends agree: there are safer ways to get strong.*

Beer Belly? No Way!

If you can no longer see your belt because of that growing belly, it's time to take action. Men are more prone to visceral fat, which is deep abdominal fat that wraps around your organs and dramatically increases your risk of heart disease, stroke, and diabetes. Whether or not you actually drink beer is irrelevant. Extra weight in your hips or thighs isn't nearly as dangerous, but belly fat? That stuff can kill you. So, use The Formula, commit to all Four Pillars of Fitness, and watch your waistline reappear as you tack years onto your life.

Ticker Tune-Up

Since your most important muscle is your heart, and I just shared the scary stat that heart disease is the #1 killer of men, let's talk about how to beat the odds. Fill your plates with produce, whole grains, and lean proteins instead of highly processed, fatty, or sugary junk. The bad stuff raises your cholesterol and clogs your arteries—like the pipes under a fry kitchen sink. Limit alcohol. Do not smoke *anything*. Manage stress and get quality sleep.

Sex is great for your cardiovascular system, so have lots of it! Whether you're with a partner or flying solo, both options are beneficial. Make it a priority to visit your doctor annually for blood pressure, cholesterol, and triglyceride checks. I hate to generalize, but I will: guys are typically not great about checkups. Catching problems early can save your life. Let your doctor spot red flags before they become emergencies.

De-Gunk Your Junk

Your entire body suffers when your blood vessels are clogged with gunk: high blood pressure, lousy cholesterol, and poor circulation. And yes, that includes your Johnson, which is home to the penile artery, which, if clogged and blood can't flow freely, neither can the magic. Clogged arteries are one of the top culprits behind erectile dysfunction. Many men have no idea that the reason they can't get it up is a result of poor nutrition and heart disease. This is a red flag sitting at half-mast. Take care of your ticker, and the rest of your body will dazzle.

Sleep, Sex, and Stamina

If your health is good, you'll sleep well and shine in the bedroom. But if you're not sleeping well, you're less likely to exercise, testosterone levels may drop, and your sex drive could tank. The good news? Your libido can bounce back with better circulation, confidence, and hormone balance, all tied to your fitness routine. Better sleep = better fitness = better sex = better sleep. Win. Win. Win.

Stiffy of Stone

Kegels are essential exercises for the pelvic floor muscles, which support your bladder, bowels, and prostate; they can also enhance sexual performance. If you train them as aggressively as you train your biceps, you'll be less likely to leak urine or stool (ack!), and hopefully avoid those little blue pills. Kegels involve flexing pelvic floor muscles for a few seconds at a time, ideally in sets of 10-15 reps. You can do them fully clothed anywhere and at any time. Supercharge your shlong with a set while waiting for a red light to turn green, reviewing a contract, or camped out on the couch watching baseball. No one will know what you're up to, so don't worry about earning "creeper status."

I'm guessing that you already love your mini-me, but if you want it to truly stand tall as the most powerful pecker on the planet, Kegels are the key to earning that crown. And if you're in a romantic relationship with a woman, encourage her to do Kegels too; the benefits for both of you and your uber-fit particulars will be extraordinary!

If you can't tell, I'm having endless fun with these weiner, wang, and willy references. Step back into the Full Throttle Femininity chapter for some classic Vajayay bits. Patting myself on the back. Giggling.

Easy, Cowboy

I want you to train aggressively but not recklessly. There's a big difference between hardcore and irrational. Focus on proper form, lift appropriate weights, warm up thoroughly, stretch often, and make room for recovery. You probably don't have a redshirt season left, so take care of yourself. Use the massage guns and foam rollers, and embrace active rest days like a pro.

Dad Bods

This is trending right now, and to be honest, I'm not even sure what officially qualifies as a Dad Bod. What I *can* tell you is this: your body is yours, and the best thing you can do is take great care of it. The Four Pillars of Fitness and The Formula are your recipe for success, regardless of your shape. Also, let's be real: dads are hot. Seriously. Men who support, coach, and nurture children? Very sexy. So if someone says you've got a Dad Bod, take it as a compliment, and then keep working on the strongest, healthiest version of you.

Play Time

Men rule this category. You guys have this magical, unspoken ability to just jump into a pickup basketball game anywhere, anytime. We gals don't really have that. This is a superpower you should take full advantage of. Sports are fun, stress-relieving, and they boost your social life. Whether you're good or not, joining a community softball, kickball, or flag football team will give you something to look forward to and a great reason to move more.

Downtime for Dudes

If you're feeling crushed by the weight of work, family, or life in general, it's time to hit the brakes. Stress isn't just a buzzkill; it's bad news for your heart, your hormones, and your head. While grinding 24/7 might sound noble, it can quietly wreck everything you're working for.

Make rest a part of the plan. Build in downtime, the little daily breathers, and the bigger, more intentional breaks. Get outside for some fresh air. Go fishing. Try acupuncture. Play your drums. Take a dang bath. Yes, men can take baths, too; your man card's safe.

Protecting your peace isn't lazy, it's strategic. Every minute you invest in mental health pays dividends in physical health. Recharge like a champ so you can come back stronger, sharper, and happier.

Sports Should Make You Fitter, Not Fatter

Whether you're watching your favorite teams live, at a sports bar, or from your couch, don't let those elite athletes become your excuse to binge on pizza, beer, and wings. You absolutely can enjoy the game without inhaling 3,000 calories. And if you truly love football or baseball, go outside and throw the ball around with your buddies. Play for Pete's sake! If Patrick Mahomes knew you were using him as a reason to gain weight and get worse, he'd probably be pissed. Instead, use your favorite athletes and love of sports as inspiration, and commit to getting fitter each time you watch a game.

Superhero Status

Whether you're a dad, uncle, boss, brother, coach, son, or friend, your actions influence the people around you. Be the role model someone might quietly need. The better you are at keeping your health and habits in order, the more you'll uplift the people in your circle. Demonstrate strength, discipline, consistency, and determination. Of course, your health is about *you*, but it just might improve the lives of everyone around you, too.

Strong men aren't just built in the gym, they're forged through discipline, fueled by purpose, and powered by the choices they make every damn day. From your heart to your hormones, your muscles and more, control what you can, when you can, and enjoy all the greatness that comes with being a M-A-N!

Chapter 22

SUPERCHARGE YOUR FAMILY

You. Supercharged!

If you're at the helm of a little tribe of humans, I'm excited to help you supercharge your entire crew. Fit families have more fun, adventure, and overall success than those who don't prioritize health. Trading screen time for outdoor activities and/or fast food for tending home grown gardens sounds nice, right? Of course! Wouldn't it be cool if you were all at your physical and mental best? You'd probably get along even better if you were venting stress through exercise and getting enough sleep! There's so much to look forward to.

Before we move forward, I want you to know something: you do not have to be like the family you were raised in. Unless, of course, they're in fantastic shape and doing everything right. The number of people who believe they are overweight or out of shape simply because their parents, siblings, or grandparents are is disturbing. Let me be clear: you do not have to be like them! If you are a "too-big" person in a "too-big" family, it is not because you are genetically predisposed. It is because you've adopted their atrocious habits. They likely taught you how to overeat and skip out on exercise, and you've been carrying on that legacy. It ends with you. That's right. You're the wise one who picked up this book, and let me fill your brain with everything you need to know about living better and longer inside a healthy body.

Chapter 22 | Supercharge Your Family

If you didn't absorb it fully the first time you read it, I'll repeat myself. You do not have to be like them! I want those words to stick in your head because they will give you control. You are not a victim of genetics. You are not destined to be overweight. With the Exact Formula and a commitment to exercise, nothing prevents you from dropping weight, changing your life, and creating a new legacy for your family, especially the generations to follow.

It's okay to love your people and choose a different lifestyle. You don't have to disregard them or rub your success in their faces. Instead, focus on what you put in your mouth and how you move your body. Politely decline unhealthy dishes when your family gathers; instead, show up with a healthy dish to share. Do not lower your standards for them, as their standards have already put you in a difficult position. Remember, you are the only person responsible for you. But know that your success may inspire them to do the same. Some relatives may mock you for eating wisely and exercising because jealousy and embarrassment often inspire mean words. Others may peek at your plate, listen to how much fun you're having with your new fitness club, and seek advice on getting started and sticking with it. After you point them toward this book, invite them to exercise with you or share a favorite recipe. Even small bits of encouragement can make a significant impact.

Your decisions and discipline have the same chance of impacting future generations as those before you. Your children would be so fortunate if you gave them the knowledge, passion, and habits of good health.

Raising a Fit Family

Many of you may be parents, and while I'm talking to parents, this message also applies to grandparents, aunts, uncles, teachers, coaches, and anyone who has the privilege of nurturing children.

Guiding and loving children is a tremendous responsibility and a valuable opportunity. Their well-being relies heavily on it, and the following principles could improve their lives.

Longevity: The Ultimate Goal

No parent wants to outlive their child. That nightmare alone should motivate us to take steps toward ensuring their long, healthy lives. Ask yourself: Are the habits you're instilling in your children setting them up for longevity? If the answer is "no" or "I'm not sure," it's time to make changes.

The benefits of exercise, healthy eating, and proper sleep are extraordinary. They can prevent numerous diseases, including type 2 diabetes, heart disease, certain cancers, and obesity, while promoting mental well-being and longevity. Fitter kids also perform better in school, sports, and life. Let's help them thrive.

Starting the Conversation

Be honest with your children. If you've been inspired to make changes, explain it to them. Say, "I love you, and I've learned some things that can help us all live healthier lives. We're going to make gradual changes together. Let's explore foods and activities that make us feel great." Avoid terms like "diet" or "fat"; this isn't about appearances: it's about health and happiness.

Nutrition: Foods That Help vs. Foods That Harm

Divide foods into two categories: those that help and those that harm. Encourage more of the former while reducing the latter. For example:

- **Helpful:** Vegetables, fruits, lean proteins, whole grains, and low-fat dairy.

- **Harmful:** Sugary drinks, processed snacks, fried foods, and excessive sweets.

Start with simple swaps. Replace soda with water or unsweetened tea. Choose baked potato chips over crackers. Opt for skim or vegan milk instead of whole milk. Gradually incorporate more produce and proteins, aiming for a colorful variety to cover different nutritional needs.

Make Mealtime Manageable

Healthy eating doesn't have to mean elaborate meals. Parenting, working, keeping a house tidy, exercising, and shuttling everyone to various activities can feel chaotic. Don't guilt yourself into making casseroles. Instead, keep it simple:

- Serve mix-and-match meals with protein, produce, and a healthy starch.
- Use frozen vegetables for quick preparation.
- Meal prep by cooking nutritious foods in bulk to serve throughout the week.
- Offer fun presentations like party platters with assorted fruits, nuts, and cheeses.

Encourage kids to try new foods by presenting them in creative ways. Remember, it can take multiple introductions for a child to accept a new food.

Beverages: Choose Wisely

Teach kids to prioritize water and calorie-free drinks. Don't serve soda, sugary juices, or unnecessary electrolyte beverages unless they're actively engaged in endurance sports. Reserve sugary drinks for rare occasions, and make water their primary hydration source.

Active Play: Fun Comes First

Children are naturally active and playful, let's encourage that. Whether wrestling, playing tag, or dancing, movement should feel like fun, not a chore. Choose active video games for tech-savvy kids. Technology isn't always bad; you just have to choose the way it's used and the amount of access kids have to it. I loved watching my kids get sweaty playing dance games and other sports. Ideally, tech activities will be limited to a small percentage of their playtime. The rest should include fresh air and hopefully friends or family to play with.

Sports offer structured opportunities to develop teamwork, leadership, and resilience. Let your children explore various activities to find what they enjoy most. Avoid overloading them with a laser focus on one sport to prevent burnout and overuse injuries. Balance is key.

Role Modeling

Leading by example is the most effective way to convince them that healthy habits are essential. Talk to them about your workouts and get active with them. Regularly tell them why health and fitness are important to you, and let them see you partake! Share how wonderful it makes your body feel, even though it can be challenging, and how it benefits your mind. Get them involved in your workouts at home, have a family member bring them out to celebrate you crossing a finish line, and take classes together.

Younger children can join in bodyweight exercises or stretches. For teens, gradually introduce gym equipment or fitness classes. Make it a family affair, play, train, dance, hike, climb, and grow stronger together. At a minimum, your kiddos should know when you exercise, why you exercise, and how much you value the benefits. The same thing goes for nutrition! Don't tell them to eat okra while you gobble up cheesy crackers and down beer or soda. You may not even realize how closely they watch you. Show them the way by regularly choosing quality foods. You don't have to be perfect, but you should demonstrate high standards.

Take Your Active Lifestyle with You

Consistency is key! Instead of dumping healthy habits every time you do something special or outside the norm, maintain them wherever you are. It's unfair to confuse kids by acting like exercise and nutrition only matter sometimes. Sure, you can splurge for a caramel apple at a theme park or a box of popcorn at a baseball game. Hopefully, the meals surrounding splurges are nutritious and beneficial to their growing bodies. Many theme parks and family-focused event centers have upgraded menus to provide healthy options. Stick with them. You can also plan vacations and special events around fun physical activities like swimming, skiing, hiking, and exploring new places.

Take Ownership

It's never too late to make changes, even drastic ones. If your child's habits have veered off track, address them calmly and sincerely. Own it if you've taught them less-than-stellar habits so far. Apologize for making mistakes and explain that when you know better, you must do better. Now that you have a clearer understanding of the importance of health, commit to making positive changes and involve your family in the process. Seek support from their pediatrician if needed, as professional advice can reinforce your efforts. Instead of making drastic changes immediately, gradually exchange unhealthy foods and drinks for better options. Trade screen time for time outdoors. Keep things positive, let them choose from various healthy choices, and progress will come.

Love Them Enough

Nobody wants to talk about this, but it's not okay for children to be overweight or obese. Not for their physical or mental health. Moms, dads, and grandparents, I'm talking to you. It's not cute or funny. It's dangerous. Excess weight puts them at risk for heart disease, joint pain, type 2 diabetes, digestive problems, depression, and more. Overweight kids are often the victims of intense bullying, and regularly mock themselves to diffuse the attention of other children. It's heartbreaking! Overweight kids usually become overweight adults with a lifetime of consequences, or worse, become adults who die young.

Instead of shrugging this off, it's time to have a serious conversation with your child's pediatrician and make concrete plans to help them achieve a healthy weight. Just as I've steered you away from diets, your child should avoid them too. Instead, stock your fridge and cabinets with nutritious foods, and trash the harmful stuff. Switch sodas, juices, and energy drinks for water and sugar-free options. Get active as a family, encourage participation in at least one sport, and pursue fitness classes they'll enjoy. Exchange rewards of fried foods and ice cream for adventures like mini-golf, skating, bowling, or paintball.

Have a heart to heart conversation with your child immediately to apologize for allowing things to get out of control, and promise to support them with all your love and resources. A counselor may be a fantastic asset in this process as well. Ask your kiddo what the supercharged version of them looks and feels like, and then love them enough to help make this change. If you think the burdens that come with being overweight as an adult are tough, know that they're tenfold for children. They may resist your efforts at first, so please love them enough to do what it takes to get them healthy!

Chapter 22 | Supercharge Your Family

Winning

Kids who aren't considered athletic should participate in some form of organized physical activity. It's a great way to keep them active and challenge their bodies in various ways. They'll learn to be leaders, followers, humble winners, and graceful losers. Sports provide valuable lessons in teamwork, self-discipline, stress management, and a positive community. Whether they choose dance, lacrosse, volleyball, cheer, karate, swimming, football, or speed skating, sports provide endless benefits to a child's body, mind, and future. Start them young. Nothing is more fun than watching a bunch of three-year-olds play soccer.

Your job as a caregiver is to preserve and protect your children's lives. Be a role model, set standards, and create an environment that fosters health and happiness. Make movement and nutrition a priority, and remember: small changes today can lead to lifelong benefits for your entire family.

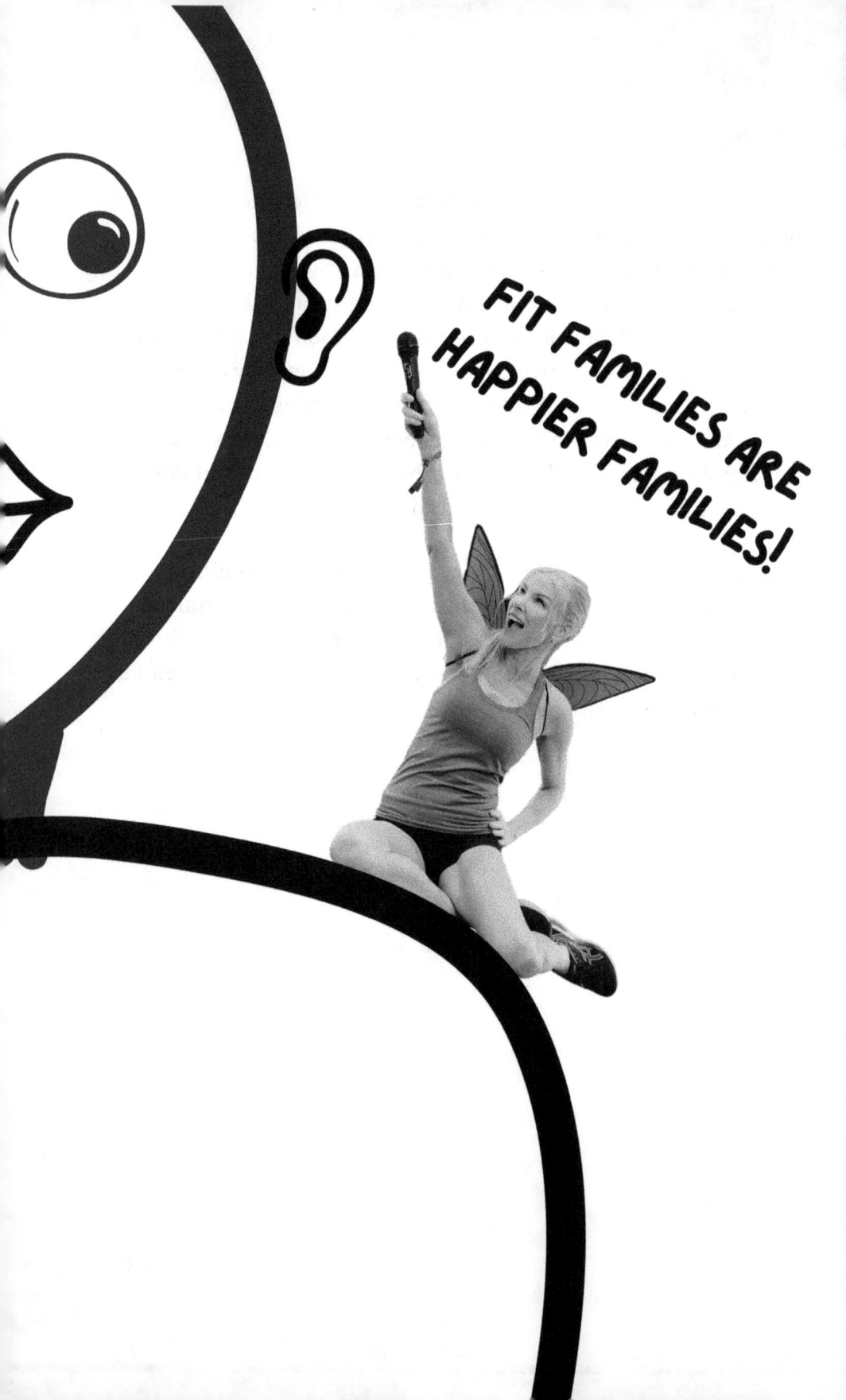

Chapter 23

BUILT TO LAST: AGING LIKE A BADASS

You. Supercharged!

Would you rather be the person who complains about feeling old at 35, or do what it takes to become the one who raves about feeling so youthful at 70? Aging is an absolute privilege! I'll say it again, aging is a *privilege*, and we should be grateful for every single year, day, and second we get. Birthdays should be celebrated, not dreaded, because far too many people have far too few. Half of my mission as a fitness pro is to help people live *longer*. I'm obsessed with tacking on extra years; more time for adventure, chasing dreams, loving your people, learning, laughing, and simply *living*. The other half? Helping people live *better*. Because without quality, what's the point of quantity? Think about it. Do you really want extra years if you're riddled with pain and prohibited from engaging in your favorite activities? Nobody wants to even think about that! So, prepare right now to ensure your golden years truly sparkle.

While many people joke that they don't want to live very long, I'd love to live beyond 100. This is one of the reasons I'm so committed to my health today. Each workout and nutritious bite I take is an investment in supercharging my future as the noisiest running, dancing, and traveling centenarian!

You have the power to extend your life through the smart, healthy habits we've covered in this book, building a body that's vibrant

Chapter 23 | Built to Last: Aging Like a Badass

and powerful from the inside out. You can prevent disease. You can dodge injuries. The amount of control you have to upgrade your life, right now and in the years ahead, is extraordinary. That said, while aging is a privilege, it comes with biological changes that challenge us in different ways.

Before the age of 20, we're practically invincible. Most of us could survive on junk food and soda, pull off acrobatic stunts, recover from injuries overnight, and still feel unstoppable.

From 20 to 50, we (ideally) start maturing. With a magical mix of wisdom and ambition, many begin phasing out bad habits and embracing the good. We start choosing better foods, moving more intentionally, and for many, that first twinge of back pain becomes a blaring wake-up call to join a gym. Career growth, marriage, and parenting push some to pursue peak performance, while others buckle and let their health decline.

Even though plenty of people believe "their best athletic years are behind them," the truth is that many of the world's finest athletes are in this age group. From football to triathlon, boxing to ballroom dance, grown men and women around the globe are *killing it*. They've dedicated their bodies and brains to physical greatness, and the results are extraordinary. You could be in that group, too.

These may very well be your most demanding decades, between professional responsibilities and family obligations. Prioritizing sleep will increase your odds of exercising often and choosing the right foods. You should also commit time and effort to active recovery methods like physical therapy, acupuncture, yoga, foam rolling, and massage. A little TLC goes a long way.

Between 50 and 70, hormones decline, and we naturally lose muscle mass. This is your cue to *fight like hell* to keep it.

Why? Because muscle isn't just for looks, it's strength, stability, posture, metabolism, energy, and confidence. No matter what your past looked like, now's the time to double, maybe *triple*, down on strength training. Do that, and you'll be the supercharged one walking tall while your peers slouch, slow down, and suffer the consequences of neglect.

Your maturity, life experience, and growing value on health should now be working in your favor. Prioritize clean, consistent nutrition, and develop the discipline to manage your intake. Carve out "me time" as a top priority. And if you're partially or fully retired? You've got the gift of time, use it wisely.

Too many people think they can't be super fit with strong pliable muscles at this age. If you think so too, you're wrong. You just have to put in the effort. Tom Cruise was strong and agile enough to crawl across the exterior of an airplane in flight at 62 for a film. He's not actually a superhero. He simply works really hard to stay fit. There's no insurmountable difference between a person like him and you. Your body will respond if you put in the work.

Don't forget, your brain needs a workout, too. Stay sharp by learning new skills, engaging in meaningful conversations, reading, playing games, or picking up a new hobby. A strong mind keeps life exciting and helps delay cognitive decline.

After 70, fitness becomes more important than ever. You're no longer training for spring break or swimsuit season, you're training for *independence*. For doing the things you love: golfing, gardening, dancing, and chasing your grandkids around the yard. Instead of letting your posture deteriorate, your steps slow, or your stability vanish, stay active and agile. Strength, cardio, flexibility, and especially balance training can keep you out of hospitals and nursing homes, and in your own home, doing what brings you joy.

Chapter 23 | Built to Last: Aging Like a Badass

Falling is one of the leading causes of preventable senior deaths. So get serious about staying upright. Add balance-focused activities like Tai Chi and senior-specific fitness classes to your routine. And for the record, as someone who's announced hundreds of running events, I've seen hundreds of men and women in their 80s and 90s cross my finish lines, from 5Ks to full marathons. So yes, sports may *still* be on the table. And if spring break calls, I hope you rock that new swimsuit with pride.

Surround yourself with good people. Laugh, share meals, join clubs, or volunteer. Friendships fuel your soul, and loneliness is toxic, so make human connections part of your health strategy.

From your first day to your last, prioritize exercise, nutrition, sleep, and stress management, and you will dominate each decade. They say time flies when you're having fun, so make your first 100 years so full of joy, laughter, and physical greatness that they *fly right by*.

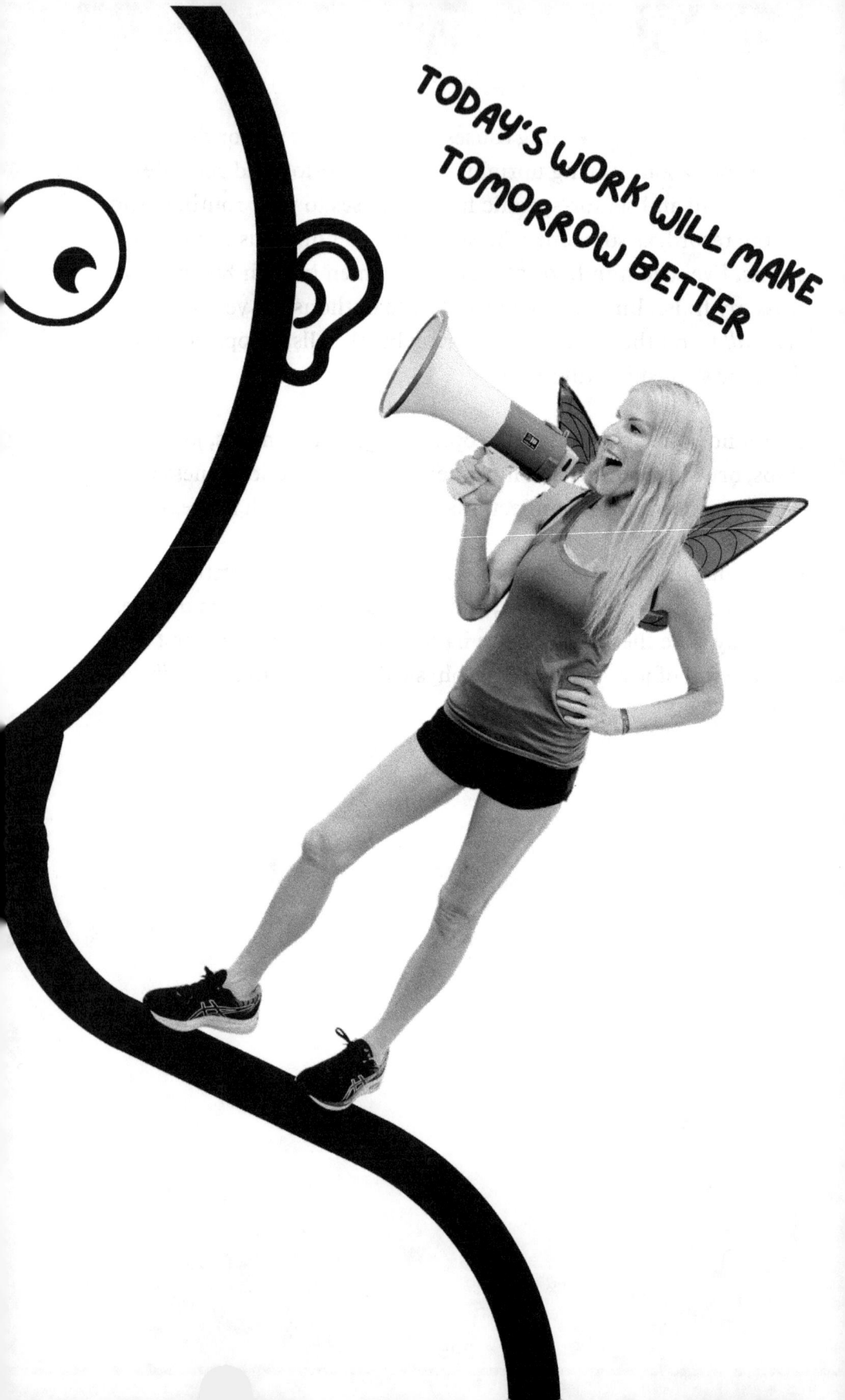

Chapter 24

SO BUSY YET SO SUCCESSFUL

You. Supercharged!

We all get the same 24 hours in a day. If you're telling yourself you're too busy to exercise, I challenge you to rethink that. Let's talk about some of the busiest people on the planet, the presidents of the United States. With the weight of the world on their shoulders, they still find time for fitness. While holding office as the "most powerful men in the world," George W. Bush regularly cycled, Barack Obama shot hoops, and even Bill Clinton made time to exercise (though he had a soft spot for fried food). If these world leaders can prioritize their health, so can you. This book wasn't out when these men were POTUS, but I bet they knew they needed to be supercharged to accomplish everything on their agendas.

Time is What You Make of It

Waiting for the perfect time to exercise? Guess what, it's not coming. Life is busy, work piles up, and family obligations take over. But here's the good news: you don't need hours to get a good workout. Even one minute counts. Can't make it to the gym? Fine. Do a minute of jumping jacks, burpees, or push-ups. String together a few mini-sessions throughout your day, and you'll have done more than most people. You don't need a magical two-hour window to appear. Got five minutes before a meeting? Do some squats. Waiting for your coffee to brew? Knock out some lunges or do a few laps around the office. If you're committed to your fitness, you'll find ways to weave it into your life, no matter how full your schedule is.

Flexibility is Key

Parents, this one's for you. Shuttling kids between sports practices and school events doesn't mean you're sidelined. Walk laps around the field while watching your kids play. Keep a resistance band in your car for quick workouts during their practice. Or stash workout clothes, sneakers, and even a yoga mat in your car, so you're ready to move no matter where you are.

One of my favorite things is seeing people in business attire and running shoes walking on a treadmill during their lunch breaks. They're prioritizing their health without letting a busy workday be an excuse. I've also found that walk-and-talk meetings are a fantastic way to multitask. Whether on a business call or catching up with a friend, you can walk while you talk. The longer the conversation, the more steps you'll take.

Make Up for Missed Days

We all have weeks where work deadlines, family events, and travel fill every moment. If you know what's coming, plan ahead. On Sunday, carve out extra time: an hour of cardio, an hour of strength training, and maybe 30 minutes of stretching later in the day. You can make up for missed days by going harder when you have time. But don't fall into the trap of being a "weekend warrior" who tries to cram it all in. True fitness is built through consistency.

Eating Habits Stay Consistent

No matter how busy you get, your eating habits should never fall by the wayside. It doesn't matter if school is back in session, you're on vacation, or it's the holidays. You are always in control of what you put in your mouth. Don't use a packed schedule as an excuse to abandon your healthy eating habits. You're the one fueling your body, and that's a responsibility you can't afford to neglect.

Have a Plan for When You Slip

Slacking off on your workouts or the Exact Formula may happen on occasion. Of course, we both wish it wouldn't, but that's not reality for most. So it's wise to have a plan in place in case you do. This is when discipline trumps motivation. For the undisciplined person, a loss of motivation can yield catastrophic results. What took a year to build in fitness can vanish in just three months of neglect. Prepare for that. Start by acknowledging your behavior change and consider what will happen if you don't get back on track.

Instead of justifying your poor eating habits or lack of fitness training, write down the reasons you committed to fitness, nutrition, and The Formula in the first place. Embellish that list with all of the positive things you have already accomplished. Once you've declared what you've gained and have to lose, immediately get back to work. Get some sort of exercise and start tracking your Exact Formula immediately. The less time that passes before you recommit, the better.

Reach Out for Support

The other meaningful move you can make is to reach out to friends and ask for encouragement, especially if you both have fitness goals in common. My free online training group is filled

Chapter 24 | So Busy Yet So Successful

with thousands of wonderful, like-minded grown-ups committed to supporting and celebrating each other with fitness. Sometimes a member who has lost a ton of weight and becomes really fit disappears, slides backward, and doesn't reach out for help until they've packed on 75 pounds. If only they asked for help when their good habits started turning bad. If only they spoke up after only gaining five pounds. We could have helped prevent the dramatic backslide. All they needed to do was speak up.

I beg of you, please reach out for support when you need it. If you don't have your own posse, join mine. The Hottie Body Fitzness Challenge Group on Facebook is a powerful place where good people accomplish great things. You can also reach me at Fitzness.com.

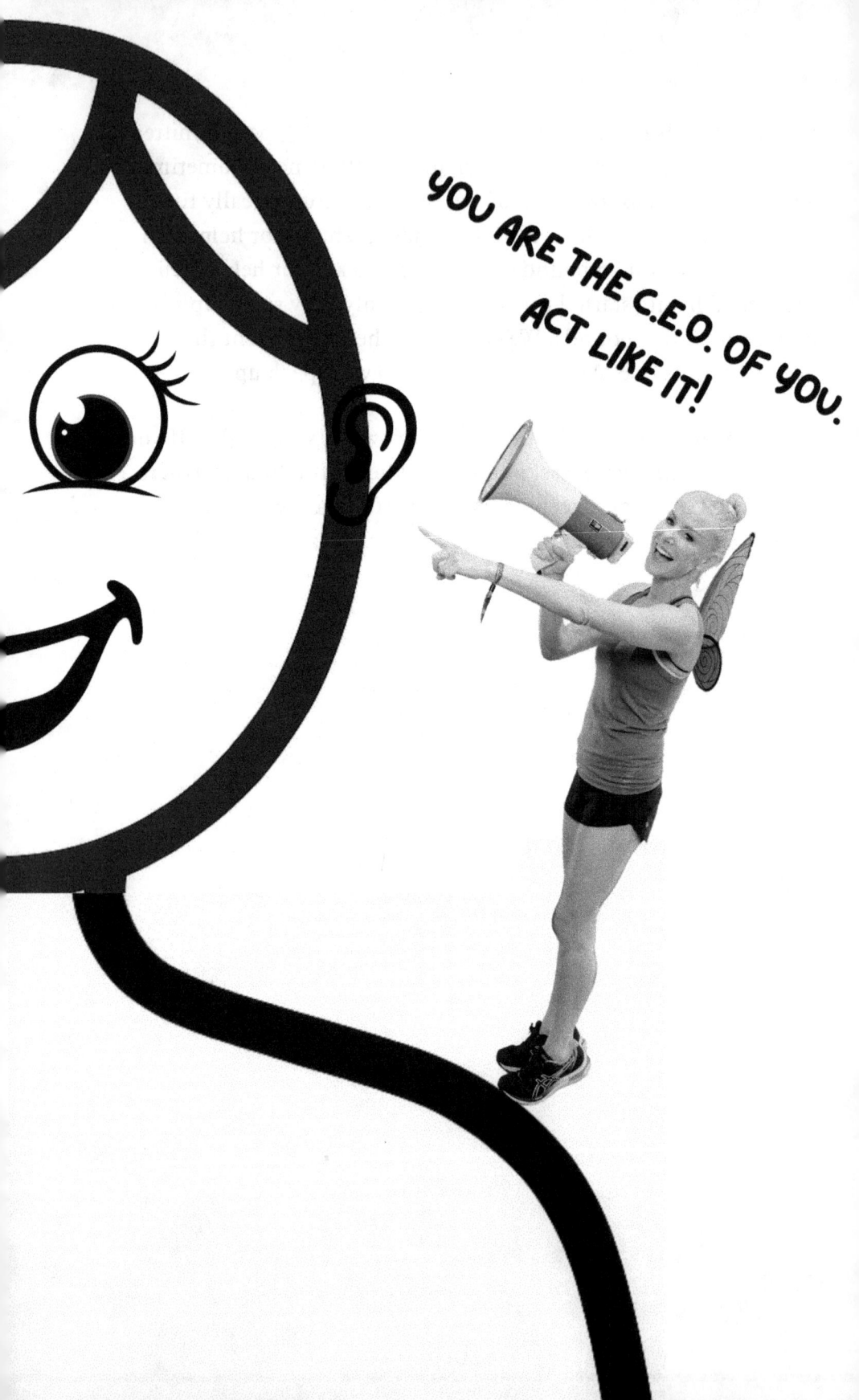

Chapter 25

HIGH TECH HEALTH

You. Supercharged!

Using Social Media & Fitness Tech for Good, Not Evil

Yes, social media can inspire hours of mindless scrolling, isolation, and inactivity. But if you're wise, it can become a powerful force for good, helping you improve your fitness, build healthy habits, and connect with incredible people worldwide. Instead of letting your devices drag you down, let's flip the script and use them to level up your life.

Guidance, Ideas, & Free Workouts at Your Fingertips

There's an app, article, YouTube video, or TikTok for everything, from creative workouts and healthy recipes to expert advice and motivation. Apps are a super source of reminders, step counting, calorie tracking, and even encouragement. Many are free, while others require a small investment. Ask friends for recommendations, read reviews, and try a few free trials to find what works for you. Following @Fitzness on Instagram and YouTube.com/Fitzness is the perfect start. I've created endless amounts of content just for you!

If you prefer to train at home, solo, or on a budget, you'll find free instructional videos for any workout style and fitness level. Whether it's Zumba in your hotel room, yoga on the beach, or strength training in grandma's garage, you can bring an instructor anywhere.

Accountability, Support & Community

Social media isn't all doom and gloom. If used intentionally, it can keep you consistent and connected.

- Proof-of-Effort Posts: Sharing sweaty selfies daily isn't bragging, it's your public form of accountability. The folks in my *Hottie Body Fitzness Challenge* Facebook group post proof after workouts because they know it's expected. These posts create positive peer pressure and inspire others to get moving.

- Supportive Communities: Online groups filled with like-minded folks can be a game-changer. My Facebook group includes thousands of the nicest people on earth who encourage one another through comments, challenges, and genuine friendships. Many have met in person for races, adventures, and meals. These connections have led to genuine friendships, romantic relationships, and even marriages. Most importantly, they've been a force for fitness and health.

- Inspiration & Motivation: From success stories to transformation photos to motivational posts, social media can keep your fire lit, especially on tough days.

Mapping, Tracking, and Progress

Keeping track of your fitness efforts has never been easier. Use apps and wearables to monitor:

- Miles, Steps, and Reps
- Calories (just for tracking, not advice!)
- Nutrition & Sleep
- Workout Frequency
- Transformation Photos

Many gadgets will track and save your stats to show where you started and how far you've come. Just remember that most of these tools are not entirely accurate. Don't rely on them to tell you how many calories you've burned or how much you should eat. Stick with *your Formula*. Use the tools for accountability, not instruction.

Bonus: Want to go hiking, cycling, swimming, camping, or mountain climbing? Apps will show you what's nearby, map your route, track your progress, and even tell you what other users thought of the experience. Seriously, how did anyone manage to do this stuff before?

Sleep Tracking for Sweeter Dreams

The watches and apps that track sleep are mind-boggling. They can tell you how long you slept, which stages you were in, if you were restless, if you snored, and more. For those who struggle with sleep, this info can be shared with a doctor and used to prescribe real solutions. It's like a mini sleep study, on your wrist.

Cool Gadgets Worth Owning

Let's talk about tech. Here are some of the most popular and powerful tools to support your health and fitness journey:

- Watches: Modern fitness watches track steps, monitor heart rate, assess sleep, map workouts, play music, and remind you to stay active. Look for features tailored to your lifestyle, such as waterproofing for swimmers or extended battery life for endurance athletes.

- Fitness Rings: Sleek, lightweight rings worn on your finger that monitor sleep, stress, activity, and more, perfect for those who don't love wrist-wear.

- Heart Rate Monitors: Whether worn as a chest strap, wristband, or watch, these tools help you train smart by measuring how hard you're working. Push harder or ease up with real-time data.

- Pedometers: Prefer to keep it simple? This old-school step counter does the job without all the bells and whistles.

- Smart Scales: Track your weight, body fat, and more. Sync with your apps to monitor trends over time, but don't obsess over daily fluctuations.

- Smart Jump Ropes: Count your jumps, track your speed, and link to apps for an upgraded cardio experience.

- Connected Home Gym Equipment: Bikes, treadmills, and fancy fitness mirrors offer virtual coaching and real-time feedback, right from your living room.

Supercharged Sound

Quality earbuds can make or break your workout. Choose what fits your style:

- Inner Ear: Classic fit, snug in your ear canal.
- Open Ear: Allows outside noise to enter and is safer for outdoor workouts.

- Bone Conduction: The sound connects at your jaw and vibrates through your skull, allowing your ears to remain open. Sounds weird, but the quality is excellent. You'll be more aware of your surroundings.

- Wired: Harder to lose, no charging needed.

- Wireless: Total freedom to move.

- Noise Cancelling: Drowns out distractions.

- Waterproof: Ideal for swimmers and water sports enthusiasts. I use a wireless pair with built-in music storage, which keeps my phone dry and my laps energized. Once I had music to keep me entertained and motivated, my swimming time doubled.

Focus on sound quality, comfort, and durability. Read reviews and shop smart; options exist for every budget.

Safety First

If you're exercising outdoors or alone, make safety a priority by being aware of your surroundings. I recommend skipping music altogether, using only one earbud, or choosing a bone conduction music source. Both men and women alike have been assaulted or struck by vehicles while exercising outdoors, so please don't hinder your hearing, which could alert you to danger. On that note, avoid running in dark places or alone in isolated locations, too. It's just not worth it.

Technology isn't the enemy, it's a tool. And social media isn't inherently evil; it's how you use it that matters. When you scroll with purpose, share with intention, and track progress with perspective, you're putting your devices to work *for* you, not against you.

So go ahead. Post that sweaty selfie. Join that challenge group. Track those steps, laps, reps, and miles, and let your gadgets help you stay on course toward a stronger, healthier, more connected you.

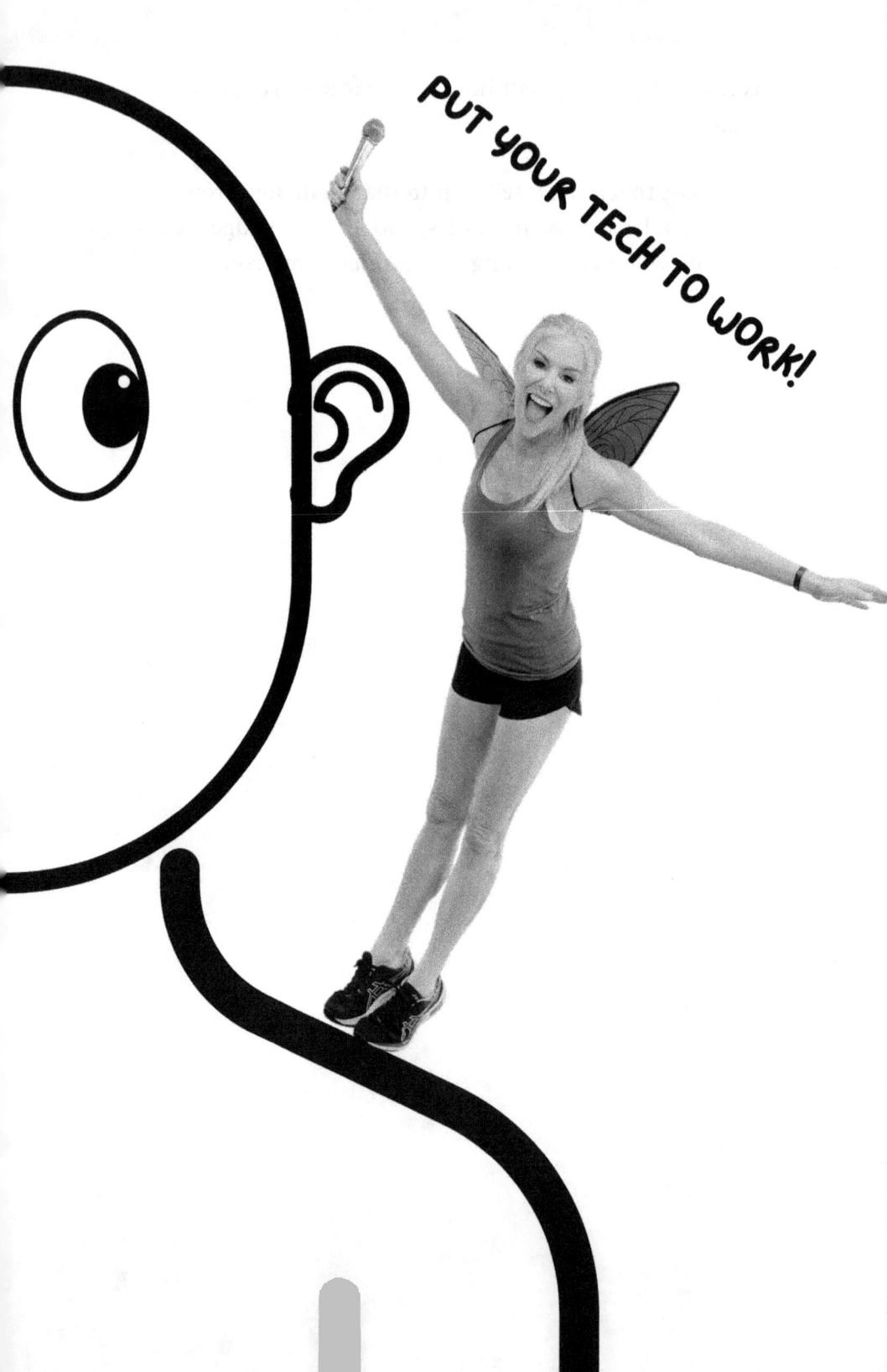

Chapter 26

WORKDAY WORKOUTS

Millions of folks with full-time jobs are also healthy and fit, and you can be one of them. In fact, I'd wager that if you're gainfully employed, you already have the discipline it takes to earn and maintain a supercharged body. You prove that every day you show up on time and do what you're paid to do. That same discipline is the key to regular exercise and to the fit, vibrant body that comes with it.

Now, imagine if your actual job was to work out. You'd get it done, right? Well, the rewards you'll reap from consistent exercise are even more valuable than a paycheck. But why not have both? Why not enjoy the incredible benefits of a healthy body *and* a healthy income? In truth, being fit can *increase* your earning potential. Fitter folks tend to snag the job, keep the job, and climb the ladder. They're sharper, more energetic, more confident, and more creative. And let's be real, strong posture and a glow of vitality are hard to ignore. Healthy employees take fewer sick days and get more done. That's money in the bank for everyone.

If you're currently unfit or overweight and yelling at this page, "I *am* focused! I *am* creative!", maybe so. But the truth is, you'd be *even* more effective if you took better care of your body and mind. And that's what employers want: supercharged humans bringing their A-game to the table. Do you know that people form first impressions within seven seconds? That doesn't leave any room for your résumé or charming anecdotes. When someone sees you for the first time, whether it's a client or a hiring manager, do they think, "Hot damn! That one's got energy, drive, and stamina!" Or do they question your ability to keep up?

Look, you might think I'm being harsh. My editors certainly do, they've been begging me to tone it down. But someone has to tell you the truth. You're not a fragile flower. You're a grown-up with a job and a future to build. The fitter you are, the better your shot at success. This has nothing to do with being an athlete or a supermodel, it's about being *your best*. And when you're operating at your best, you'll blow past obstacles and unlock the kind of greatness most people only dream about.

So let's stop using employment as an excuse to be unhealthy. Use your skills, smarts, and discipline to fit workouts and clean eating into your workday.

Exercise Before Work

Set your alarm earlier. Get it done before the day has a chance to derail you. A morning workout fires up your brain, energy, and focus, and nothing that happens at 3 PM can rob you of a workout already completed. I recommend laying out your clothes the night before to save time and energy in the morning.

Exercise After Work

Stash a change of clothes in your car, desk drawer, or gym bag. Meet a friend at the park or hit the gym on your way home. Unless you're fighting fires or delivering babies, there's rarely a good excuse to skip your sweat.

Exercise On the Way

Walk, bike, skateboard, or rollerblade to work if you live close enough. The fresh air and physical activity are a perfect pairing. Toss some wipes and a fresh outfit in your bag to freshen up once you arrive.

Exercise During Work

Every bit counts. Walk-and-talk meetings? Yes, please. Take the stairs, two at a time. Pace while on calls. Knockout push-ups, squats, or lunges in your office or an empty conference room. Squeeze in ten one-minute workouts a day. If your job includes physical activity, appreciate the built-in perks!

Pack a Lunch Box

Throw it back to elementary school. A cooler bag with healthy snacks, a protein-packed entrée, and a fun design can upgrade your day. Watch your coworkers get jealous.

Dine Like a Boss

Eating out? Go for the grilled protein, veggies, sushi, or quinoa bowl. Order like the champion you're becoming.

Limit the Booze

At conferences or client dinners, you don't need to lead with liquor. And if you're negotiating, know this: your opponent *wants* you to drink. You'll be easier to beat. Don't hand over your power for a glass of pinot.

Chapter 26 | Workday Workouts

Conference Food

Breakfast? Choose eggs, fruit, and Greek yogurt. For lunch and dinner, opt for lean proteins, soups, salads, beans, and veggies. Skip the sugar bombs and white bread.

Explore Corporate Perks

Smart companies aren't just investing in productivity, they're investing in people. A healthy workforce is profitable, and many businesses have finally caught on to that simple truth. Whether you work for a global corporation or a small local business, there may be more wellness perks available than you realize. The catch? You have to ask. Chat with someone in HR, peek at your employee portal, or bring it up at the water cooler, and you might uncover a treasure trove of support and savings.

On-Site Fitness Centers

If your workplace has a gym on the premises, you're sitting on a goldmine: use it. No excuses about traffic, childcare, or weather: it's right there. You could fit in a workout before your shift, during lunch, or right after work without ever leaving the building. That's time-efficient, cost-effective fitness at your fingertips.

Shared Spaces

No full gym? No problem. Many companies have multipurpose rooms or shared spaces stocked with basic equipment, such as yoga mats, resistance bands, stability balls, or dumbbells. Pop in for a few rounds of squats or a quick stretch between meetings. If they're not already stocked, put in a friendly request. "Hey, we've got a closet full of dusty filing cabinets, how about a wellness corner instead?"

Fitness Funding

Plenty of employers will subsidize or fully cover a gym membership, especially if it keeps you healthier and reduces insurance claims. Whether it's a big-box gym, a boutique studio, or even virtual workouts, it's worth asking if there's a reimbursement plan. Even better? Some plans include classes like yoga, spin, martial arts, or Pilates. Get fit on the company dime!

Incentivization Plans

Some businesses straight-up bribe their employees to stay healthy, and we love that. Incentives might include gift cards, extra PTO, cash bonuses, or even discounts on insurance premiums for doing things like logging workouts, losing weight, quitting smoking, or completing wellness challenges. If you're competitive (or just like free stuff), this is your playground.

Corporate Challenges

Step challenges, hydration goals, meditation streaks, stair-climbing contests, these are all common in companies that care about wellness. Not only do challenges make healthy habits more fun and engaging, but they also build camaraderie and positive peer pressure. So sign up, show up, and maybe even win something cool.

Equipment Subsidies

Believe it or not, some companies will help you build your own home gym. They may offer stipends, interest-free loans, or discounted partnerships with fitness equipment providers. Want a treadmill, rower, standing desk, or Peloton delivered to your door without wrecking your budget? Ask your employer. You might be surprised what's possible when you speak up.

Chapter 26 | Workday Workouts

Presentations

Some businesses bring in outside experts (like me!) to fire up the workforce, teach simple and powerful wellness strategies, and motivate teams to take ownership of their health. These sessions can be game-changers. If your company hasn't hosted one yet, be the spark, suggest it to HR or your boss. You might just be the catalyst for a fitter, happier workplace.

Techy Tactics

Fitness trackers, pedometers, and heart rate monitors are small but mighty tools. And companies often hand them out as part of wellness initiatives. They're not just gadgets; they're accountability buddies on your wrist. Tracking your steps, heart rate, and sleep can lead to major gains in health and performance, both on and off the clock.

Team Sports

Workplace kickball team? Yes, please. Company softball league? Even better. Many businesses organize intramural teams for employees, and participating is a fantastic way to blow off steam, bond with coworkers, and sneak in a solid workout. There's something special about wearing your company logo while crushing it on the field. Bonus points if your jersey has a fun nickname like "Boss Buns" or "Cardio Queen."

Coworker Collaboration

Even if your workplace doesn't offer official wellness perks, your coworkers might be just as eager to get moving. Start your own lunch-hour walking group, challenge each other to planking contests, or train together for a local 5K. Start a softball, volleyball, or basketball team and challenge some local businesses to a tournament! Shared goals = shared accountability = shared success.

Bottom line: If your employer offers free or discounted ways to be fitter, healthier, and happier, TAKE THEM UP ON IT. These programs are designed to improve your life, and they work. If they do not offer perks for healthy behaviors, be the squeaky wheel and start the conversation. Corporate wellness begins with people who care, and that's you.

Having a job or owning a business proves that you can make plans and get things done. Instead of using your career as an excuse, make it a motivator. You'll never know how far up the totem pole you can go or how much money you can make unless you're energized, focused, and physically at your best.

Chapter 27

TRAVELING FIT

Whether traveling for work or vacation, eating wisely and staying active are possible no matter where you go. Whether it's domestic or international, healthy food options are always available. Fruit, vegetables, whole grains, and lean proteins are available almost everywhere, and water is easy to find anywhere you go. Airports, train stations, bus terminals, and even gas stations offer healthier choices, too. Salads, fresh fruit, and nutritious snacks are available; you just have to choose them.

Planning ahead makes all the difference. When traveling by air, car, bus, or train, it's easy to pack simple, nutritious snacks. Tossing a banana, tangerine, apple, or some nuts into your bag before heading out sets you up for success. It's just as important to think about your return trip. If your hotel provides breakfast, grab some fresh produce to take with you for later. Many hotels keep fruit baskets at the front desk or in their fitness centers. Don't hesitate to take advantage of these offerings. If not, stop by a grocery store or have healthy options delivered to your hotel using a shop and delivery app. The goal is to avoid relying on vending machines or fast food, both of which tend to be less nutritious.

If you were traveling with an infant, knowing that a hungry baby is a very cranky baby, there's no way you would leave home without formula or baby food. Know this: Hangry (hungry/angry) adults become cranky, too. You need healthy foods just as much as those cute but noisy babies. So, instead of leaving nutrition to chance, prepare! Pack snacks for yourself, with or without a cooler bag.

Staying fueled is just one piece of the puzzle. The other? Staying active, even when you're on the go. Whether you're exploring a new city, commuting between work meetings, or spending hours on a train, there are countless ways to stay active. Every country, state, and town on earth offers free sidewalks, parks, and outdoor spaces perfect for walking, running, or even a quick set of push-ups. The great outdoors is the most reliably accessible fitness facility because it's always open.

Hotel fitness centers are the best, even if they're the worst. These little gyms might not always be top-tier, but a 30-minute workout, whether on a dated treadmill or with bodyweight exercises, is still better than nothing. For extra flexibility, pack light fitness gear like resistance bands or a jump rope, which are easy to carry and great for quick, effective workouts wherever you are. With so many online resources available, it's easy to find workout videos or apps to follow, regardless of location. Fitzness.com is jam-packed with free workout videos and advice. I'd love to exercise with you! Make it a habit to pack sneakers, sports bras, and swimwear.

Consider stopping at safe rest areas or parks for a quick walk or stretch when traveling by car. Take advantage of stops or layovers on longer train or bus rides by moving around, stretching, or walking in place. Airports are the perfect place to get some steps in, especially the large ones. Walking as much as possible before your flight boards instead of just sitting at your gate is a brilliant choice. I've been known to cover more than three miles in large and small airports by walking through each nook and cranny available. A light backpack or wheeled carry-on makes this easier.

Mile-High Movement. Staying active mid-air helps maintain energy, prevent stiffness, and reduce your chances of developing blood clots. When possible, book an aisle seat so you can get up and down without disrupting anyone else. Plan to move about the plane for five minutes each hour you're in the air. I frequently head to the bathrooms on flights, and often stretch while I'm in there, or even as I wait in line to enter. If you're worried that a bunch of strangers you'll never see again will think you're a weirdo, don't. Your health trumps their unimportant opinions.

Reinventing Vacations. The idea of "getting your money's worth" at an all-inclusive all-you-can-eat resort or on a cruise is a common trap. The truth is, no matter how much you eat, it's unlikely you'll consume the cost of your entire vacation in food. Overeating only leads to feeling bloated and sluggish, and it's hard to enjoy your trip if you're feeling weighed down. Returning home in worse shape can be defeating as well.

Adventure Time! Vacation is an opportunity to step out of your comfort zone, try something new, and create lasting memories. Hike a woodsy trail or through a national park, bike through the countryside, snorkel in tropical waters, kayak down a river, or try zip-lining through the rainforest. Supercharge your mind, body and soul with activities that leave a lasting impression, with memories you'll look back on with a smile. You'll never get emotional reminiscing about the countless meals consumed at forgettable restaurants.

If you've had a recent armpit injury or skull replacement, it makes sense if you'd prefer not to sled down a mountain. However, you can cover a ton of mileage and get a bunch of steps in sightseeing on foot. Walking is a wonderful way to tour a new place while benefiting your body, whether you're touring the Colosseum in Rome, the rainforests of Costa Rica, or small-town America.

Hold the Hangover. Alcohol can be a major travel trap. A cocktail here and there is fine. But a weeklong binge-fest? It's counterproductive, especially for those who care about their health. Enjoy a drink in moderation, but don't let it overshadow the experiences that truly make a vacation worthwhile.

Focused Free Time. You can't claim to have no time for exercise when vacation, by definition, is free time. Freed from the daily grind, you should have even more time to move your body. Whether it's a quick morning workout or building an entire day around physical activity, the time is there if you prioritize it. Do not be confused. This is all about mindset. If you are determined to maintain healthy habits at all times, you will. If not, you won't.

Ultimately, traveling is about exploring, experiencing, and enjoying life. Instead of focusing on food and alcohol, shift your attention to the places you'll go, the activities you'll do, and the memories you'll create. Live in the moment, discover new things, and return home feeling better than when you left.

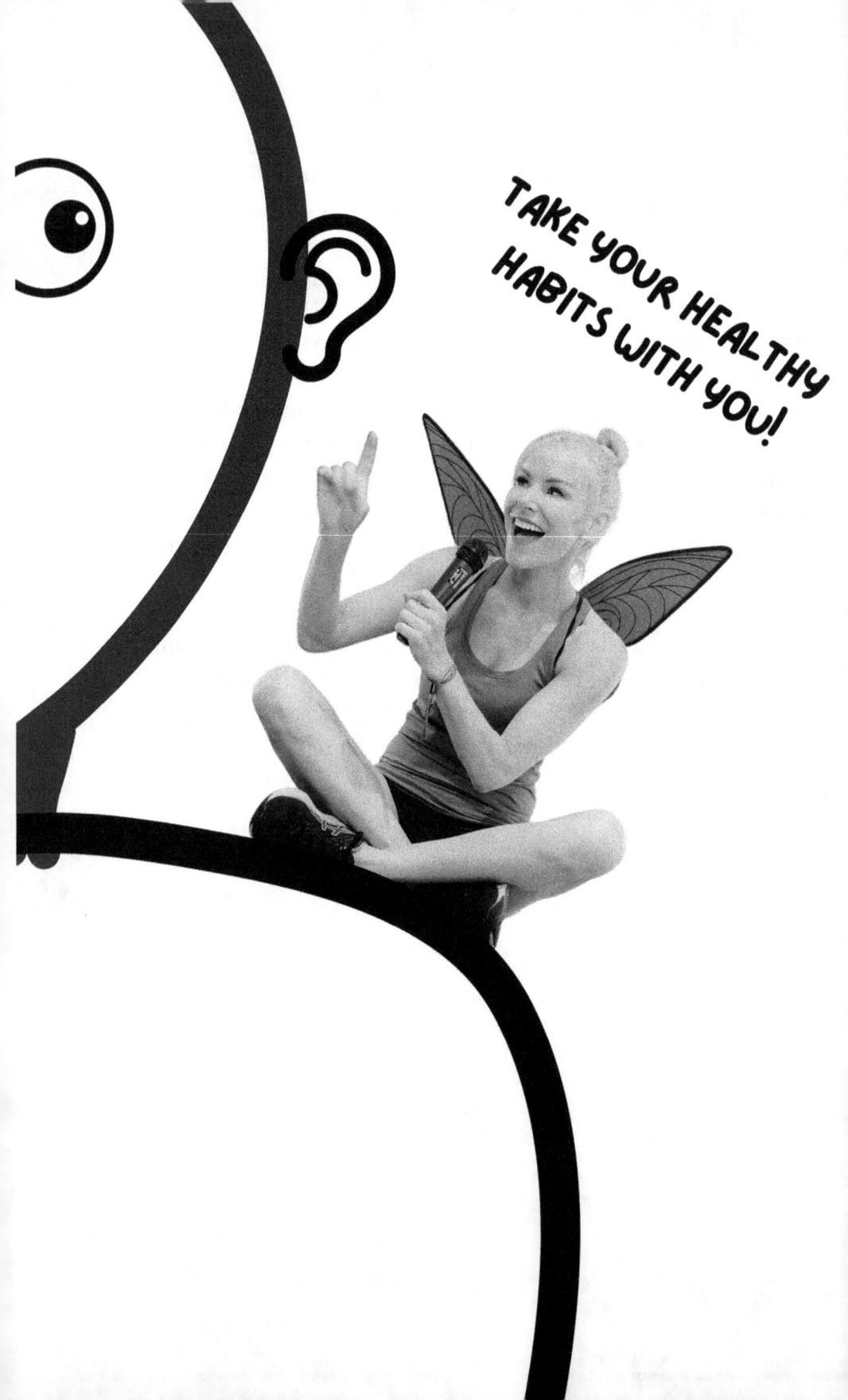

Chapter 28

HOLIDAY HACKS

You. Supercharged!

It's the most wonderful time of the year, fa-la-la-la-la-la-la-la-la. It's also one of the most challenging. Holiday weight gain is a real thing, and while there are some obvious reasons for that, overcoming them is not as hard as one might think. It just requires some know-how, creativity, and discipline. It's said that first-worlders gain between five and eight pounds during the holiday season. Whether that number is accurate or not, it's clear that many of us find it all too easy to pack on some extra weight during this festive season. This happens when we allow our discipline to go "on holiday" and succumb to culture. We're surrounded by parties packed with delicious food, sweets, and cocktails. People are gifting junk food left and right, and with all the holiday activities, exercise often takes a backseat.

So, what can you do to enjoy the season without earning a Santa-esque bowl full of jelly? I've got a stocking full of options to help you enjoy the holidays without regret. With the right strategies, you can fully embrace the festivities and still start the New Year feeling strong and energized. Let's dive into some game-changing holiday hacks!

Supercharged Strategy Sesh

What do you want to achieve by January 1st? Start with a game plan and a snapshot of where you're beginning. Step on the scale,

Chapter 28 | Holiday Hacks

take measurements, and jot down key fitness goals, whether it's losing a few pounds, gaining muscle, or improving endurance. Also, note your energy levels, mood, and stamina for a more holistic approach to health. Tracking progress isn't about pressure; it's about empowerment. Think of this like setting a destination in your GPS; if you don't know where you're headed, you can't map the best route. Define what success looks like for you on January 1st so you can chart a clear path forward.

Exercise Daily

You've set your goals, now it's time to bring them to life. The best way to stay on track? Move daily. Let's take exercise from 'most days' to every day! Carve out time in your schedule for at least 20 minutes of physical activity daily. This could be anything from punching a heavy bag to walking on your lunch break. Daily exercise is a strong defense against holiday weight gain and depression and a powerful tool for stress management, so make it happen.

Stick to the Exact Formula

Your caloric budget should stick with you year-round. Remember? It's not a diet, gimmick, or quick fix. It's your ultimate commitment to managing your intake, earning, and maintaining a healthy weight forever. The Formula doesn't disappear for the holidays; it helps you through them! The beauty of The Formula is that it empowers you to pick and choose your holiday indulgences without going overboard. I promise you that if you stick with The Formula, you'll be able to enjoy the holidays without stressing over unwanted weight gain. Yes, you can have some fruitcake and eggnog if that's your jam, as long as they fit into your daily caloric budget. Isn't that fun? Knowing you can indulge in some fun treats without paying a lengthy price for it should be extremely comforting. Enjoy your favorite treats guilt-free, knowing you're in control. That's what makes The Formula so powerful, it works in every season. Ho! Ho! Ho!

Challenge Accepted

Wouldn't setting yourself up with an athletic challenge make you merry? As Frosty might say, 'Now that'd be cool!' Signing up for a New Year's 5K with a specific time goal would be the perfect way to keep you pushing your limits in fitness, with a laser focus on performing your best. You could also sign up for an indoor swim meet, a ballroom dance competition, or a cross-country skiing race. Whatever your age, there is an opportunity for grown-ups to compete in all categories of sport. Find an event that excites you and commit now!

The Rule of 7

Holidays can get pretty crazy, especially if you work at a school, police department, or office with many people. It may seem like a constant barrage of cookies, brownies, candies, and specialty desserts is attacking you. Sure, these treats come from a generous heart, but do the givers realize how hard it is to stare at a massive tin of specialty popcorn all day without diving in? Talk about temptation! Their thoughtfulness sure does make life difficult for people who struggle with weight.

Unfortunately, I don't forecast an end to the holiday cookie crisis; so instead, I will coach you on how to handle it. Commit to saying 'no thank you' to the first seven treats offered to you each day. Every time you reject an unnecessary treat, your confidence will increase, and politely declining will become less challenging. By the eighth offer, pause and ask yourself: Do I really want this? Is it worth it? Does it fit into my Formula? If yes, enjoy in moderation.

If not, say 'no' again and move on! Remember, you, not the cookie tray, are in control. Small, mindful choices add up to big wins!

Pre-Party Like the Fittest Rock Stars

Not sure your White Elephant party will have healthy options? Eat a nutritious meal beforehand so you're not stuck with foods you'd rather avoid. Take charge of the menu! Bring a fruit tray, salad, shrimp cocktail, or guacamole, so you know there's at least one healthy option.

The Mashed Potato Method

Did you know that you don't have to overeat just because it's a holiday? Technically, you can enjoy any holiday favorite whenever you want! Knowing this takes the pressure off, making it easier to eat a reasonable amount and stop before you regret it. Maybe it's the Irish in me, but I get really pumped about eating mashed potatoes on Thanksgiving. Giddy, even. I think about them, talk about them, and light up like a disco ball when I see them. But even with all of the joy and excitement they bring, I rarely overeat. Why? Because I know that I can eat more every other day of the year. That's right! I can get mashies whenever I want. The same goes for pie, turkey, stuffing, and cranberry sauce. So, instead of giving myself a tummy ache by gobbling up too much, I eat a reasonable amount and then stop. Crazy, right?

And that's the Mashed Potato Method. You can still experience intense enthusiasm for your favorite holiday foods and bliss as they cross your lips. But when the time comes, exercise willpower and put your fork down before you feel sick. Your stomach only holds about a quart of food comfortably, so why push it? Enjoy every bite, but remember, true satisfaction comes from savoring, not stuffing.

Invisible Fences

Resist the temptation to bring holiday goodies into your home. If something is gifted to you, enjoy it in moderation or regift it, but don't keep it around the house. It's easy to stick to a bite or slice of cake and pie when you're at the office, a restaurant, or a party. However, restraint may become exponentially more difficult if a basket, box, or tray of decadent yumminess lands on your kitchen counter. Military strategists know that it's always better to do battle on someone else's land. The same thing goes for you and your efforts to achieve a healthy weight and become fitter. Do not bring sugar bombs into your home. It's not sacrilegious to throw desserts in the garbage. They're just a combo of sugar, butter, oil, refined flours, and dye. Instead of worrying about trashing unhealthy foods, concern yourself with the potential for these unhealthy concoctions to trash your body. Create an invisible dome around your home to keep temptations out. Be a good little toy soldier, and let me hear you: "Ma'am, yes, Ma'am!"

Bake Wisely

I know, I just said to keep tempting treats out of the house, but baking is different. I'm not a Scrooge! Holiday baking is about tradition, creativity, and joy. The key? Make healthier versions and share the love instead of stockpiling sweets at home. Replace butter with applesauce, sugar with stevia or monk fruit, and refined flour with whole wheat. You may even replace the oil in your brownie recipe with black beans (seriously! It's delicious and protein-rich). Small tweaks have a big impact! Oh, and if you're making potato latkes, go easy on the oil or cook them in an air fryer, and please, oh please, send some to me. I'm obsessed. Most importantly, wear a cutesy apron, play some festive music, gather a giggly group of friends, make an enormous mess, and have funzies. When you're done, package all but a few of your extraordinary edibles and spread the joy, because nothing tastes better than sharing!

Family Time

The holidays are about gratitude, celebration, and time with loved ones, so why not make movement part of the fun? Take an after-dinner stroll, play a backyard game, or a round of Twister. Staying active isn't a chore, it's just another way to make memories. And if all else fails? Crank up some holiday music, turn your living room into a dance floor, and try Rockin' Around the Christmas Tree.

Track Your Progress Weekly

Step on the scale once weekly, not as a punishment, but as a checkpoint. Celebrate progress, and if you notice changes, tweak your habits accordingly. And don't just track your weight, log your steps, strength training, and workouts to see how far you've come. Your progress is more than just a number on the scale. Whether it's lifting heavier, cycling farther, or feeling more energized, tracking helps you stay on course and motivated throughout the season!

Put a Bow On It

If you've met your goals by the time the New Year rolls around, take a moment to celebrate. A healthy body and mind are gifts in themselves, but there's nothing wrong with rewarding your hard work. Whether it's a spa day, a new outfit, or an adventure you've been eyeing, choose something that feels meaningful and reinforces your success.

Supercharge each holiday season to feel jolly and bright. With your strategy set and Fitzy, the bossiest little elf on your shoulder, you've got a clear path for getting to New Year's Day, fitter than you were in October. Stick to your plan, stay mindful, exercise daily and enjoy your favorite treats in moderation. These strategies won't take the fun out of the holidays; they'll help you enjoy them without regret. That way, when the clock strikes midnight on January 1st, you'll be toasting to your success, not scrambling for a reset. Cheers to that!

Chapter 29

RUNNING, WALKING, AND RACING

You. Supercharged!

Left foot, right foot, left foot, right foot ... doesn't seem like it could be such a big deal, but holy hell, it can be life-changing! Running, walking, and racing are getting their very own chapter in this book for a few reasons (cyclists, swimmers, dancers and lifters, please know I love you all the way too). My commitment to and enthusiasm for this type of exercise have monopolized an enormous portion of my career, personal fitness, and the lives of so many I guide and support. Excuse me if I seem like I'm playing favorites. I am.

Running and walking are spectacular choices for cardiovascular fitness because they are skills most able-bodied people have, and very little instruction or equipment is required. Could you run barefoot and naked if a cranky moose were chasing you? Indeed, you could. And that is precisely what makes these activities a superb choice. When we remove the need for equipment, rhythm, skills, coaching, and expertise, we remove almost all our excuses not to exercise.

The other tremendous gift that comes with these simplistic forms of exercise is the opportunity for friendship, travel, athleticism, and competition. While it becomes increasingly more difficult to join a cheerleading or lacrosse team as we age, though not impossible, you can run, walk, and race until you're dead, even if you live past 100. Through my work as a professional race announcer, I have seen thousands of incredible folks in their 80s, 90s, and a few beyond 100 cross finish lines. Plus, the community is incredible! We're friendly, supportive, silly, and sometimes travel worldwide to race.

In 2011, I launched a before-school walking and running program called The Morning Mile, which has since been implemented at more than 400 schools across America and several countries. Why did I choose walking and running when I could have created a program for kids to play games or sports? Because I crave mass impact. My specialty is getting enormous numbers of people to move and keep moving. Can everyone play soccer, and will they want to? Does everyone have equipment? Figuring that out could get complicated. But with The Morning Mile, we provide a 30-minute window for kids, their families, and the faculty to show up and do an exercise they already know how to do. They can wear what they want and go at whatever pace makes them happy. Want to walk really slow in your cowboy boots and dress while chatting with your besties? Fantastic! Want to run really fast in sneakers and your school uniform? Cool. Coaching isn't even encouraged at The Morning Mile. The only thing we encourage is moving forward. And the beauty of that is these kids can continue this habit they've learned at school into their 20s, 50s, and 90s.

Schools that implement The Morning Mile often have over 100 participants each morning and surpass 90% participation throughout the school year. That's because it's fun, everyone knows how to walk or run, there's no pressure, and the reward system is fantastic. I like to "keep it simple stupid," and this simple turnkey program has yielded millions of miles. Morning Milers aren't just fitter, they learn and behave better too. Proof that starting each day with exercise can enhance our entire day. Oh, and if you had any idea how many parents, teachers, and bus drivers have benefited from this school program, you'd fall over. It just works!

Did you know that running is the largest participation sport in the world? And even with that, the number of people who walk for fitness is three times larger. The National Football League (NFL) is proud to squeeze 60,000 fans into their stadiums to watch about 100 athletes mix it up on Sundays each fall. Many road races worldwide have 60,000 or more athletes show up at the start line. Can you imagine if every person in each stadium were actually there to compete? I can, because road racing is enormous and I've been a part of those massive events. Of course, the NFL is a magical, money-generating spectacle that brings endless joy and excitement to millions. Still, the running industry is comparatively colossal when it comes to players playing. The NFL has about 1,700 active athletes on their roster annually. That amount would be considered a small event for just one race taking place in one town, and hundreds of races take place each weekend throughout America alone.

Globally, it is estimated that 600 million adults run and several billion walk for exercise. Hopefully, these ginormous numbers encourage you to join us. If you are looking for a simple cardio workout that you can do anywhere and anytime for zero dollars, running and walking are for you. Prefer a gentle workout? Walking is one of the best. Want to increase your cardiovascular fitness while burning a ton of calories? Running will make you huff and puff in a big way. Hoping to improve your bone density? Both are great options.

Even though running was something we did as children for fun and play, grown-ups often begrudge it. I hear you. Running is challenging. It can make you feel winded and weak, fatigue your legs, and tax your will to keep going. Those things are also why running is wonderful. You know how to run, and that's a way

Chapter 29 | Running, Walking, and Racing

better start than if you were to try fencing or ballroom dancing. The hard part is what makes you better, physically and mentally. Instead of shying away from running because it's challenging, pursue it to take your physical and mental health to the next level. Even with its formidable reputation, running can be fun! Remember running in the rain? When's the last time you bolted across a parking lot in a storm to avoid getting soaked? It was exhilarating, right? If doing that has ever made you giggle, you're likely one of us.

Can't run because you have some sort of knee, spine, or foot condition that permanently prevents you from doing so? Fine. Walk! Walking is terrific and can be incredibly challenging, too. If you pick up the pace or walk up an incline, you can turn this low-impact activity into a serious sweat session, entirely dictated by your own pace.

Let's talk about pace. Whether you are walking or running, your speed is your business. Seriously, whatever pace makes you huff and puff is the perfect pace. Who cares if you are as fast as you or your friends were 10 years ago? That's not the point! You exercise to challenge the body you have today, not to outdo some rando on the treadmill next to you. That would be odd. Having said that, if you have a competitive streak and can use it wisely to make you better, more power to you. Just don't allow a lack of speed to prevent you from getting going. Some of my favorite running groups have adopted turtles and sloths as their mascot. Their slower paces do not prevent them from covering an incredible number of miles. On the flip side, you could totally be a badass speedster at any age. With the proper training and quality nutrition, you could begin running at any age and become one of the best, at least in your age group. Runners are generally judged against their peers in five to ten-year age brackets.

Racing, and I use that term loosely, is something you should consider. I know it can sound intimidating, but I'm confident that you'll take more interest once you understand who the "racing" community is. Racing can be serious, like the Boston Marathon or the Carlsbad 5000, where major prize money is awarded for speed. It can also be exclusively for fun and/or fundraising, like a local 5K where nobody gets a shirt or medal, and no winners are declared. The great majority of races are of the casual, unserious variety. But even with most of the bigguns, almost everyone can register, and running is not required.

Common race distances include the marathon, half marathon, 10K, 5K, and one mile. Note that the ONLY race that should be called a "marathon" is one that covers 26.2 miles. Period. A 5K isn't a marathon. A half marathon is 13.1 miles, you guessed it, half the distance of a marathon. 10K is 6.2 miles. 5K is 3.1 miles. And I have no idea why the world has chosen to flip-flop between miles and kilometers for distances, but they have. It's confusing and weird, and I apologize for whatever weirdos made this decision. An ultramarathon is any distance over 26.2 miles, and yes, many folks test their physical and mental limits with 100- and even 250-mile races. Also, you may stumble across random distances like 6K, 8K, 10-miles, 18-miles, and more. Race organizers can make up their own fun, and I encourage you to try it all. Why not?

More things you should know about racing:

You Don't Have to Run. That's right. Many people do run, but an equal number exclusively walk. It's common for many to alternate between running and walking. If you want to walk, go ahead and walk. Walkers are welcomed, wanted, and celebrated. Period.

Chapter 29 | Running, Walking, and Racing

It's Social! Whether you put some miles in with a friend, join a run club, or attend races, you're bound to make new friends.

Travel to Travel. Flying or driving somewhere to traverse on foot is a stellar way to see the sights. Once folks get comfy racing at home, they often branch out to do so in a new place. Many totally "normal" people, I point this out because you may think I'm talking about Olympic superstars, make destination racing a big part of their lives. Mid-race, many even stop to take pictures. Some commit to running a race in all 50 American states or all seven continents. There's even a challenge where you can run seven marathons on seven continents in seven days. These commitments are a clever way to fill your life with exercise and adventure.

Goal-Setting Gold Mines! Registering for a race of any distance is the perfect way to commit to regular training. Keeping a race on your calendar will add structure to your workouts.

Walking Events. Did you know that some events discourage running? These events are usually focused on raising funds for a special cause, and you might feel silly if you do run!

Age Group Awards. Although races that give prizes recognize overall winners, most will recognize champions for both genders and age group speedsters in five- or ten-year brackets.

Causes and Community. If you're not inclined to race for your own health and enjoyment, perhaps you'll do so to support a cause that's near and dear to your heart. Whatever inspires you to get involved, the benefits to your body and soul are the same.

Party in the Back, and the Front! Believe it or not, racing is also the silliest sport on earth. Many run in crazy costumes such as princesses, pirates, tacos, and bananas. Some races have wild themes like the Zombie Run, Mrs. Roper 5K (everybody runs as old ladies in house dresses), and Santa Runs.

Spectating is a Sport, too. Race fans are serious. They set up party tents along our courses, pass out snacks (sometimes alcohol), and make and wave funny signs for all. "Worst Parade Ever!" is one of my favorites.

Obstacle Course Racing (OCR). Combining walking, running, mud, and obstacles is a thrilling way to test your talents in fitness. It's also an insane amount of fun. There's never a monotonous minute in an OCR because your course is broken up by walls to climb over, nets to crawl under, and muddy ditches to wade through. Some are designed with a high level of physical strength required, and some focus on silliness with bounce houses and other inflatables to navigate. No matter which you choose, you can always try an obstacle; if you can't conquer it, move along to the next. Participants are encouraged, never shamed. And my favorite part? The giggles and belly laughs! OCRs are packed with fun, whether you can or can't do a challenge, they're always a great time.

If you're convinced to try running and walking or you're already deeply embedded in our community, I'm shaking my big pink cowbell for you. Now here's some advice: Don't just run. That's right. I've spent multiple pages telling you how much I want you to run and walk, but that can't be all you do. Sadly, runners tend to only run. Walkers tend to only walk. No matter how serious you decide to be about it, you MUST work on the other three Pillars of Fitness: strength, flexibility, and balance. If you don't do so, you will eventually pay the consequences of lacking true fitness or suffering injury.

Putting in many miles has many benefits, but it can also yield real consequences if you're not smart. Common runner issues like IT

Chapter 29 | Running, Walking, and Racing

band syndrome, piriformis syndrome, and plantar fasciitis often stem from overuse, tightness, and weakness. If you stretch often, you will not be tight. If you strength train, you will not be weak. You won't deal with overuse injuries if you manage your miles wisely and complement your training with other cardio options like cycling and swimming. If you balance train and miss a step, you'll be less likely to eat the pavement.

The Everything Exercise chapter has a ton of strength, stretching, and balance exercises for you. I'd also like for you to do my Strength Training for Runners workout, which you can find on the cover of Fitzness.com and on my Fitzness YouTube channel. It's free, it's about 12 minutes long, and was specifically designed to help you run further, faster, and pain-free. If you were on a collegiate running team, you would have a strength and conditioning coach who would make you do the exercises I demonstrate in this video. If you do not do them now, you will eventually be instructed to do them by a physical therapist. Skip the pain and suffering and do the work upfront.

Running and walking should be one of your supercharging staples—your go-to, your lifetime backup plan, the failsafe. Do it outside to get fresh air, or inside on a treadmill when the weather is foul, the sky is dark, or you just need to be in. Let it be a source of alone time, adventures with your dog, new friends, competition, socialization, and travel. A tremendous form of cardiovascular and bone-building fitness, the challenge of taking on miles or time on your feet will test your will, determination, and ability to celebrate your accomplishments. Speaking of celebrating your achievements, I'd love to be a part of that. When looking for races, visit Fitzness.com and check out my race announcing schedule. Wouldn't it be fun if the Lil Fitzy on your shoulder came to life, and the real Fitzy was able to give you some noisy love and a finish line hug? I think so.

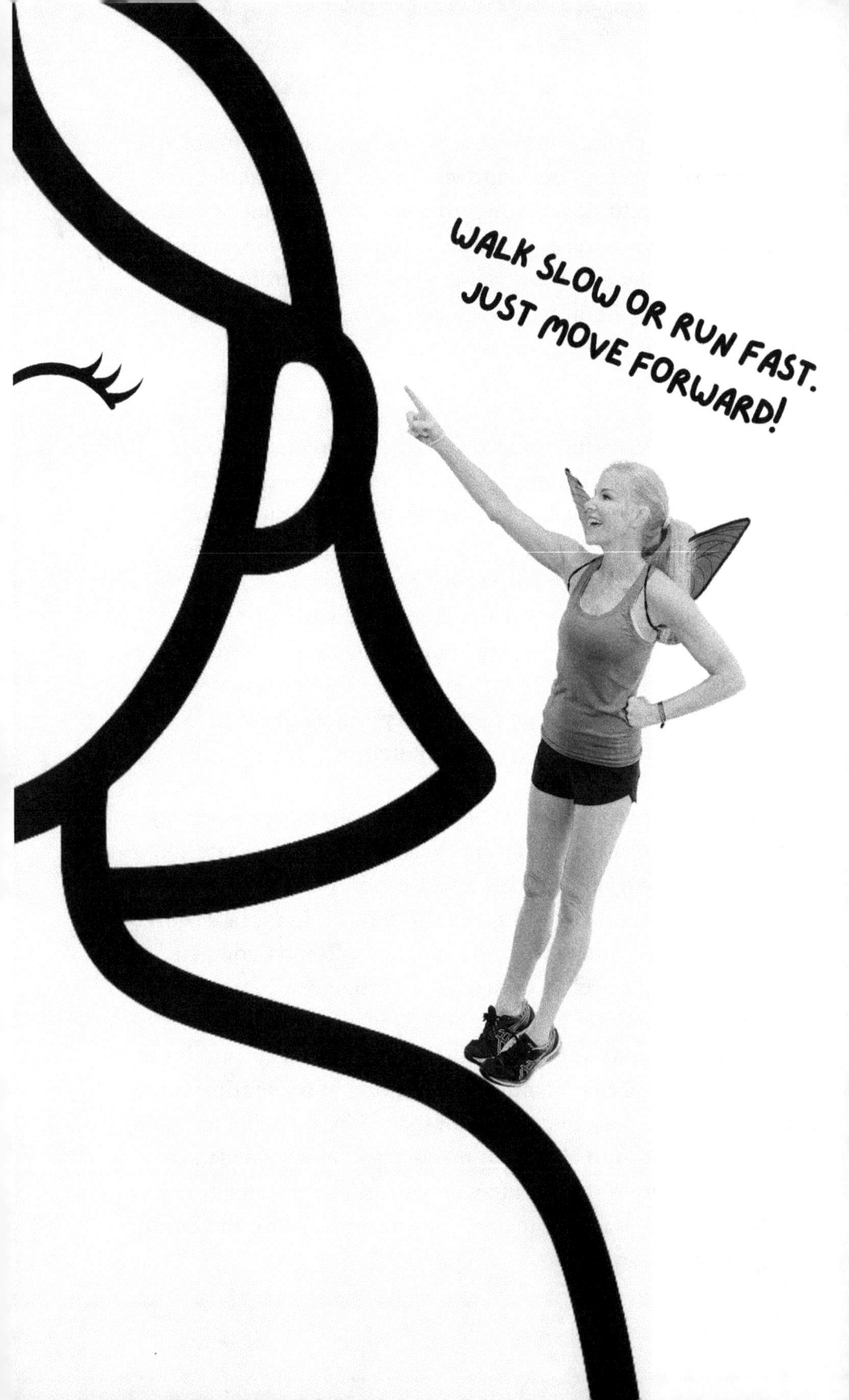

Chapter 30

WHY YOUR EXCUSES ARE LAME

I've heard them all. Every freaking excuse on the planet has passed through my ears, and I've got to tell you, only one in a thousand has been legit, if that. Folks, if you sincerely want to supercharge your body and mind, you will always find a way. If you're half-hearted about it, you will find an excuse. Sure, life can be difficult. Stuff happens. None of it is a valid justification for neglecting your health, though, because there is no overlap between being a supercharger and an excuse-maker. You are either one or the other. So if lame excuses start swirling through your mind or floating out of your mouth, brace yourself: Lil Fitzy will be winding up to smack you on the back of the head to pop that nonsense out of you.

As we review some favorites, I have tried not to be too abrasive. But if I have failed to coddle you enough, #SorryNotSorry. If you're disappointed that I'm not being snarky enough, you can enjoy my full wrath by listening to my podcast, *The Fitzness Show*. Nobody edits my big mouth but me.

I've got no time to exercise.

We all have 168 hours in a week. You're not too busy. You're just prioritizing other things over your health. Let's be honest: if you have time to scroll social media or watch TV, you have time to move. Think about it: you brush your teeth every day, no excuses.

Chapter 30 | Why Your Excuses Are Lame

Your smile is important, sure, but you can live without perfect teeth. You can't live well with an unhealthy heart. If you wouldn't skip brushing, why would you skip caring for the one muscle that keeps you alive? If you can make time for dental hygiene, you can make time for your physical health.

Thirty to 90 minutes is ideal, but even if you don't have a big chunk of time to dedicate to fitness, you can build in small increments of exercise throughout your day. For example, 90 seconds of push-ups or burpees can be incredibly challenging and effective. If you don't think so, pause, put this book down, and try 90 seconds of either. Now, apologize for doubting my advice! You owe me a hug.

The all-or-nothing mindset, thinking that if you can't do a long workout, it's not worth doing anything at all, is nonsense. Small efforts count. You can fit in exercise by making an appointment with yourself and sticking to it. Put it in your calendar, set an alarm, and don't let anything interfere unless it's a true emergency.

If you're out walking and someone calls, make it a walk-and-talk meeting. Multitask if needed, but keep your body moving. The reality is that time is not an excuse. Even the busiest people on the planet, CEOs, world leaders, and doctors, make time to work out because they know it makes them sharper, stronger, and more effective. If they can fit it in, so can you. No more excuses. It's time to move.

I'm too tired.

Too tired to exercise? That's exactly why you need to do it. Feeling drained usually isn't a sign to skip movement. It's a symptom of not moving enough. The irony is that exercise itself builds energy by releasing adrenaline and endorphins. Think of yourself as a solar panel, and exercise is your sunlight. Like solar panels need the sun, your body needs movement to stay powered up. The more you move, the more energy you generate. If you sit still too long, you'll feel drained, sluggish, and stuck in low-power mode. And don't overthink it. Just move. Get up, lace up your shoes, and go. Within minutes, you'll start to feel energized, and that burst of ZING will carry you through. The first few workouts might be difficult, but soon, your body will start to crave exercise, and skipping it will feel worse than getting it done. So stop waiting to 'feel' energized. Move first, and the energy will follow. Also, if you're tired because you ran your first marathon or did two boot camp classes in a row, it's fine to take a day off or at least have an easy day.

I don't know how to exercise.

Come on now. If you can learn to fix a random car part on YouTube, you can learn how to exercise. There's a video tutorial for just about everything, and plenty of people dishing out free advice on every topic imaginable, including me! Not sure where to begin? I've spent decades building a free fitness library at Fitzness.com. Whether you need to tighten your core, decrease hip and knee pain, or learn an entire strength training for runners workout, you'll find step-by-step guidance at Fitzness.com. If I disappear tomorrow, you'll still find everything you need, including thousands of articles, fitness videos, recipes, success stories, and more. So, if you're saying, "I don't know how to do that," look it up! You can learn from books, podcasts, and friends. Ignorance isn't an excuse anymore. The knowledge is out there; you have to be willing to look for it. Have I told you how happy I am that you're reading this book?

I can't afford a gym or a trainer.

But you don't need those things. You can stand up and do jumping jacks right now. That's exercise! You don't need a gym, and you

Chapter 30 | Why Your Excuses Are Lame

don't need a trainer. Sure, they have their perks, and spending money on your health is never frivolous. Consider a $7 latte frivolous. On the other hand, fitness is an investment in your length and quality of life, and it's something worth prioritizing.

But let's be honest, we all have budgets. The sidewalk? Free. The park? Free. Push-ups, burpees, and lunges, all free. It doesn't matter how much money you have; some of the fittest people in the world live in poor countries, running barefoot and still staying incredibly fit because they prioritize it. And on the flip side, some billionaires are morbidly obese. So, no, money isn't the issue. Use the ground beneath your feet, the free, accessible space around you, and get moving. You don't need a gym membership to take control of your fitness.

It takes too long to grocery shop and prepare healthy meals.

Oh, please. Do you know what the quickest, most uncomplicated food is? An apple. It takes no time at all. You can even grab one at the gas station while you're filling up. Eating healthy doesn't have to be time-consuming. In fact, nothing is quicker than raw produce. You can also throw together the simplest meals with any combination of raw or cooked fruits and veggies, canned beans heated in the microwave, and a side of instant whole-grain rice. Boom! Dinner.

On busy days, I eat what I call "counter food," which consists of the stuff I leave on my kitchen counters. Bananas, tomatoes, potatoes, nuts, and other simple grab-and-go foods. Is it fancy? Nope. Is it all healthy, quick, and convenient? Damn right. Simplicity is key, but you can easily mix things up with various fresh or frozen fruits, vegetables, proteins, and whole grains. Use simple cooking techniques like the toaster, roaster, steamer, air-fryer, and microwave to cook hot food in a hurry. If shopping feels like too much, invest in a grocery or produce delivery service subscription and let a professional shopper drop the good stuff right at your door. Eating healthy can always be fast, easy, cheap, interesting, and delicious!

My friends are overweight, so it's okay if I'm overweight too.

Be the reason your group gets healthier, not heavier! It's easy to feel better about bad things when you are sharing the experiences with friends. But the risks of obesity don't disappear just because others around you are facing them, too. The threats to the quality and length of your life do not diminish just because you feel more comfortable amongst your larger peers. Instead of blending in, lead the way by making positive changes for your health, achieving your ideal weight, and inspiring your pals to do the same. Invite them for workouts and trade dinners for bowling or painting dates. You can create a circle of support where everyone lifts each other up.

My friends are tiny, so I need to be tiny.

Nonsense! Fitness is not about being tiny; it's about being the healthiest version of yourself, regardless of size, and being tiny does not necessarily equal healthy. Whether your build is tall, short, slight, or strong, being healthy isn't about a number on the scale; it's about fitness, energy, and being mentally well. Your health should be about how you feel in your body, not how it compares to someone else's. I'm sure you and your friends have some far more exciting qualities in common, such as your hobbies and sense of humor. If you are at your healthy best and are bigger, don't starve yourself into their weight category; just offer to open the pickle jars when necessary.

My family is overweight, and that's why I'm overweight.

It's easy to think that if your family is overweight, it's just part of your genetic destiny, but that's not true. Obesity is not inherited,

Chapter 30 | Why Your Excuses Are Lame

it's learned through habits. Yes, body types can be passed down, but the habits that lead to obesity can be changed. You CAN and SHOULD adopt different habits than your loved ones. That's clearly on your agenda because you're reading this book, but it's imperative that you understand how much control you have. If you adopt The Formula, pursue quality nutrition, and exercise wisely and religiously, your body will have no choice but to respond. You can change more than your fate with this effort, too. Improving your fitness and achieving a healthy weight will prove to your relatives and future generations that they are not destined to be overweight either. You will prove that a fit body can be achieved with an intelligent plan, determination, and consistency.

I can't get fit because I have kids.

Let's change this to "I have to become and remain fit because I have kids." Those fabulous humans you've created or adopted should be your incentive, not your excuse! I know it's not easy. Between your job, caring for your kids, and all the other responsibilities, it can feel like there's no time for anything else. But taking just a few minutes a day to prioritize your health can make a huge difference, for you and your family.

I know you want to live up to your obligation of providing care, support, and guidance for them as long as possible. You cannot ignore your health because the consequences are guaranteed to impact your children negatively. The most shocking excuse I hear is when parents say, "I can't exercise because I have kids." Seriously? Blaming your kids for your lack of fitness? That's not fair to them. Imagine them spending their childhood hearing, "I'd be in shape if it weren't for the kids." Then, one day, you drop dead at 45, and your kids think, "Oh, it's my fault. Mom couldn't exercise because of me." Cruel.Flip the script. Say, "I have kids, a spouse, or elderly parents I love, so I need to take care of myself to be here for them." Use your family as motivation! You love your people, right? So do whatever you can to grow old together. If you keep putting off your health, you risk your ability to enjoy years of meaningful moments and memories. Depriving your family of your energy, presence, or life because you're "too busy" is not okay.

Let me tell you about a woman I know who didn't let her family stop her. Her husband had a serious injury, and instead of saying, "I'm his caregiver, so I can't exercise," she went and got herself three gym memberships. Yep, three. That way, no matter what medical appointment he had, whether it was physical therapy or a hospital stay, she found a way to exercise. She knew that to take care of him, she had to be in the best shape of her life.

You also bear the burden of being a role model, so commit to fitness and get your family involved. Make physical activity and healthy eating a family activity. Play Frisbee, wrestle in the living room, go swimming, and prepare nutritious meals together. You can change your family tree. If you come from a family with unhealthy habits, stop that cycle immediately. Most families aren't genetically predisposed to obesity, they've just passed down bad habits. Poor eating and lack of exercise are what leads to relatives suffering from diabetes, heart disease, and other health issues.

Be the one to slam on the brakes. Don't tolerate obesity or bad health in your family anymore. It's your job to lead the way and make a U-turn toward health. I'm excited for your entire clan!

I'll do it tomorrow.
No, you won't. Tomorrow's workout rarely comes, so get to work today. What you need right now is discipline. Instead of doing it by yourself, put me on your shoulder and let me help. That's right. Imagine a mini-Fitzy sitting on your shoulder, a little voice of reason reminding you that every moment counts. When that lazy voice says, "I'll do it tomorrow," mini-Fitzy chimes in with, "No, you won't, get moving now!" Skipping today means tomorrow's

Chapter 30 | Why Your Excuses Are Lame

workout might feel tougher, and each day you put it off makes it harder to get back on track.

Put on your shoes. Walk the dog. Dance in the kitchen. Head to the gym. Whatever it is, get your body moving. Lil Fitzy is a pro at the P.I.T.A. treatment, reminding you that each day matters. You've got 24 hours in this day, and if you're not actively working on your fitness, guess what? You might be falling behind. Maybe your back's a little stiffer, your calves a little tighter, or you've lost some endurance. Lil Fitzy won't like that, and neither will you.

By staying consistent, you'll see improvements in strength, flexibility, and energy levels. And the best part? Every day you commit makes tomorrow that much easier. Your future self will thank you!

P.I.T.A. = Pain in the Ass

I'm too sore to exercise.

Severe soreness is a legitimate reason to dial it back, but more importantly, it's a reminder not to go overboard. Doing too much too soon or trying to impress others with your workouts is foolish. I know it can be hard to gauge how much is too much, but you should at least try, and use this hard lesson learned for the next time. If you can't sit on the toilet or brush your hair without pain, take the day completely off or do gentle activities like swimming, walking, or stretching.

I can't exercise because I work the night shift.

Are you suggesting that humans cannot exercise between midnight and 8:00 a.m.? That's strange. So, your schedule is different from the norm, you still have the same 24 hours in a day as everyone else. Make time to exercise in large or small chunks before, after, or during whatever hours you work. You may have to find a 24-hour fitness center or other safe places to exercise during late-night hours, but there are always plenty of options, including your home. Night shifts can be tough, and adjusting your sleep and exercise schedule might take some time. But you can start small, perhaps a 10-minute workout when you wake up, or stretching and walking after your shift. You still have 24 hours in a day. Make the most of them.

I'm too embarrassed to go to the gym.

If you're genuinely concerned about what people think, how about you work to impress everyone with your commitment? Honestly, shame has no role in fitness, but this comment tells me you're prioritizing the wrong things. Whatever your fitness level, know that you instantly become part of the cool club when you enter a fitness center. Your mere presence earns you the respect that comes with being part of the group of people who care about their health and are doing something about it. Fit people wish everyone would give exercise a try. Also, most folks in the gym are busy worrying about their own workouts to concern themselves with anyone else. Nobody has the time or interest in stalking you. So take a deep breath, walk into that gym, and watch your life change for the better.

I don't have exercise clothes.

Fitness apparel can make exercising more comfortable; however, it's rarely a requirement. One of my favorite things to see at the gym I attend is busy professionals walking on a treadmill in a suit and sneakers. It shows an absolute commitment to fitness, which I adore. I also see a few cowboys in jeans and boots lifting weights on occasion. So cool! Instead of letting fashion delay your fitness training, show up wearing what you have. Sweats, t-shirts, leggings, shorts, or even jeans. If you can eventually put a few dollars aside for exercise clothing, hit up a local thrift store, and then feel free to wear the same outfit religiously. Exercise is more important than what you wear doing it.

I can't lose weight because I have big, heavy bones.

OMGosh. I love this one because I have the absolute craziest information to share with you. Do you know how much an adult human skeleton typically weighs? Five to 12 pounds! Seriously, that includes tiny to very large adults. Therefore, the size and weight of your bones are not the cause of your struggles with weight. Now that we have cleared that up, let's take ownership of the parts of our bodies we can affect with exercise and nutrition.

I can't exercise because I hate to run.

If I had a penny for every time someone told me they'd like to get fit and lose weight but they "hate running," I'd have a lot of dirty pennies. Who cares if they or you hate running? Is running the only exercise on earth? You've heard of dancing, karate, swimming, pickleball, skiing, and basketball, right? Fitness requires effort in the Four Pillars, but how you pursue each pillar is your call.

Friend, you have a way better chance of sticking with any exercise if you enjoy it, even slightly! And if you're sitting there thinking you don't enjoy any sort of exercise, you're lying to me and lying to yourself. I promise, you just haven't found the right one yet. Remember, you don't have to be great at anything; you just have to move. Start by doing things that are comfortable and not so hard, and then increase the frequency, intensity, and time as you progress. Once you're moving comfortably, start trying things that might be enjoyable. Why is the world obsessed with pickleball right now? Because it's fun! Most people love the social aspect as much as the game itself. But guess what? They're still getting fit in the process. So stop stressing about what you think exercise should be. Just get moving and let the rest take care of itself.

I'm not good enough to do that workout or sport.

Comparing yourself to others is a waste of time. You are not them, and they are not you. It's okay to garner motivation and inspiration and share tips with friends, but your fitness will rely on your abilities, skills, and desires. Not theirs. While it's natural to notice what others are doing, remember that their journey isn't yours. Be inspired, but don't get caught up in comparisons, especially if your neighbor is Tom Brady! Instead of worrying about how you stack up against others, focus on your progress. Set your own goals, celebrate your wins, and keep moving forward. That's what really counts.I've seen endless numbers of real people turn their lives around, going from sedentary, unfit, and unhappy to vibrant, active, and confident. That's why I love teaching fitness. It's not about plaques on the wall or titles. My success is seeing you succeed, getting those messages that say, "I did it. I finished my first 5K!", "My back no longer hurts," or "I feel amazing in my jeans again."

I believe in you, and it's time for you to believe in yourself.

Whenever those silly excuses creep in, picture a little Fitzy on your shoulder, reminding you how far you've come. She's poking you in the cheek, shouting, "You've got this, one step, and one choice at a time!" Because the truth is, even when you hear my voice in your head, it's really your own. And you have complete control over it. I want to be there for you, but you must take me along. Let's do this together!

Chapter 31

QUESTIONS AND ANSWERS

Even though we've covered most of these topics throughout this book, I'm revisiting many of the most common questions to ensure the answers are seared into your supercharged skull.

Question: What's the best way to set my goals?

Answer: Goals should be specific and target the way you look, perform, and feel. Set far-reaching goals that will take significant time and effort to conquer, along with smaller ones that can be achieved quickly.

For example, if your big goal is to climb Mount Everest, your short-term goal could be climbing 90 steps without getting winded. Maybe you'll aim to climb the Empire State Building next. Or if you want to lose 100 pounds, focus on the first 10. Once you achieve that, celebrate, not with an eating party, but with something that acknowledges your success.

Track your progress regularly, as data is a clear indicator of progress. When you hit your milestones, celebrate in a way that supports your journey. Non-food rewards are ideal. Treat yourself to a massage, a spa day, a night out, or maybe a fun adventure like zip-lining. You can invest in fitness gear, take a weekend getaway, or enjoy some quiet time alone. Rewards should motivate you without sabotaging your progress.

Chapter 31 | Questions and Answers

Remember, the reward should uplift your health and mindset, not undermine it. So, skip the "Friday night feast" or drinking binge just because you reached a goal. Instead, focus on things that enhance your well-being and make you feel genuinely good.

In the end, it's about building the life and the body you want, one small goal at a time. Stay focused, track your wins, celebrate them, and keep moving forward.

Question: How do I know what to wear for exercise?

Answer: It depends on what you're doing. Most activities require specific apparel, made with fabrics and fits for comfort, movement, and support. You'll need proper swimwear like trunks, a bikini, or a one-piece if you're swimming. There are running shorts, basketball shorts, bike shorts, boxing shorts, and board shorts. Jog bras and yoga bras. The key is to dress for each activity; most have a typical wardrobe.

You can always research options online or browse in-store, but the main goal is functionality. Loose, baggy clothes may seem comfortable, but they can be a hassle for certain activities like yoga. You're upside down half the time, and your shirt might ride up or your pants shift around, making it harder to focus. That's why tighter, more form-fitting clothing is common for activities that require a lot of bending.

However, comfort goes beyond just fit, it's about choosing fabrics that make sense for the conditions. Moisture-wicking materials are great because they pull sweat away from your skin and help keep you cool. Yet, I often see people running in 85-degree Florida heat wearing long black tights. Why? Most of the time, it's because they're self-conscious about their legs or knees. I know it's easy to feel self-conscious, but trust me, most people are too focused on their own workout to notice. And even if someone does see your knees, so what? Your comfort and performance matter more than their opinions. In hot weather, you should wear something light, like shorts and a tank top. You'll feel better, perform better, and be less likely to suffer from heat-related illnesses.

I even have a "tank top mandate" in my *Hottie Body Fitzness Challenge* Facebook group during the summer. No sleeves in the heat! At first, many people hesitate, leery of displaying their arms for all to see. But once they give sleeveless a try, they realize how much more comfortable and energized they feel. It's a small but powerful step toward feeling proud of your body.

You should be just as thoughtful when dressing for cold temperatures and snow sports. Layering is key, but make sure your base layer wicks away sweat. Wet clothes in the cold can make you even chillier. And don't forget safety gear like helmets for anything involving wheels, high speeds, or contact sports.

Lastly, it's okay to want workout clothes that make you feel good. My daughter, for example, asked me to buy her some cute new workout outfits after seeing her friends in them. I was happy to splurge a bit to encourage her to exercise. Guess what? It worked. She hit the gym the next day in her new gear and has remained consistent. Fitness apparel you feel fabulous in can be a real motivator, and you don't have to spend a fortune on it. Great workout clothes come at all price points. Whether it's high-end or budget-friendly, what matters most is that it fits, feels good, and allows you to perform at your best.

Question: How do I choose the right footwear for exercise?

Answer: Footwear should always be chosen based on your activity. Shoes are designed to offer specific support, flexibility, and structure in different areas of the foot and ankle. The soles are also made for varying levels of traction. For example, a smooth sole allows for easy twisting and sliding, which is great for dancing or court sports. On the other hand, shoes with thicker treads or cleats are designed to grip surfaces like grass or turf, preventing you from slipping. Choosing the wrong shoe for your activity can lead to poor performance and increase the risk of injury. Take running as an example. Every time your foot strikes the ground, you absorb about three times your body weight on impact. If you weigh 150 pounds, that's 450 pounds crashing to the ground with each step. Running shoes are designed to absorb and diminish some of that shock from each impact, protecting your feet and joints. Meanwhile, basketball shoes are designed with extra ankle support to prevent ankle rolling or sprains during quick directional changes.

Specialty stores can be beneficial, especially if you're new to the activity or unsure of what kind of support you need. In a running store, for instance, staff are often trained to evaluate how you walk or run. They can help identify whether you need a neutral shoe, extra arch support, or something to correct over-pronation. This level of expertise is harder to find in big box retailers, though they often carry a fabulous selection of options. It's important to note that you can find sales, special discounts, and loyalty club perks at both types of stores.

Don't feel tied to a specific brand just because your friends are wearing it or you liked it in the past. Be open to trying new styles or brands, and don't be afraid to return shoes if they're not a good fit. Many stores allow you to test shoes and return them if they aren't comfortable or cause problems after a few wears. Note that even the best shoes will wear out eventually. Most running shoes last about 300–500 miles. Other types of training shoes should be replaced if the cushioning, support, or tread wears down. Proper footwear isn't just about comfort, it's about protecting your body and helping you perform at your best.

If you want to save money on footwear, I recommend shopping for last season's model. Shoe brands rarely make significant changes to the structure of a shoe style but regularly release new colors. So, if you can live with the colors that launched a few months ago, you're likely to find them on sale. Lastly, if you fall in love with a shoe and it really adds to your performance, buy an extra pair.

Question: How do I break a plateau?

Answer: Plateaus happen because your body adapts to repeated movements and eating habits, making progress stall. You break a plateau by shaking things up, adding variety, going a bit harder, and keeping your body on its toes. If you've been walking day in and day out, try something completely different. Take an innovative dance class, give CrossFit a go, or try Pilates. Your body will start responding, thinking, "Whoa, this is new!" Boxing, for example, is a unique challenge for your body compared to other activities, and that shake-up forces your body to adapt and improve.

Sometimes, it's not just about the workouts, it's also about what you're eating. Eating habits can get just as stale as workout routines. People tend to stick with what works, but then hesitate to make changes because they fear it'll mess up their progress. Maybe you need to clean up your eating habits a bit. Try eating more vegetables instead of loading up on starchy carbs, or mix in some plant-based meals for a while.

If you're feeling stuck and haven't been as disciplined with your caloric intake, tighten things up! To look and perform like an athlete, you need to act like one. Athletes break through plateaus by pushing harder, getting creative, and trying new things. Sometimes, a plateau is more mental than physical. Setting a new challenge, like a race, competition, or personal best, can reignite motivation. So, step out of your comfort zone, throw in something fresh, and watch your body start making progress again.

Question: Is there really a benefit to taking group classes?

Answer: Absolutely! Taking new classes comes with several fantastic benefits, and if you're worried about trying something new, many offer free trials, and instructors are there to help beginners feel comfortable. You don't have to be an expert to start! First, paying for a class in advance helps ensure you'll show up and make the most of your investment. Additionally, classes introduce variety into your workout routine, which can challenge your body in new ways. This variety often increases intensity, as the group setting can motivate you to push harder. Moreover, classes allow you to expand your social circle by connecting with like-minded individuals who share your fitness goals.

If you're used to working out alone, joining an instructor-led class can be a refreshing change. For instance, you might find yourself using diverse equipment like rowing machines, battle ropes or slides, or doing unique exercises like angry-ups and alphabet shoulders. Starting with a beginner class is a smart move, even if you're already fit, as it allows you to learn the basics before moving on to more advanced challenges. My friend Jennifer tries new classes frequently, but tries to hang near the door so she can leave if she doesn't like it. Beyond physical benefits, taking a class can boost your confidence and help relieve stress. The structured environment and group energy can be a great mental reset.

Classes also offer a chance to meet new people and potentially make new friends who are into similar activities. If your current social scene isn't supporting your fitness goals, this can be a great way to connect with others who share your aspirations. Plus, the commitment to a scheduled class can be as motivating as having a workout buddy or personal trainer. So, why not sign up for a trial class this week? You might find your new favorite workout!

Question: What is the worst piece of equipment in the gym?

Answer: Without a doubt, the worst piece of equipment in any fitness center is the one you're not using! Varying your workouts to include different movements and equipment is essential for continued progress. If you only do what you can already do, you will hit an impasse. But if you constantly change things up to challenge your body in unique ways, it will continue to show progress. Make a habit of veering into the uncharted sections of the gym you usually avoid and give at least one new move or machine a try.

Question: How do I stay active and exercise when the weather is too hot, cold, rainy, or snowy outside?

Answer: The key is to adapt and use every situation to your advantage. When it's sweltering outside, head indoors or dive into water-based exercises like swimming, snorkeling, paddle boarding, or canoeing. Summer doesn't have to mean sitting around lazily; take advantage of the heat and stay active in the water! If the weather turns cold, embrace it! Cold weather can be invigorating for activities like running or hiking as long as you're dressed appropriately. For someone like me, who's used to Florida's warmth, the cold can be a bit daunting, but it's also an opportunity to try exciting activities like snowboarding, skiing, or snowshoeing. So don't let the seasons dictate your fitness routine.

In extreme conditions, safety comes first. Stay hydrated in the heat, wear moisture-wicking layers in the cold, and watch for icy or slick surfaces. Remember that you can always work out indoors! Whether it's storming outside or you're stuck at home with little ones, there are countless indoor exercise options. Set up a home

Chapter 31 | Questions and Answers

gym with equipment like a treadmill, bands, dumbbells, and kettlebells, or follow workout videos. You can also hit up a fitness center if that's more your style.

Never let the weather or seasons be an excuse to skip your workout. Be creative, go with the flow, and adjust your routine to fit the conditions. Whether it's finding ways to adapt outdoors or making the most of indoor options, staying active is always possible. And hey, thank goodness for air conditioning, right?

Question: Should I exercise if I'm sick?

Answer: It depends how sick and what kind of sick! If you've got something serious like a stomach bug, pneumonia, or the flu, stay home and get some rest. If you've got the common cold, make a grown-up decision for yourself. It's possible some mild or moderate exercise might feel good, if you're nursing something simple. If you can go for a walk, do leg lifts in bed, or stretch in the shower, you should! If exercise makes you feel worse though, wait another day and try again. Lastly, if you're contagious, keep your germs to yourself. Don't attend a Pilates class and give your health-minded peers the plague. Do Pilates in your living room using an online instructor instead.

Question: How do I continue to find motivation?

Answer: Motivation starts from within. You've got to reach a point where you're sick of the status quo and ready for change. True motivation comes when you're fed up with being out of shape, dealing with pain, or lacking energy. It's not about external pressure or what others think, it's a guttural need for personal improvement.

To keep that fire burning, set clear goals and keep them visible. Write them down, pin them to your wall, or get a neon sign if that helps. Make your goals public, too, tell everyone you know. This adds a layer of accountability because your ego will push you to follow through.

Celebrate your progress with both small and big rewards. Whether it's a social media post, a movie night, or a new outfit, these celebrations help keep you motivated. If you have a big goal, like running a marathon, commit to it by registering and paying for it. This financial investment makes you more likely to stay on track.

Use technology to your advantage. Track your progress with apps, wearables, or fitness trackers. They can help you monitor your steps, workouts, and health metrics. And don't forget to use online resources like MyFitness.com for recipes, workout videos, and guidance.

Consider hiring a trainer. A good trainer can guide, challenge, and keep you accountable. Get recommendations from friends and make sure they're well-reviewed.

Join fitness classes. Commit to a set number of classes and make sure you show up to get your money's worth. Partnering with a workout buddy can also be motivating, as having someone to meet can be a powerful incentive to get up and exercise.

Explore clubs and teams. Whether it's a local running club, dance troupe, or corporate team, these groups offer support and camaraderie. They keep exercise fun and engaging and remind you that being active can be a social and enjoyable part of your life.

Find one new way to boost your motivation this week, whether it's setting a goal, finding a workout buddy, or trying a new class. Keep pushing forward!

Chapter 31 | Questions and Answers

Question: What do I do when I reach my goal?

Answer: Celebrate, of course! We've talked a lot about celebrating achievements, and that's crucial. But don't stop there, look forward! Your next goal could be running a 10K, mastering pull-ups, or trying a new sport. Keep attacking a better life with vigor. Remember, fitness has no finish line!

Let's say you're 40, and you've hit your target weight and built strength and flexibility. Do you just coast from here? Nope. If you do, all the hard-earned benefits can slip away. Have you decided you're okay with being out of shape when you're 60 or 70? I hope not!

So keep pushing forward. Work hard and continually set new goals for yourself, whether for tomorrow, next month, or next year. Celebrate your success, find that next challenge, chase it down, and never stop improving!

Question: What do I do if my spouse eats poorly?

Answer: Ah, the classic case of "my spouse's food choices are driving me crazy." I get it: it's hard when someone you love doesn't share your healthy eating habits. But sadly, you can't change them by force, bullying, or nagging, nor can you allow them to sabotage your efforts. You can't control what another adult chooses to eat, no matter how tempting it might be to try. If they choose indulgent foods like creamy pastas and desserts, that's on them, not you.

So, you do you. If you're the one cooking, cook healthy foods in a healthy way. Perhaps your honey will eat what they're fed. If they're cranky about it, feel free to whip up their guilty pleasures, but make sure you're also creating something nutritious for yourself. And when dining out, don't feel pressured to order the same as they do. Choose something that aligns with your goals and tastes.

If you feel comfortable, talk to your spouse about your goals and how their food choices impact you. It might not change things overnight, but a little understanding goes a long way. Ultimately, you're in charge of your own plate. Let them enjoy their choices while you stick to yours. Consistency is key, so keep up your healthy habits, and don't let anyone or anything derail your progress.

Chapter 32

DO'S AND DON'TS OF SUPERCHARGING

You. Supercharged!

Do know who you want to be and make a plan to become the supercharged version of yourself!

Don't operate without a clear destination and path forward.

Do aim high! Instead of striving for mediocrity to avoid failure, set yourself up for a rigorous road of challenges that actually make you better.

Don't settle. What a terrible way to live.

Do pursue all Four Pillars of Fitness: strength, cardio, flexibility, and balance.

Don't be a one-trick pony, only relying on one type of fitness training.

Do take two steps at a time while climbing stairs; it's great for your glutes and legs!

Don't take the elevator unless you absolutely need to.

Do utilize the Exact Formula for Weight Loss. It's simple and effective, can get you to a healthy weight, and keep you there for life.

Chapter 32 | Do's and Don'ts of Supercharging

Don't diet or rely on quick fixes for weight loss. They'll only yield temporary results and will likely make you miserable.

Do get 80-90% of your calories from highly nutritious whole foods prepared in a healthy way.

Don't overindulge in highly processed, high-sugar, trans- or saturated-fat-laden foods.

Do prioritize reasonable portions. Eating too much leads to weight gain, even when eating healthy foods.

Don't feel pressure to be perfect. You can get away with eating not-so-healthy foods if you consume small amounts of them.

Do drink lots of water, with some low-calorie alternatives on occasion.

Don't overload on sugary, highly caffeinated, or alcoholic beverages.

Do commit to drinking far less alcohol or none at all. These useless calories can negatively affect your body and mind while sabotaging your efforts in fitness.

Don't trick yourself into believing it's okay to drink alcohol daily, drink more than a couple in one sitting, or as a crutch to decompress.

Do put your knowledge into action, it's time for progress!

Don't play dumb. By this point in the book, you know 95.7% of everything you need to improve your health dramatically.

Do take ownership of your mind, body, actions, and professional and personal success. You are not a victim, and you are not helpless.

Don't blame anyone or anything for your lack of success. Lack of accountability is a common trait among failures.

Do pursue activities you are bad at. A new challenge will serve your body and mind in wonderful ways.

Don't talk yourself out of trying new things. As long as it's safe, take risks and expand your horizons.

Do vary your workouts by trying new classes, sports, exercises, and equipment. Each will challenge your body in unique ways, forcing it to adapt and improve.

Don't do the same thing every time; your routine should never become routine.

Do surround yourself with positive people, both in person and online, who can guide, support, and celebrate your efforts.

Don't let unhealthy people with bad attitudes drag you down. Negativity is contagious; distance yourself if you can't convince them to change their ways.

Do participate in sports. Whether competing against others or trying to best yourself, step into an arena or onto a field or court! Working with teammates or against opponents can be exhilarating, narrow your focus, and expand your social circle.

Don't fear losing. Unless your match is televised with a million-dollar prize purse, you're not likely to suffer any consequences from a loss other than a twinge of disappointment. Who cares if you lose?

Chapter 32 | Do's and Don'ts of Supercharging

Do commit fully. The results come fast and hard when you dive into fitness, nutrition, and other healthy habits. Immediate benefits include adrenaline rushes, increased energy, mouthwatering flavors, and stress reduction.

Don't be half-assed. Major progress awaits if you go full throttle on your efforts to become one percent better daily.

Do understand what benefits your insurance provider and employer offer. You may be entitled to a free gym membership, a consultation with a registered dietician, massage, or acupuncture treatment. Perhaps you can score discounts on fitness classes, exercise equipment, or tech.

Don't shy away from challenges. If you're incentivized to take a certain number of steps, complete various workouts, or lose a bit of weight, go for it! Even if you are not the overall winner, making strides in health is always a win. Note that the healthier you are, the more productive and less costly you'll be to your employer. This is why I do so many corporate keynotes. Their investment in me is an investment in the overall health of the organization and the financial bottom line.

Do pursue as many free trial classes as you can until you discover challenging workouts you like.

Don't sign up for too much of anything. You don't need to commit to a two-year membership. Sign up for two months or 10 classes. Having an extended financial commitment won't actually make you show up.

Do multitask! Walk and talk meetings are genius. Put your earbuds in, cell phone in your pocket, and crush a couple of miles while you're chatting with your sales team or bestie. Use a treadmill desk or replace your office chair with a Swiss ball to keep your core engaged.

Don't settle for being sedentary. Get creative and force movement into each day.

Do encourage your family to be healthy. Every generation has room to improve, inspire, educate (gift them this book), plan, and role model healthy habits, which can be contagious.

Don't allow poor influences or indignation from your family to ruin your efforts. You're in charge of your kids, but if your spouse, siblings, parents, or cousins aren't into it, don't let them sabotage your success.

Do be the judge of your success. Know what it looks like to you, and monitor your progress.

Don't worry about what others think. Everyone's got an opinion, and theirs is none of your business.

Do make time for rest, relaxation, and rejuvenation with meditation, late mornings in bed, great books, concerts, coffee dates, and playtime with your pets.

Don't act like a martyr. You're a human. Your body and mind need time for rest and recovery. Pushing yourself until you're sick, physically or mentally, is foolish. R&R is an important part of health.

Do plan out meaningful rewards for your successes, from spa days to new training gear or event registrations. Set each bar high, and when you reach them, celebrate appropriately.

Chapter 32 | Do's and Don'ts of Supercharging

Don't fail to recognize your efforts. Patting yourself on the back while taking pride in your outcomes will keep your internal fire burning.

Do find a way to follow through on your workout plans and healthy meals. When obstacles pop up, go over, under, or through them to achieve your goals. Be the "make shit happen" person!

Don't make excuses. As we've discussed, they're totally lame. Turn obstacles into opportunities. You're too clever and disciplined to let anything stand between you and your goals.

Do take immediate action. Figure out what you can do right now to improve one percent and do it.

Don't procrastinate! Don't you wish you had reached your fitness goals last year? Ten years ago? Twenty years ago? If you've been putting it off, you're probably not so pleased with yourself. Know this. Someday equals NEVER! You could have done it before, and if you did, everything would be better. You would look better, feel better, and perform better. Regret sucks, so don't waste another day.

Do change the voice in your head. The new voice is hyper-confident, creative, and disciplined. It tells you why you should and how you can, and harps on how awesome you are for following through.

Don't ever speak negatively of yourself. The voice in your head should be talking you up instead of putting you down. You deserve love and support, and that's got to start internally.

Do put Lil' Fitzy on your shoulder. I'd love to go everywhere with you, giving you cute but annoying little pokes in the chest.

If you allow me into your head, we can take you further and faster together.

Don't ignore me because I'm a pain in the ass. I harass you because I love you. You should also feel me hugging your giant neck with my teeny arms each time you succeed.

Chapter 33

GET IT TOGETHER! THE TOUGH LOVE CHAPTER

You. Supercharged!

My editors have begged me to soften my tone in every chapter. And I've mostly complied, so you wouldn't slam the book shut and sprint away from fitness forever. But mincing my words has been exhausting. I'm a straight-shooter who loves poking people I care about in the chest, especially you.

Over the years, my blunt delivery has worked wonders because people know it comes from a place of love. My words may sound harsh, but they're always delivered with a smile. My editors worry that strangers might think I'm a jerk. That's possible. But I've decided to reserve one glorious chapter, this one, to go full-throttle Fitz Koehler for those who can handle it. If you're hyper-sensitive, skip ahead. If you're ready for a love-filled kick in the can, buckle up.

Friend, it's time to get your shit together. None of us are getting any younger, and if you want to feel and look great in your 30s, 60s, and 90s, you need to put in the effort right now. Look around! Too many people have destroyed themselves and are living their absolute worst lives because they simply refuse to exercise and watch what they put in their mouths. And that's just asinine.

Seriously! Could the luxury of being a slacker and eating whatever you want really be worth the price of having a body that makes

Chapter 33 | Get it Together! The Tough Love Chapter

you mentally and physically miserable? I don't think so. They say, "Nothing tastes as good as skinny feels." Okay. I'd rather flip that. What tastes so good that it's worth chronic back pain, type 2 diabetes, heart disease, or sudden death? Or even worse, a long, drawn-out, excruciatingly-painful and scary death? I'm pretty sure the answer is nothing, but millions of people make that trade and it pisses me off. Why? Because life can be spectacular, and the suffering brought on by these lifestyle-related ailments is extreme.

Commit! That's right. Don't half-ass commit and eat garbage 50% of the time while downing cocktails every night. Commit for real. I've only asked you to make quality food choices 80-90% of the time. You have wiggle room, and I've specifically encouraged you not to be perfect. So any claims that anything in this book is rigid just won't hold up. Just decide what your caloric budget needs to be using the Exact Formula and stick with it. It's almost mindless, and it works every single time. You just have to use it.

Here's a little inside scoop from a gal who's guided millions: Men generally tend to hear The Formula, nod, and say, "Cool, I got this." Then they *follow* it. Women, on the other hand, my beloved, amazing women, hear the same thing and say, "That's simple!" Then, they get derailed by girls' night out, stress, or something hormonal.

Guys tend to be more robotic and solution-oriented, while women tend to be more emotional. So, ladies! My girls. My besties. Please do better and prove me wrong. I'd love that. Stick with your Formula, and you WILL succeed, no matter what drama is distracting you. You'll never get where you want to go if you make too many excuses.

No matter where you are or where you're going, you can always find healthy food. And if you're concerned that you won't, bring some. If you had a baby, you wouldn't leave home without bottles or baby food for fear of a meltdown. Well, guess what? Grown-ups are just big babies; when we get too hungry, we melt down, too. So pack healthy snacks or an entire cooler. Never pretend that the only choice you have is to eat processed nonsense from a vending machine, because that will rarely be the truth. Prepare in advance, and you won't be left gnawing on a bag of fried sugar.

And I'm going to sound like a judgey ass, but so be it! This is my judgey asshole chapter. Alcohol doesn't need to be a daily part of your life. Blah, blah, red wine has antioxidants, blah, blah. I've heard it! You can relax and unwind in so many different, fully productive ways. If you drink any sort of alcohol daily or almost daily and swear it's not harming you, take an entire month off, that's right, 30 days with zero alcohol. When you get to the end, you'll probably notice that your pants are looser, your head is clearer, your energy is higher, and you've been sleeping better. And if you're not? Fine. You win, do what you want.

And for those of you who pride yourself on juggling all the balls and being the martyr in your family, being at the end of your rope isn't something to be proud of: it's a red flag! Instead of letting your life get willy-nilly out of control because you're trying to be everything to everyone, learn how to let things go. Learn how to say "no." And don't blame anyone else for the stress in your life. You are not a victim! And the victim mentality is gross. Ewwww. You are capable and responsible for your own success. Nobody can prevent you from exercising, eating wisely, or sleeping well. If you prioritize your health, you'll make progress. If not, you won't.

When it comes to exercise, you've just got to do it. Thinking about it and talking about it won't accomplish jack. You've got to get started, even if you're not as fit as you used to be. Even if you can't run a marathon, and even if you don't have a gym membership. The floor you're standing on right now is a freaking fitness center if you drop and do some crunches, push-ups, or planks. So shut

Chapter 33 | Get it Together! The Tough Love Chapter

that namby-pamby voice inside your head up and replace excuses with exercise. I've only asked that you commit to getting one percent better daily. You can totally do that.

You'd be surprised how many people have come to me for advice, and once I start to give it, they tell me how they were a star athlete decades ago in high school. How is that relevant now? Unless you're 19, it's not. It doesn't matter who you used to be. All that matters is who you are now, what you know, and what you're doing. So stop rehashing ancient history and comparing yourself to it. It's irrelevant. Eyes forward! No matter what kind of shape you're in, it can and should be improved. Why not? Go from sickly to bad, bad to good, good to great, or great to excellent!

If you spend your time complaining about why you can't get fit, you won't. You definitely won't. And that sucks. Because being weak and tight with poor stamina and crappy balance sucks. Sleeping poorly and roaming around all day without energy sucks. Dealing with constant digestive issues because your body is revolting against the food and drinks you're feeding it sucks. Missing out on dates, jobs, raises, and other opportunities because you slouch, lack confidence, and give off less-than-awesome vibes totally sucks.

What if you were continuously having success and people were magnetically drawn to you? What if you walked into rooms and future clients, bosses, or romantic interests thought, "Hot damn, I need to know more!"? There's a real chance you could be making more money, more friends, and enjoying a slew of interesting added opportunities if you were fitter, stood up straighter, and exuded more confidence. People would trust you more and take more interest. Not because your waist was smaller or you look great in a thong, but because you ooze vibrancy and confidence. You'll be surprised how many doors will open for you as your body, poise, and energy change for the better. When you supercharge yourself, everything you touch becomes supercharged too.

If you spend your days making a series of little and large efforts toward health, you will continuously improve. Tiny steps in the right direction will eventually turn into giant leaps and drastic upgrades to the way you feel, function, and flourish. If you stick with it long enough, you'll become one of those people who exercises because you know you'll feel bad if you don't. You'll eat mostly the right amounts of the right foods for the size you like to be because you enjoy being at your best. Without a doubt, there is a more fantastic version of your already awesome self available. You just have to force the issue.

I'm laying into you because I love you. I'm desperate for you to do what it takes to live better and longer. To make every single day more joyful, peaceful, and powerful. I've spent my career fighting for that. Whether cheering enthusiastically or swinging a sledgehammer, I'll do whatever it takes to reach you. Cause I know what you're capable of. I hope you do too!

Chapter 34

YOU DID IT! NOW WHAT?

You. Supercharged!

Halleh-freaking-lujah! You're finally in a body you feel great about. Your body works well, you've erased most or all of your pain, and you feel good about what you see when you look in the mirror. **YOU. ARE. SUPERCHARGED!** I'm jumping up and down for you, because this moment deserves celebration. Now, I'm guessing you didn't just "poof!" magically transform over the few days it's taken you to read this book. But I hope you'll return to this chapter when you get *there*, to the place you programmed into your GPS. The place you mapped out when I asked you, "Who do you want to be?"

Many people go through life never reaching their full potential, falling short of goals of all sorts. But not you! You had a vision for yourself, your body, mind, and your quality of life. Badass! I want to eat you up because driven, disciplined, and successful people are the most delicious. Yummy!

So now what? Keep going! You double down on the great decisions and habits that brought you this far. I hate to move the finish line on you, but it gets even better than this! That's right, you can be stronger, firmer, with greater stamina, flexibility, and balance. You can sleep better, think better, and have even more energy. Am I blowing your mind? You made it to the promised land and now the bossy lil' Fitzy on your shoulder is poking you again? She sure

Chapter 34 | You Did It! Now What?

as hell is, because you've proven yourself, and you are capable of so much more!

Whoosh. This is fun. So instead of stagnating and backsliding, keep moving forward. Remain proud of who you've become and use this confidence to fuel future endeavors. Wanna play Michelangelo and sculpt your body even more? Go for it! Do you want to become more competitive in a sport? I think you should. Considering an adventurous vacation or getting certified to teach Pilates? Go for it! Go for it all. Use your new zest for fitness and life and push every limit you can.

Now, I'm going to rudely interrupt this celebration with some guidance I wish I didn't have to give.

You worked hard, lost weight, and expected applause. Instead, you got judgment, side-eyes, and a flood of unwanted opinions. Welcome to the bizarre world of weight-loss criticism. I hear this all the time, and I've lived it myself. Whether rooted in genuine concern or bitter jealousy, it's tough for some to accept their once-overweight friends' slimmer, healthier bodies. Where were these people when your overweight body put you at risk for diabetes, heart disease, and stroke? I bet they were silent. Strange that they're showing concerns now, right? Conversations about weight are tricky, but ignoring the health risks associated with being overweight isn't kindness, it's avoidance. Extreme weight loss can sometimes be a concern, but that's far from the norm. In my decades of experience helping thousands of people lose weight, losing too much hasn't been something I've seen more than a few times.

I was a heavier teen, wearing some pretty big sizes. In college, despite teaching 10 advanced exercise classes a week, I was overweight because my eating habits were abysmal. But no one mentioned my weight or unhealthy lifestyle; nobody expressed concern. Eventually, I decided to clean up my eating with less beer, beef, fried foods, and sweets, and started focusing on water, vegetables, grilled chicken, fruit, and whole grains. I stopped coating everything with butter and started dipping my salad into dressing instead of pouring it on. I also pursued competitive kickboxing. As a result, I lost 45 pounds over a few years, earning a lean, hard, athletic body that I was proud of. I felt and looked my best. To my horror, that's when the criticism from my family started. Filled with joy and compliments from strangers on my healthy appearance, my family was ganging up on me. "You look old!" "Are you sick?" Ironically, I was eating right for the first time in my life, and it was working for me. I guess my family was just accustomed to me being a bigger girl and struggled to accept the changes. Eventually, after careful observation, my mom realized that I was eating plenty of nutritious foods and called the dogs off.

I've seen this pattern time and time again: when you're overweight, no one comments, but once you slim down, suddenly everyone has an opinion. My friend Nick knows this all too well. Over the years, he transformed his once-obese physique into a lean, muscular frame. He looks fantastic, and women even compliment his "superhero jaw." Yet, despite his impressive transformation, his father told him he needed to gain weight, particularly in his face! It's another example of how our loved ones can't always handle change, especially when we become thinner. Yet, to the outside world, we often look better and healthier.

The reality of weight loss is that it affects your entire body, your waist, thighs, chest, feet, and even your face. You get to shape yourself like a sculptor, making your body smaller, leaner, and fitter. But along with the physical transformation comes unsolicited opinions from people who are concerned, jealous, or simply uninformed. Don't let their comments derail your progress. I've seen this weight-loss backlash countless times, and rarely is it an indicator of real health danger. Some people still have

Chapter 34 | You Did It! Now What?

significant weight to lose when they start getting the "you're too skinny" remarks.

When faced with these comments, you have a few options:

- Politely say, "Thank you for your concern," and move on.
- Ask, "I appreciate your concern, but did you have the same worries when I was carrying extra weight? What makes you think I'm unhealthy now?"

Your health is yours to own. Let the skeptics talk, while you keep thriving. You don't owe anyone an explanation for taking care of yourself.

Back to the par-tay!

Your achievements in health and fitness should convince you that you are capable of making changes in all categories of your life. Use the same determination and discipline you've exhibited here to get out of debt, make new friends, learn how to do makeup, play guitar, and more. This supercharged version of you is confident, capable, and on the hunt for new opportunities to conquer. You've proven that you can do hard things. So do them!

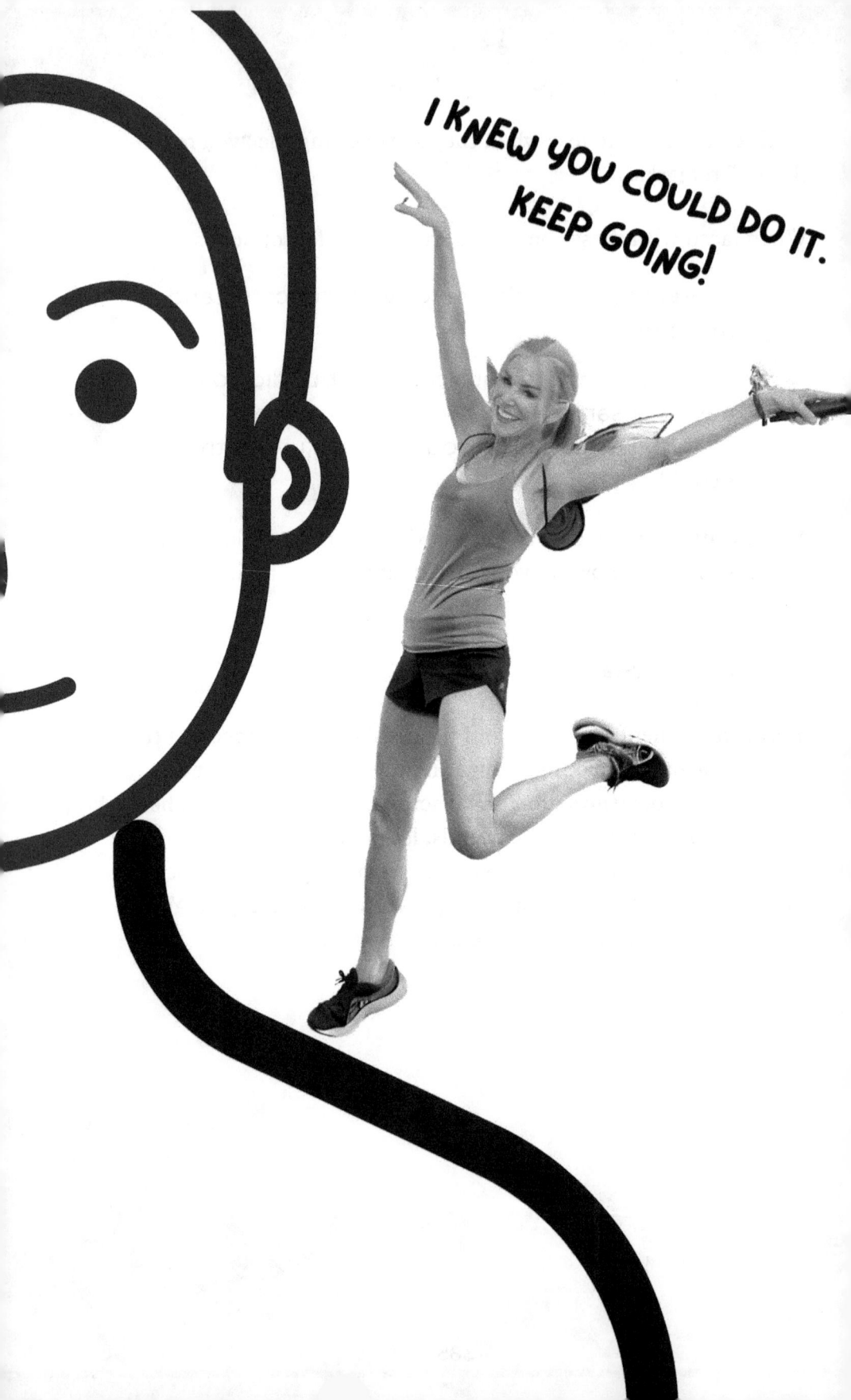

YOU CAN DO HARD THINGS!

You. Supercharged!

My Fitzness Fiends,

You are strong. You are capable. You have everything you need to take control of your health and become SUPERCHARGED. I've shared a massive amount of fitness knowledge and excuse-busting strategies with you. If you've paid attention, you know the simple science behind what it takes to succeed, and you understand the work ahead.

Know exactly who you want to be and make that your North Star. Take time to recognize your strengths. Acknowledge where you want to improve, but don't dwell on past struggles; use them as fuel. The most successful transformations come from focusing on what you can do, not what you've failed at before.

Write things down: your goals, your health stats, your workouts, and the victories you achieve along the way. Documenting your path and progress is a crucial part of the process, reminding you of where you began and how far you've come. Whether your health is dire or you feel pretty fit, there is always room for improvement. Aim high! Update and upgrade everything, and have fun with it!

I've worked hard to connect with and convince each of you, but some may slip through the cracks. After absorbing my words, most will be compelled to make positive changes. Disappointingly, some of you will receive all of this information and enthusiasm and do nothing with it. Gahhhh! That'll kill me (and possibly you). So, for the final time, I plead with you to take action to do better and be better. I promise the outcome will be worth it.

Mediocrity is no longer an option for you. You're ready to become the next best version of yourself. With the Exact Formula, the Four Pillars of Fitness, revitalized sleep, and renewed peace of mind, your days ahead will be more energetic, productive, and satisfying. Is this going to be hard? Maybe. But you are wildly capable of doing hard things. You've conquered them before, and I have complete faith you can do this too. It's go time! You've got the knowledge, the tools, and the power, now, put them to work.

Keep your bossy Lil Fitzy on your shoulder. Take me with you. Yield to my harassment and respond every time I poke you in the chest. I can continue to help and encourage you every day if you let me. I'm always accepting questions for *The Fitzness Show* podcast, so send them my way at FITZNESS.com or @Fitzness on Instagram and Facebook. And when you have reasons to celebrate, please include me. Message me to brag about your successes, so I can share in your joy.

I wrote this because I love you. Now get to work!

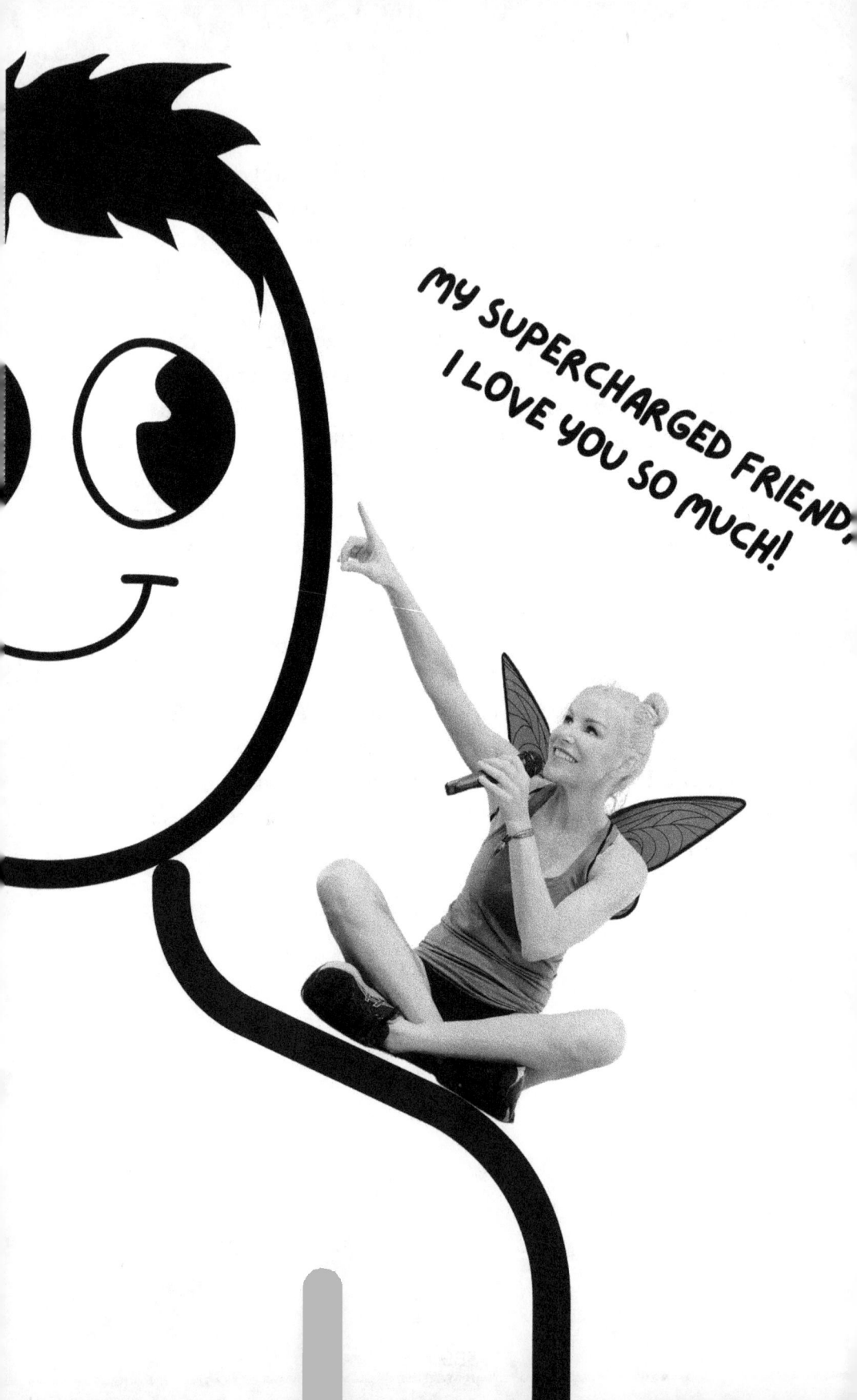

Acknowledgements

Thanks to my doggos and besties, Piper and Joey, for making my life better in every way. My 16-year-old lab mix, Piper, has served as Vice President of Fitzness since we adopted her as a puppy, helping me navigate all the big and small decisions. Joey, my four-year-old Maltese mix, is my Chief Cuddling Officer, keeping me company for hours on end outside on my swing as I've pounded away at this keyboard. Together, they keep me active, giggling, cozy, outdoors, happy, and at peace. Book-writing would be far more lonely without their support, wisdom, and unconditional encouragement.

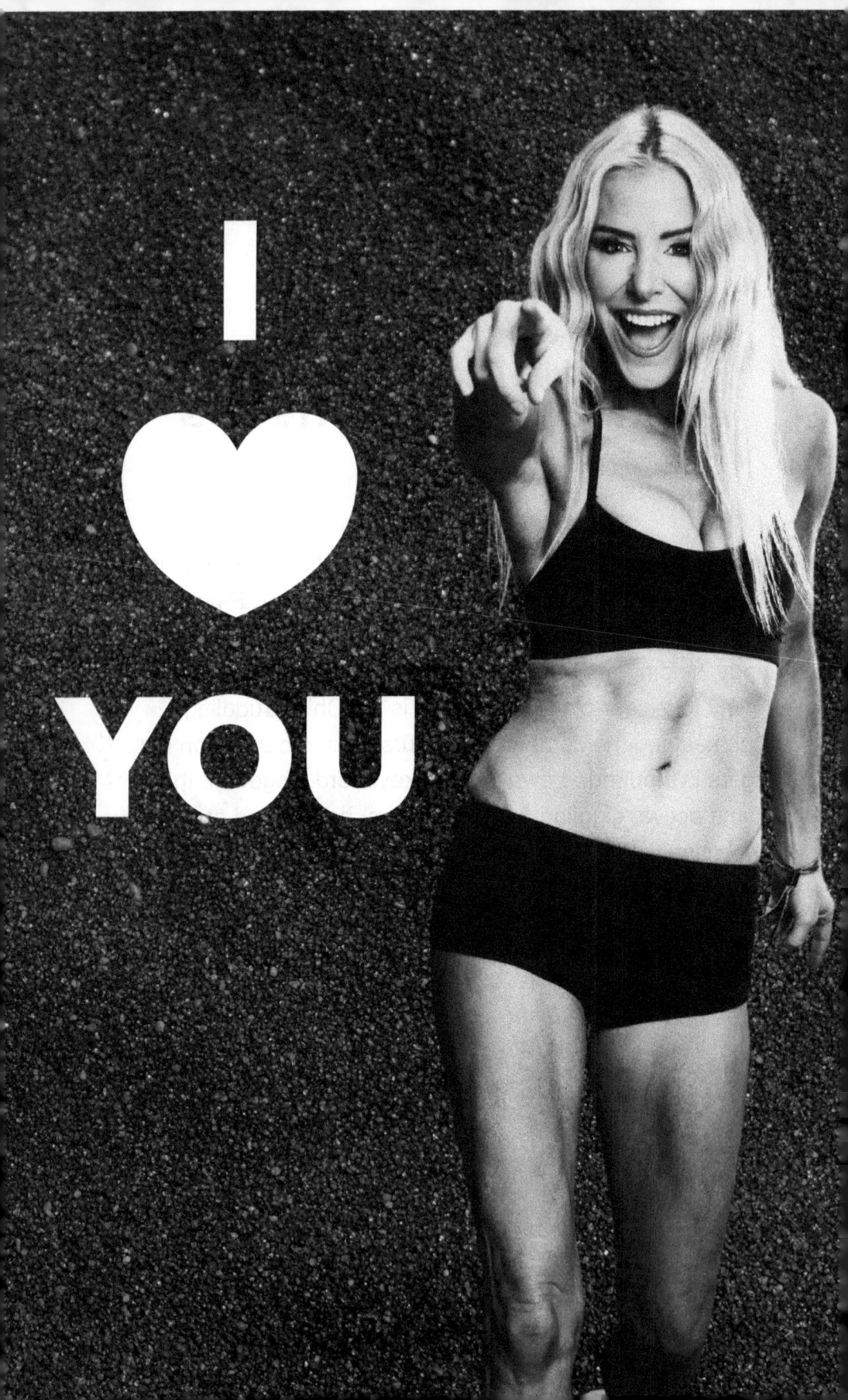

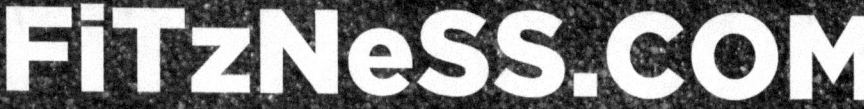

FiTzNeSS.COM

FREE WORKOUT VIDEOS
ARTICLES
TRAINING TIPS
FITZ'S EVENT CALENDAR
BOOKS
ONLINE COURSES
APPAREL
CONTACT

LIVE BETTER & LONGER

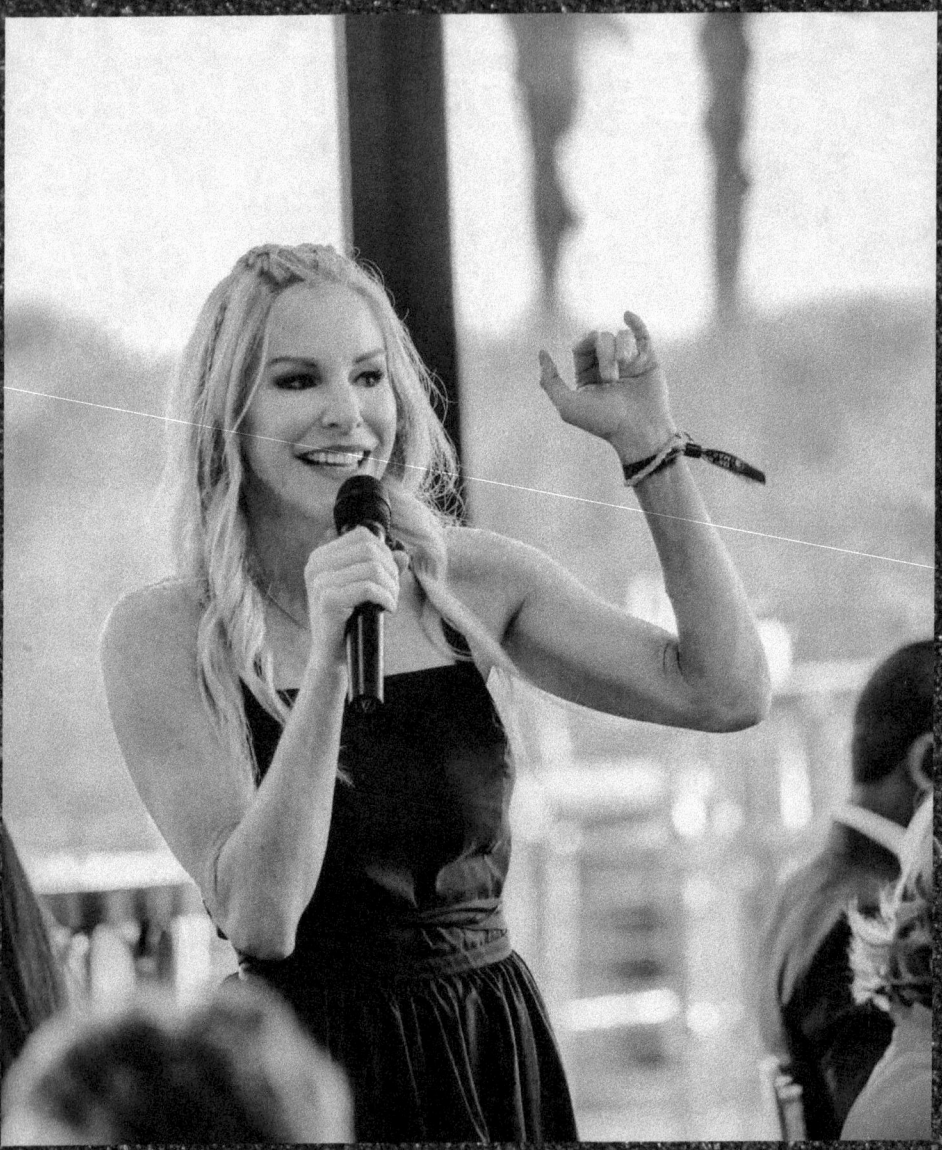

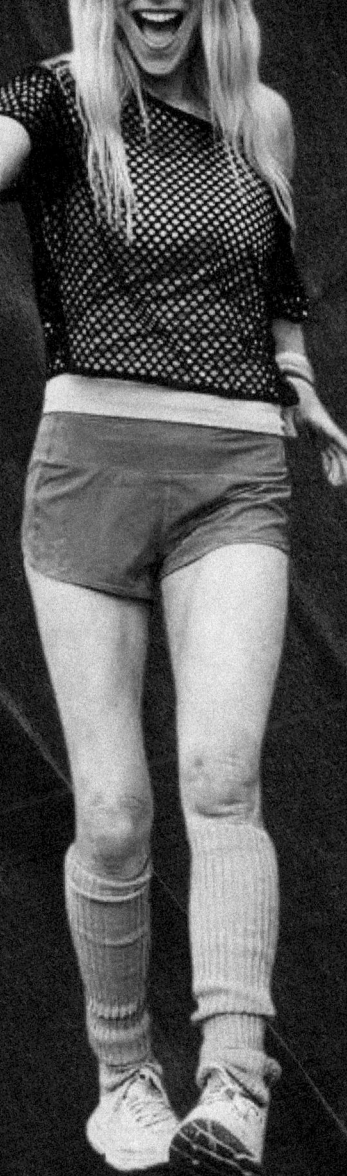

RACE WITH FITZ

CHECK OUT FITZ'S RACE ANNOUNCING CALENDAR AT FITZNESS.COM AND MAKE PLANS TO RUN THROUGH HER START AND FINISH LINES. NOISY LOVE AND SWEATY HUGS ARE INCLUDED!

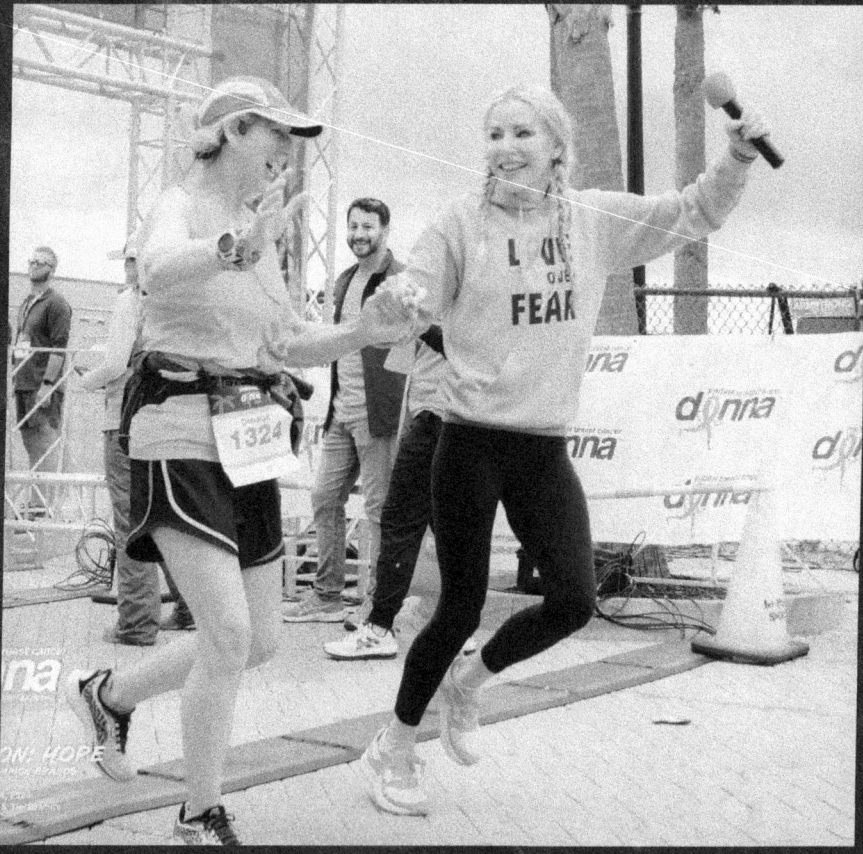

FiTzNeSS.COM

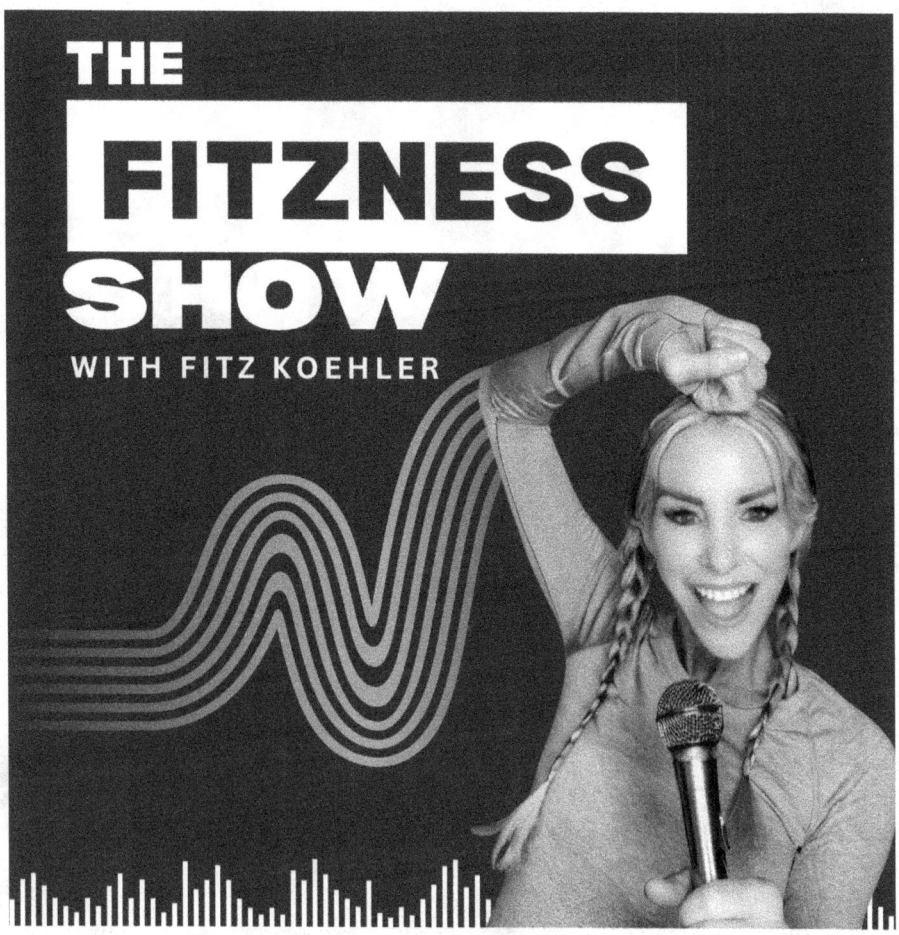

GET FITTER, STRONGER, AND FIRED UP WITH THE FITZNESS SHOW! THIS NO-NONSENSE PODCAST HELPS YOU CRUSH IT AT LIFE—NOT JUST IN THE GYM. YOU'LL GET STRAIGHT TALK, SMART STRATEGIES, AND LAUGH-OUT-LOUD HONESTY ABOUT FITNESS, HEALTH, WEIGHT LOSS, AND BEYOND. FITZ DELIVERS THE BOSSY MOTIVATION AND REAL-WORLD ADVICE YOU NEED TO DO BETTER AND BE BETTER. EXPECT CELEBRITY GUESTS, ANSWERS TO YOUR BURNING QUESTIONS, AND A SUPERCHARGED POKE IN THE CHEST THAT KEEPS YOU MOVING FORWARD, FIRED UP, AND LIVING YOUR BEST LIFE.

🎧 LISTEN ON APPLE, SPOTIFY, GOOGLE, OR WHEREVER YOU GET YOUR PODCASTS.

GOT QUESTIONS?

LET'S KEEP THE CONVERSATION GOING! SUBMIT YOUR QUESTIONS AT FITZNESS.COM OR @FITZNESS ON INSTAGRAM

LOOK FOR ANSWERS ON THE FITZNESS SHOW

THE HEALTHY CANCER COMEBACK SERIES

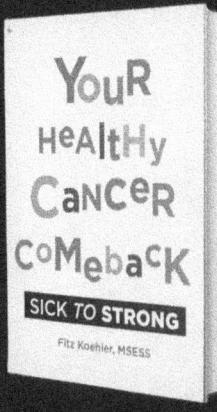 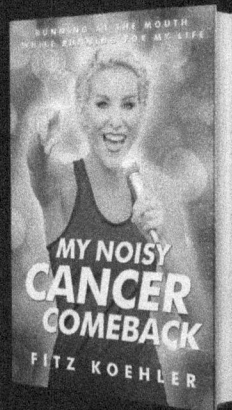 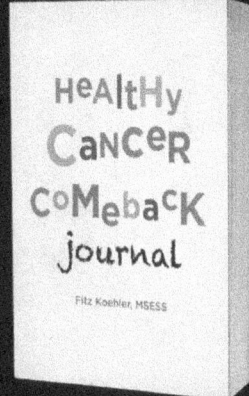

PACKED WITH THE INSPIRATION AND INFORMATION EVERY CANCER PATIENT AND SURVIVOR NEEDS TO GO FROM SICK TO STRONG! MAKES A GREAT GIFT.

ORDER SIGNED BOOKS WITH A FREE GIFT AT

FiTzNeSS.COM

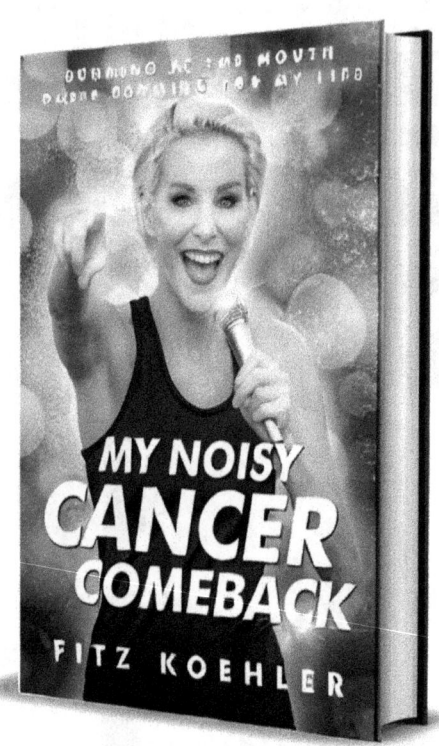

"A FUNNY, DRAMATIC, AND HONEST INSIGHT INTO ONE VERY NOISY WOMAN'S ADVENTURES AND MISADVENTURES WHILE BATTLING CANCER. IT'S THE ULTIMATE MOTIVATIONAL TOOL FOR THRIVING WHILE SURVIVING! FITZ'S STORY PROVES THAT ANYONE CAN ENDURE HARDSHIPS BETTER BY UTILIZING PERSPECTIVE, PASSION, AND POSITIVITY."

SIGNED COPIES AND BULK ORDERS AVAILABLE AT FITZNESS.COM

AVAILABLE IN HARDCOVER, PAPERBACK, EBOOK, AND AUDIOBOOK.

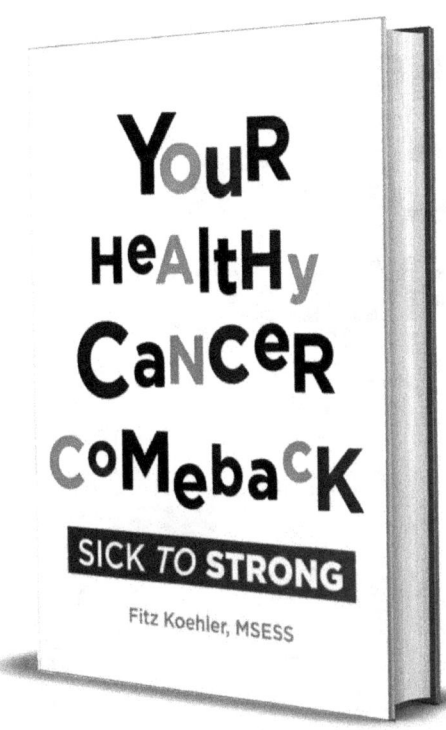

THE COMPREHENSIVE GUIDEBOOK FOR CANCER PATIENTS AND SURVIVORS TO MAINTAIN AND REGAIN STRENGTH, STAMINA, VIBRANCY, ATHLETICISM, AND HEALTH. CANCERS OF ALL TYPES AND THEIR TREATMENTS CAN BE BRUTAL. INSTEAD OF SURRENDERING YOUR HEALTH AND FITNESS TO THIS MONSTER, FIGHT BACK AND CONTROL THE THINGS YOU CAN!

SIGNED COPIES AND BULK ORDERS AVAILABLE AT FITZNESS.COM

AVAILABLE IN HARDCOVER AND PAPERBACK

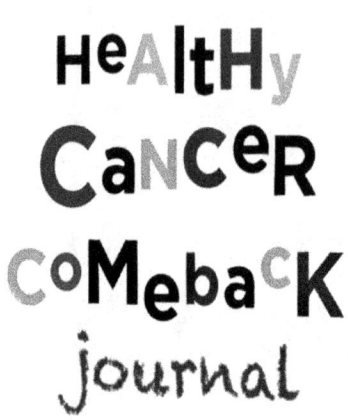

CANCER IS COMPLICATED, EMOTIONAL, CHALLENGING AND FILLED WITH UNIQUE EXPERIENCES. PACKED WITH THOUGHTFUL PROMPTS, KEEP TRACK OF YOUR EXPERIENCES IN ONCOLOGY, ALONG WITH YOUR FEELINGS, FEARS, LAUGHTER, TEARS, FAITH, AND FACTS ABOUT YOUR CARE. DOCUMENT YOUR STRATEGIES FOR EXERCISE, NUTRITION, AND PROGRESS ON YOUR WAY FROM SICK TO STRONG.

SIGNED COPIES AND BULK ORDERS AVAILABLE AT FITZNESS.COM

AVAILABLE IN HARDCOVER, PAPERBACK,

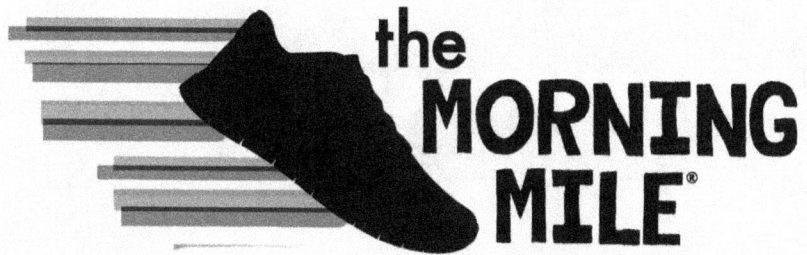

CREATED BY FITZ KOEHLER, THE MORNING MILE™ IS AN EASILY IMPLEMENTED BEFORE-SCHOOL WALKING/RUNNING PROGRAM THAT GIVES CHILDREN A CHANCE TO START EACH DAY IN AN ACTIVE WAY WHILE ENJOYING FUN, MUSIC, AND FRIENDS. IT'S ALSO SUPPORTED BY A WONDERFUL SYSTEM OF REWARDS, WHICH KEEPS STUDENTS HIGHLY MOTIVATED AND FREQUENTLY CONGRATULATED. INQUIRE TO SPONSOR PROGRAMS OR TO GET YOUR FAVORITE SCHOOLS STARTED.

LET'S GET MORE KIDS MOVING IN THE MORNINGS!

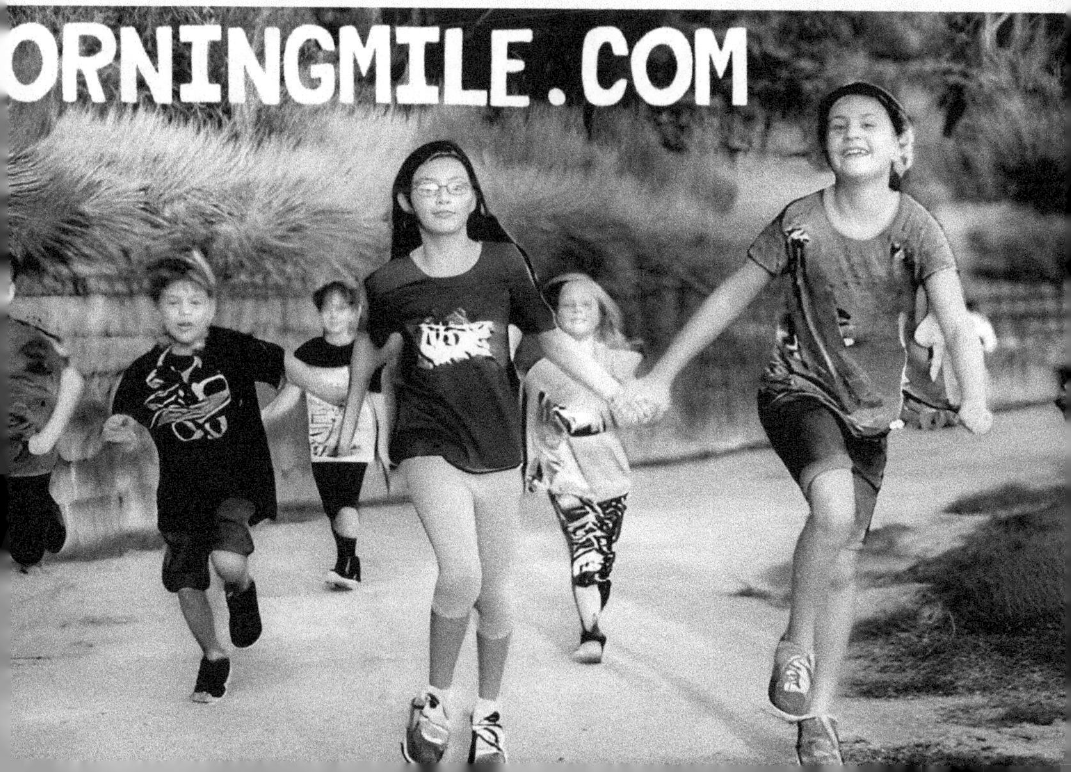

MORNINGMILE.COM

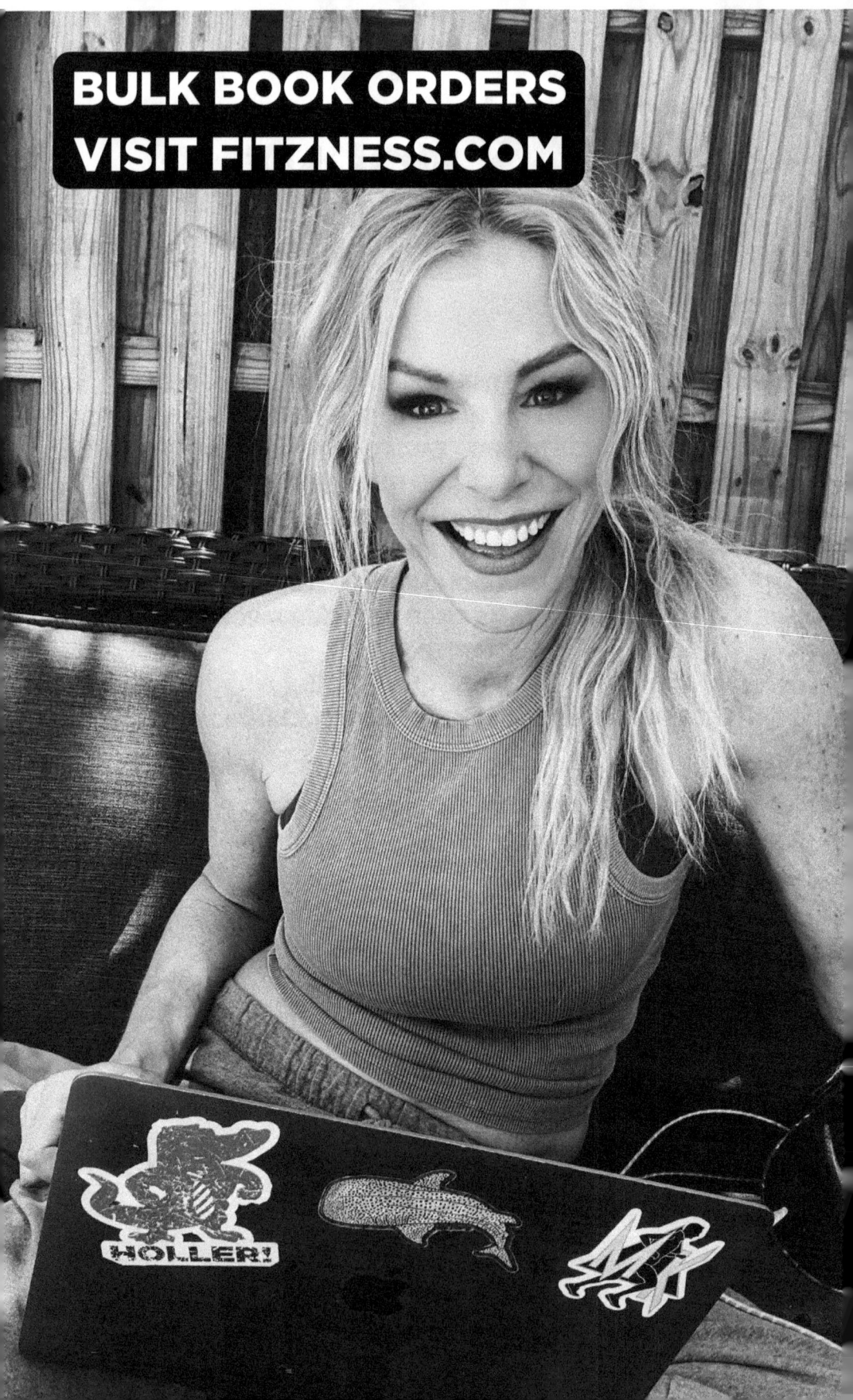

TESTIMONIALS

With Fitz Koehler's guidance, I lost over 100 pounds and completed 75 races. Her method is realistic, effective, and life-changing—proving that lasting fitness fits into any busy life. —Jonelle Cooper

Fitz's strength training plans helped me train for the Boston Marathon and recover from stage four colon cancer. I'm 50 with ripped abs and living fully supercharged thanks to Fitz! —Phil Decker

With Fitz's guidance, I've lost 60 pounds, gotten sober, and gone from completely bedridden to living a strong, vibrant, and joy-filled life! —Jennifer Sawyer

You. Supercharged! is equal parts science, sass, and serious results. Fitz delivers the real-world plan you need to feel strong, energized, and unstoppable. —Tara Collingwood, MS, RDN. The Diet Diva

Fitz's unwavering support—and her perfectly timed "kick in the pants"—helped me power through breast cancer and keep living my best life. —Tamara Milliken

Fitz's no-nonsense guidance transformed fitness into a family affair for us—we train, eat healthy, and thrive together. Her Exact Formula and tough-love approach made me, my husband, and our sons stronger, healthier, and more confident than ever.
— Elise Donabedian

TESTIMONIALS

After discovering Fitz Koehler and committing to her Exact Formula for Weight Loss, I lost 90+ pounds, gained confidence, and found new purpose. Her methods didn't just change my body—they supercharged my mindset, helping me thrive, write books, and live fully—even while battling Parkinson's disease. —Michael Jones

Fitz Koehler's guidance helped me lose 80 pounds and complete over 500 races. You. Supercharged! is the ultimate roadmap for staying strong, focused, and ready t tackle life's toughest challenges. —Sean Matlock

Because of Fitz, my abs stay hard, lean, and ready for Florida's never-ending swimsuit season. —Kristi Hill

Few people embody joy in motion like Fitz Koehler. You. Supercharged! captures her unstoppable spirit—a blend of science, heart, and fierce compassion. This book lights the path to true vitality. Read it, move your body, and feel your soul come alive.
—Dr. Dawn Mussallem at Mayo Clinic

By following Fitz's formula and workouts, I'm in the best shape of my life—crushing seven marathon PRs, three Boston qualifiers, and proudly shopping for smaller belts! —Tim Patton

BACK OF THE BOOK

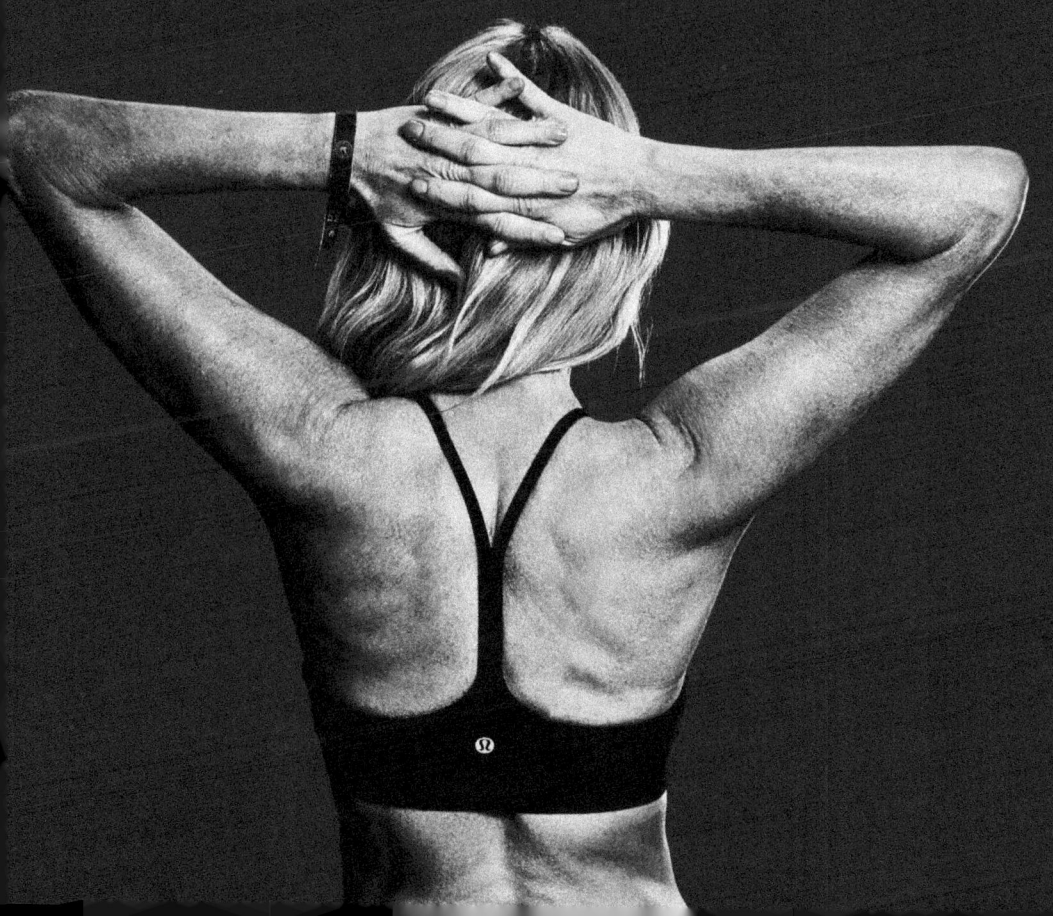

ABOUT THE AUTHOR

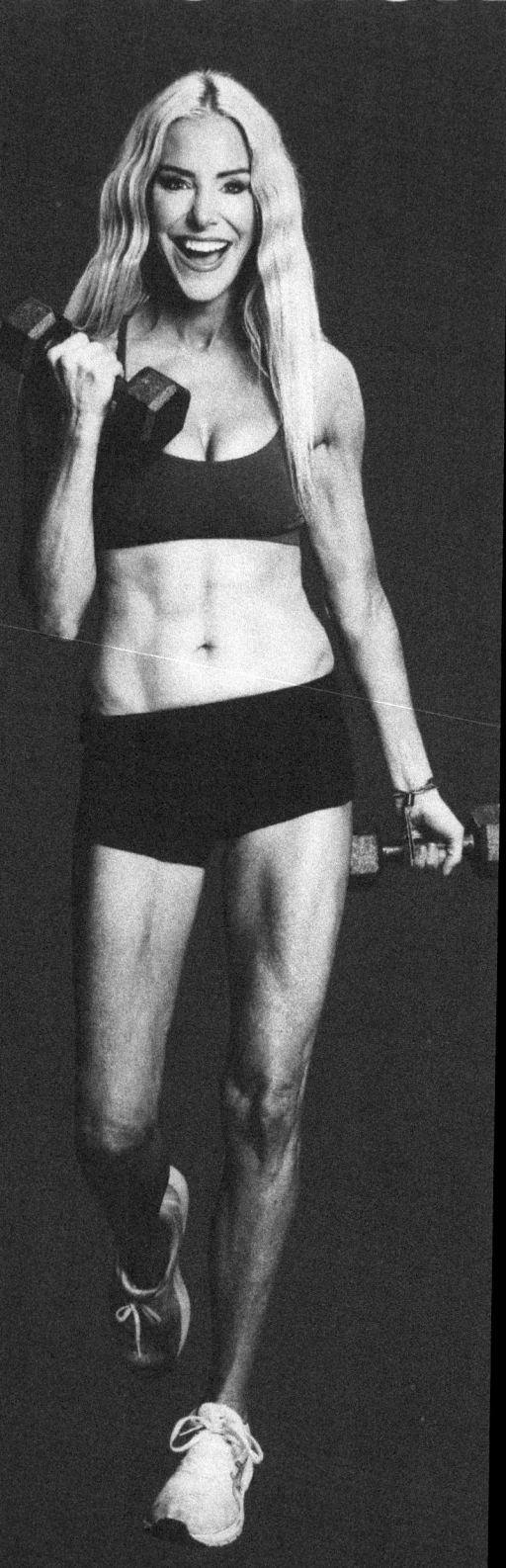

FITZ KOEHLER IS A POWERHOUSE IN THE FITNESS INDUSTRY—GRACING STAGES WORLDWIDE, FIRING UP FINISH LINES AS AMERICA'S NOISIEST RACE ANNOUNCER, AND CALLING OUT EXCUSES WHEREVER THEY LURK. SHE COMBINES HER MASTER'S DEGREE IN EXERCISE AND SPORT SCIENCES WITH A BLEND OF HUMOR, LOVE, AND BOSSINESS. HER NO-NONSENSE, GET-IT-DONE ATTITUDE MAKES HER GUIDANCE FEEL LIKE A PEP TALK FROM YOUR MOST FUN, MOST BRUTALLY HONEST FRIEND.

FITZ BRINGS THE ENERGY VIA KEYNOTES, TV, RADIO, AND HER HIT PODCAST, THE FITZNESS SHOW. SHE'S ALSO THE AUTHOR OF FOUR OTHER INSPIRING BOOKS, USING HER PERSONAL EXPERIENCES BEATING CANCER TO CREATE THE HEALTHY CANCER COMEBACK SERIES. WHETHER SHE'S GUIDING YOU THROUGH WORKOUTS, LIFE COMEBACKS, OR THE SNACK AISLE, FITZ KEEPS IT REAL—AND KEEPS IT FUN.

WHEN SHE WRITES, READERS MOVE. WHEN SHE SPEAKS, EXCUSES VANISH. AND WHEN YOU FOLLOW HER LEAD? YOU GET RESULTS.

FiTzNeSS.COM

www.ingramcontent.com/pod-product-compliance
Lightning Source LLC
Chambersburg PA
CBHW051523020426
42333CB00016B/1752